Veterinary Dentistry for the General Practitioner

Content Strategist: *Robert Edwards*
Senior Content Development: *Clive Hewat*
Project Manager: *Sruthi Viswam*
Designer/Design Direction: *Christian Bilbow*
Illustration Manager: *Jennifer Rose*
Illustrator: *Richard Tibbitts*

Veterinary Dentistry for the General Practitioner

Second Edition

Cecilia Gorrel BSc MA VetMB DDS MRCVS HonFAVD DipEVDC

European and RCVS-recognized Specialist in Veterinary Dentistry
Veterinary Oral Health Consultancy, Pilley, UK

Susanne Andersson RDN RVN

Managing Director
Accesia AB
Halmstad, Sweden

Leen Verhaert, DVM, Dipl. EVDC

European Veterinary Specialist in Dentistry
Dier en Tand
Duffel, Belgium;
Ghent University, Faculty of Veterinary Medicine
Merelbeke, Belgium

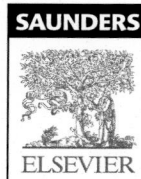

SAUNDERS

ELSEVIER

Edinburgh   London   New York   Oxford   Philadelphia   St Louis   Sydney   Toronto   2013

ELSEVIER
SAUNDERS

First edition 2004

ISBN 9780702049439

British Library Cataloguing in Publication Data
A catalogue record for this book is available from the British Library

Library of Congress Cataloging in Publication Data
A catalog record for this book is available from the Library of Congress

Notices
Knowledge and best practice in this field are constantly changing. As new research and experience broaden our understanding, changes in research methods, professional practices, or medical treatment may become necessary.

Practitioners and researchers must always rely on their own experience and knowledge in evaluating and using any information, methods, compounds, or experiments described herein. In using such information or methods they should be mindful of their own safety and the safety of others, including parties for whom they have a professional responsibility.

With respect to any drug or pharmaceutical products identified, readers are advised to check the most current information provided (i) on procedures featured or (ii) by the manufacturer of each product to be administered, to verify the recommended dose or formula, the method and duration of administration, and contraindications. It is the responsibility of practitioners, relying on their own experience and knowledge of their patients, to make diagnoses, to determine dosages and the best treatment for each individual patient, and to take all appropriate safety precautions.

To the fullest extent of the law, neither the Publisher nor the authors, contributors, or editors, assume any liability for any injury and/or damage to persons or property as a matter of products liability, negligence or otherwise, or from any use or operation of any methods, products, instructions, or ideas contained in the material herein.

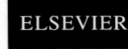 **ELSEVIER** your source for books, journals and multimedia in the health sciences

www.elsevierhealth.com

Working together to grow
libraries in developing countries

www.elsevier.com | www.bookaid.org | www.sabre.org

ELSEVIER   BOOK AID International   Sabre Foundation

The publisher's policy is to use paper manufactured from sustainable forests

Printed in China

Contents

Preface   vii

Acknowledgments   ix

1. Equipment and instrumentation   1

2. Anesthesia and analgesia   15

3. Antibiotics and antiseptics   31

4. Anatomy of the teeth and periodontium   37

5. Occlusion and malocclusion   43

6. Oral examination and recording   57

7. Dental radiography   67

8. Common oral conditions   81

9. Periodontal disease   97

10. Preventive dentistry   121

11. Resorptive lesions   129

12. Emergencies   141

13. Tooth extraction   171

14. Dental diseases in lagomorphs and rodents   191

Appendix 213

Glossary 215

Index 223

Preface

I have written the expanded second edition of *Veterinary Dentistry for the General Practitioner* with the same aim as the first edition, namely to supply the general practitioner in small animal practice with all the information required to be able to practice good dentistry. This book presents comprehensive and detailed knowledge of how to prevent, diagnose and treat common oral and dental diseases in the dog and cat. It also provides information as to the diagnosis and management of less common diseases, where the ultimate treatment will generally be performed by a specialist, but the general practitioner needs to be able to identify a problem and have a basic understanding of the pathophysiology of the tissues involved. Dental conditions of lagomorphs and rodents are also covered.

Oral diseases are common in small animal practice. Many conditions cause discomfort, and some diseases cause intense pain. Detection of pathology is often late in the disease process since our pets cannot express and describe the sensations of discomfort and/or pain associated with these conditions. Moreover, there is strong evidence that a focus of infection in the oral cavity may lead to systemic problems. Thus, prevention and treatment of oral conditions is important for the general health and welfare of our pets. It is certainly not a cosmetic issue.

Although this expanded second edition is written for general practitioners, and therefore covers common conditions in detail, it should also be of value for veterinary students, both during their initial studies and as they seek specialist qualifications.

Cecilia Gorrel
Pilley 2013

Acknowledgments

This book would not have been written or revised without the assistance of Graeme Blackwood. Thank you for your emotional support, constructive criticism and practical help.

I wish to thank Leen Verhaert and Susanne Andersson for co-authoring Chapters 14 and 1, respectively, with me. I would also like to thank Alexandra Kentsdottir for her help with illustrations.

Leen Verhaert and I wish to thank Professors Lauwers and Moens of the Morphology Department, Faculty of Veterinary Medicine, Ghent University, for allowing us to take photographs of the skulls in the Department Museum.

Chapter 1

Equipment and instrumentation

with Susanne Andersson

INTRODUCTION

A poor workman blames his tools! While there is some truth to this statement, it is not possible to perform good dentistry and oral surgery, however skilled the operator, without appropriate equipment and instrumentation.

This chapter will deal with important general considerations, some of which are often disregarded. It will also outline equipment and instrumentation requirements for general practice. The additional requirements for lagomorphs and rodent dentistry are detailed in Chapter 14. Radiography is mandatory; equipment and techniques are covered in Chapter 7. Practicing dentistry without taking radiographs would be considered negligent in human dentistry. The same applies in veterinary dentistry.

GENERAL CONSIDERATIONS

Dentistry poses a health hazard for both operators and patients. There is the possibility of both indirect contagion (hands, nails, skin, clothes, instruments) as well as the dangers associated with the bacterial aerosol created by some procedures, e.g. scaling, but also by sneezing, coughing and by the water coolant and compressed air used. Consequently, dental procedures should be performed in a separate room that is carefully designed and maintained to minimize these hazards. The room must have adequate light and ventilation. A bright light source is required. Investing in a *dental light* is mandatory. A good dental light is expensive, but definitely worth the money.

Ergonomic considerations are of paramount importance in the layout of the dental operatory. All equipment and instruments should be within easy reach of the operator. Posture is important! Ideally, the operator should be seated (Fig. 1.1).

It is essential to *protect operator and staff*. The veterinarian and the assistant should wear designated operating clothes. Moreover, facemasks and appropriate eye wear (spectacles or face shield) to protect them from the bacterial aerosol and other debris are essential. There is a risk of infection of skin wounds if the operator works in a dirty environment without gloves. The oral cavity is never a sterile site, so the use of surgical gloves is recommended. In addition, hand disinfection should be practiced frequently.

Important *patient considerations* are as follows:

- General anesthesia with endotracheal intubation is essential. This prevents inhalation of aerosolized bacteria (and other debris) and asphyxiation on irrigation and cooling fluid. Chapter 2 covers anesthesia and analgesia for the patient undergoing oral and dental surgery.
- A pharyngeal pack (Fig. 1.2) is also recommended during oral and dental treatment. Remember to remove the pack prior to extubation!
- The animal should be positioned on a surface that will allow drainage to prevent it becoming wet and hypothermic. This can be achieved by the use of a 'tub-tank' or placing the animal's head on a disposable 'nappy', which is frequently replaced. Most animals benefit from a heating pad.

Some important *equipment and instrumentation considerations* are as follows:

- There are different degrees of cleanliness required for oral/dental procedures, ranging from visually clean to sterile.

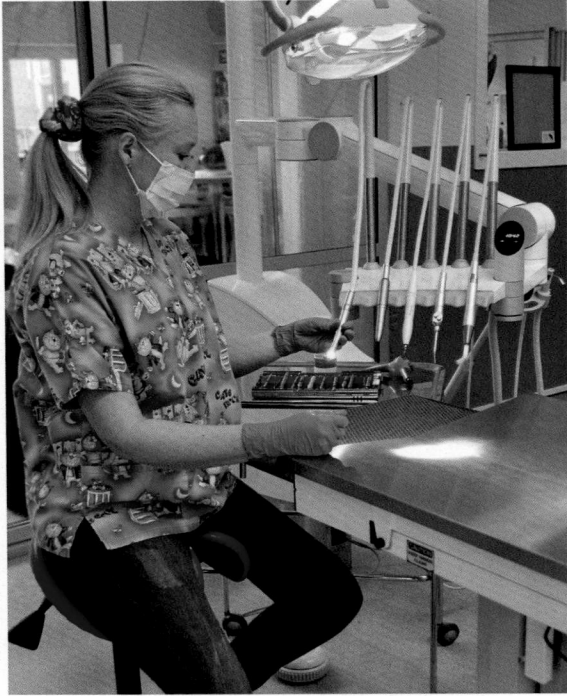

Fig. 1.1 Ergonomic considerations The operator should be seated with all equipment and instrumentation within easy reach.

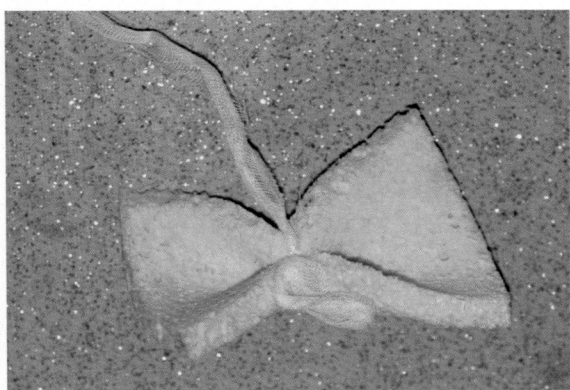

Fig. 1.2 Pharyngeal pack Pharyngeal packing should be used for greater airway security. Commonly used packs include sponge, surgical swabs, gauze bandage. Packs will become saturated with liquid during procedures and will then no longer offer adequate protection and should be replaced as required. It is imperative to remove any packing prior to extubation.

- Some equipment and instruments need to be 'clean', i.e. units, lamps, tub tables, etc., and need to be wiped clean with an all-purpose disinfectant.
- Any instrument that will be used inside the oral cavity but *without penetrating* the oral mucosa, e.g. examination instruments, burs, scalers, curettes, must be exceptionally clean, as defined by the European Standard (EN)/International Organization for Standardization (ISO), Document 15883. This degree of cleanliness is achieved by mechanical cleaning followed by heat or chemical treatment. This is best achieved using a disinfector, where both cleaning and disinfection occur automatically. Another alternative is placing the instruments in an ultrasound bath or ordinary dishwasher followed by disinfection in an autoclave. A third option is to use chemicals for cleaning and disinfection. The last option is usually limited to equipment/ instrumentation where heat disinfection is not suitable, e.g. instruments with plastic handles.
- Instruments that *penetrate* the oral mucosa or the pulp system of the tooth need to be sterile, as defined by the European Standard (EN), Document 556. This entails packaging and sterilization, as detailed by the European Standard (EN)/International Organization for Standardization (ISO), Document 14937.
- Suitable (clean, extremely clean, sterile, as required by the procedure) instruments should be available for each patient. Ideally, several pre-packed kits with the required instruments for different procedures, e.g. examination, periodontal therapy, extraction, should be available.
- Power equipment requires regular maintenance (daily, weekly) in the practice and regular servicing by the supplier. Draw up checklists for these chores. Check maintenance and servicing requirements with the supplier.

EQUIPMENT AND INSTRUMENTATION FOR ORAL AND DENTAL EXAMINATION

There is a wide selection of dental equipment and instrumentation available on the market. Our recommendation is to identify your needs and then invest in a bit more than you think you will require. The better you get at performing dentistry and oral surgery, the more demanding of your equipment you will become. There is also an element of personal preference, so test different options before making a decision. Finally, *be prepared to upgrade*.

Details of how to perform an oral examination and recording are covered in Chapter 6. The following will outline equipment and instrumentation requirements.

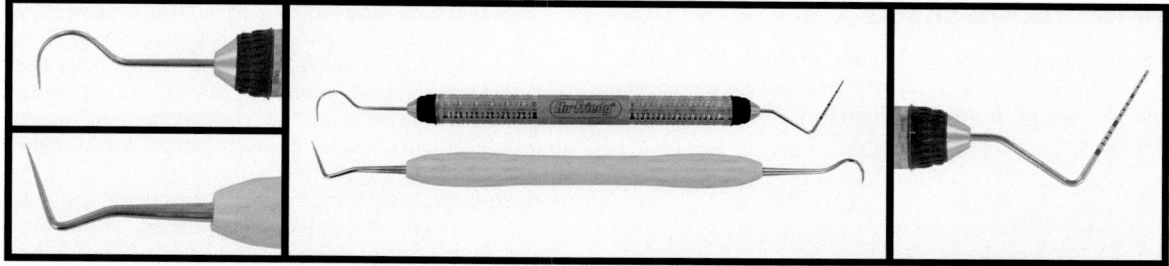

Fig. 1.3 Probe and explorer The periodontal probe is a narrow rounded or flat, blunt-ended, graduated instrument while a dental explorer is a sharp-ended instrument. Center picture depicts double-ended instruments; top is a combined explorer and probe and lower (yellow handle) is a combined curved explorer and straight explorer. On the left are close-ups of a curved (top) and straight (bottom) explorer. On the right is a close-up of a periodontal probe.

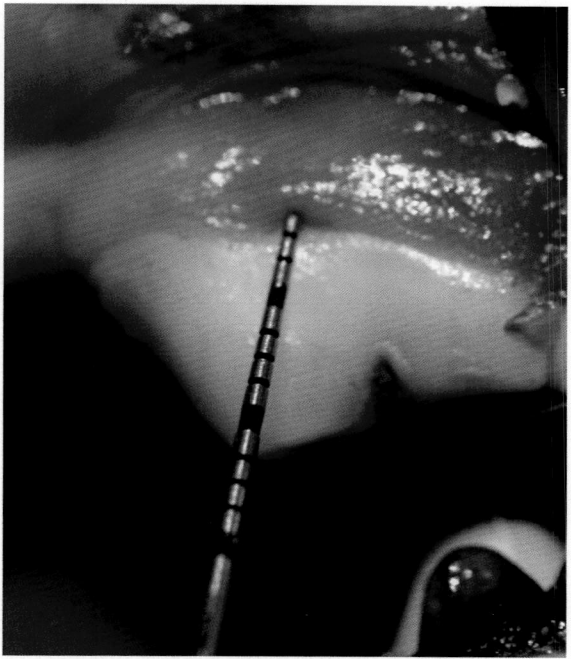

Fig. 1.4 The periodontal probe The periodontal probe is a blunt-ended, graduated instrument, which can be inserted into the gingival sulcus without causing trauma.

Personal preferences have been inserted as a guide, where appropriate.

Periodontal probe

The periodontal probe is a narrow rounded or flat, blunt-ended, graduated instrument (Fig. 1.3). Because of its blunt end, it can be inserted into the gingival sulcus without causing trauma (Fig. 1.4). The periodontal probe is used to:

- Measure periodontal probing depth
- Determine the degree of gingival inflammation
- Evaluate furcation lesions
- Evaluate the extent of tooth mobility.

A narrow, rounded rather than flat, probe is our preferred choice, as it is easier to enter the gingival sulcus without causing damage with the rounded probe, especially in cats, where the flat probe is impossible to use.

Dental explorer

The dental explorer or probe (Fig. 1.3), a sharp-ended instrument, is used to:

- Determine the presence of caries
- Explore other enamel and dentin defects, e.g. fracture, odontoclastic resorptive lesions.

The explorer is also useful for tactile examination of the subgingival tooth surfaces. Subgingival calculus may be identified in this way.

Dental explorers are either straight or curved. They are also either single-ended or double-ended, usually combined with a periodontal probe, i.e. one end is an explorer and the other end is a periodontal probe.

Dental mirror

A dental mirror is a vital, but traditionally rarely used, tool. It allows the operator to visualize palatal/lingual surfaces while maintaining posture, reflect light onto areas of interest and retract and protect soft tissue. Orientation may cause confusion and the use of a dental mirror requires practice; however, the time taken to learn how to use a dental mirror is a worthy investment. To prevent condensation occurring on the mirror, it can be wiped across the buccal mucous membranes before use. Dental mirrors can be purchased in several sizes. A small (pediatric size) mirror for cats and small dogs and a larger one for medium to large dogs should be available.

Dental record sheets

Recording and dental record sheets are covered in Chapter 6. A complete dental record is required for diagnostic and therapeutic purposes, as well as for medico-legal reasons.

EQUIPMENT AND INSTRUMENTATION FOR PERIODONTAL THERAPY

Periodontal disease therapy is detailed in Chapter 9.

Scaling

Scaling describes the procedure whereby dental deposits (plaque, but mainly calculus) are removed from the supra- and subgingival surfaces of the teeth. Scaling may be performed using a combination of mechanical and hand instruments. The use of mechanical (powered scalers) requires less treatment time than hand instruments. Moreover, mechanical instrumentation is less fatiguing to the operator than hand instrumentation. However, mechanical scalers cannot replace hand scaling. If only powered scalers have been used, post-treatment examination using compressed air to retract tissues and dry calculus demonstrates residual deposits. Occasionally, mechanical scalers will plane over the surface of a calculus rather than dislodge it. The sharpened blade of a hand instrument is more likely to break the calculus away from the tooth surface. Hand instruments should be used to remove large, bulky supragingival deposits before going on to powered scalers. Also, hand instruments are required to remove subgingival dental deposits.

Hand scaling instruments

Scalers and curettes (Fig. 1.5) are used to remove dental deposits from the tooth surfaces. Each has a handle, a shank and a working end (tip). They require frequent sharpening to maintain their cutting edges. Instrument sharpening is covered later in this chapter.

Instrument (scaler and curette) handles are available in a variety of shapes and styles. Weight, diameter and surface texture of handles are factors that need to be considered when selecting hand instruments. Round, hollow handles are recommended because they are lighter in weight, which increases tactile sense and minimizes hand fatigue. A larger diameter handle is advisable for ergonomic comfort. A handle with a smooth surface must be grasped more firmly to maintain control over the working end, leading to hand fatigue. Textured handles (ribbed, diamond-textured or knurled) allow the operator to maintain control over the instrument more comfortably. They also maximize sensory feedback.

The part of the instrument that extends from the working end to the handle is called the functional shank. Functional shanks may be angled, curved or straight. They also vary in length (short, moderate, long) and flexibility. Straight shank instruments are commonly used on the accessible anterior teeth. Posterior teeth need angled shanks for better adaptation of the working end to the tooth surfaces. Instruments with short functional shanks can be used on anterior teeth, while moderate to long shanks are needed to reach posterior teeth and to access periodontal pockets. Instruments with rigid shanks are used to remove heavy calculus deposits. Instruments with more flexible shanks (e.g. Gracey curettes) are used for removal of fine, light calculus and give better tactile sensation (feedback). The terminal shank is the smaller portion of the functional shank. It extends between the working end and the first bend in the shank. It is essential to locate the terminal shank on an instrument when you are trying to identify the working end and sharpen its cutting edges.

The working end refers to that part of the instrument that is used to carry out the function of the instrument. Working ends can be made of stainless steel or of carbide steel. The working end of a sharpened instrument is called the blade. Carbide blades may hold their cutting edge(s) longer but tend to corrode easily if not cared for properly. The blade is made up of the following components:

- Face
- Lateral surfaces
- Back
- Cutting edge(s).

The cutting edge is the line where the face and a lateral surface meet to form a sharp cutting edge. A blade designed with a pointed tip is called a **scaler**. A blade that ends with a rounded toe is classified as a **curette**. Figure 1.6 demonstrates the differences between a scaler and a curette.

Scalers are used for the supragingival removal of calculus. As already mentioned, a scaler has a sharp, pointed tip and should thus only be used supragingivally. If a scaler is used subgingivally, the pointed tip will lacerate the gingival margin. A scaler should generally be pulled away from the gingiva towards the tip of the crown (occlusal surface).

Scalers come in a variety of shapes. The most common is the sickle scaler, which can be either curved or straight. A straight sickle scaler is also known as a Jacquette scaler. A sickle scaler has the following characteristics:

- The face of the blade is perpendicular to the terminal shank
- The blade has two cutting edges
- The face of the blade has a sharp point or tip
- In cross-section, the blade is triangular in shape.

Curettes are used for the subgingival removal of dental deposits and for root planing. They can also be used supragingivally. There are basically two types of curettes, namely universal, e.g. Columbia, and area specific, e.g.

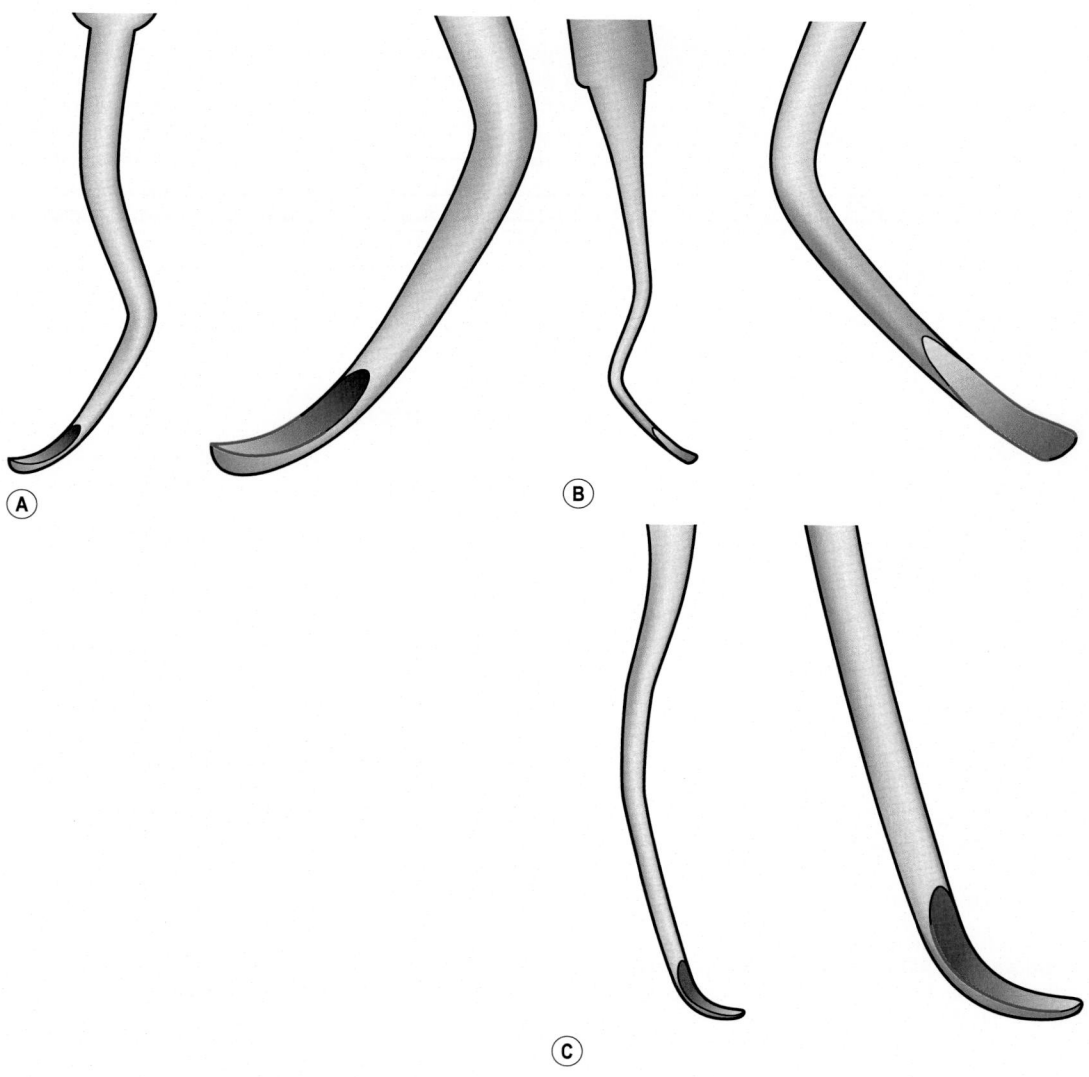

Fig. 1.5 Sickle scaler, universal and Gracey curette (A) Sickle scaler. Because of its sharp pointed tip it would lacerate the gingiva if inserted subgingivally; this instrument can only be used to remove dental deposits above the gingiva. Note the two cutting edges (highlighted in red). (B) Universal curette. This instrument also has two cutting edges (highlighted in red) but because of its rounded tip it can be used to remove subgingival deposits and restore the root surface to smoothness. It can also be used to remove supragingival dental deposits. (C) Gracey curette. This curette is considered an area-specific curette and has only one cutting side (highlighted in red).

Gracey. The working end of a curette is more slender than that of a scaler and the back and tip are rounded to minimize gingival trauma. The cutting edges curve from the terminal shank to the toe.

A selection of curettes is required for periodontal therapy. Our preferences are the Gracey 7/8 and the Columbia 13/14. We do not use a separate scaler as curettes can be used both above and below the gingiva, while scalers are limited to supragingival use.

Mechanical scaling instruments

Mechanical or powered scalers enable fast and easy removal of calculus. However, they have great potential for iatrogenic damage if used incorrectly. There are two types of mechanical scalers, namely sonic and ultrasonic. The most commonly used in veterinary dentistry is the ultrasonic scaler. As already mentioned, gross supragingival calculus deposits are best removed with hand

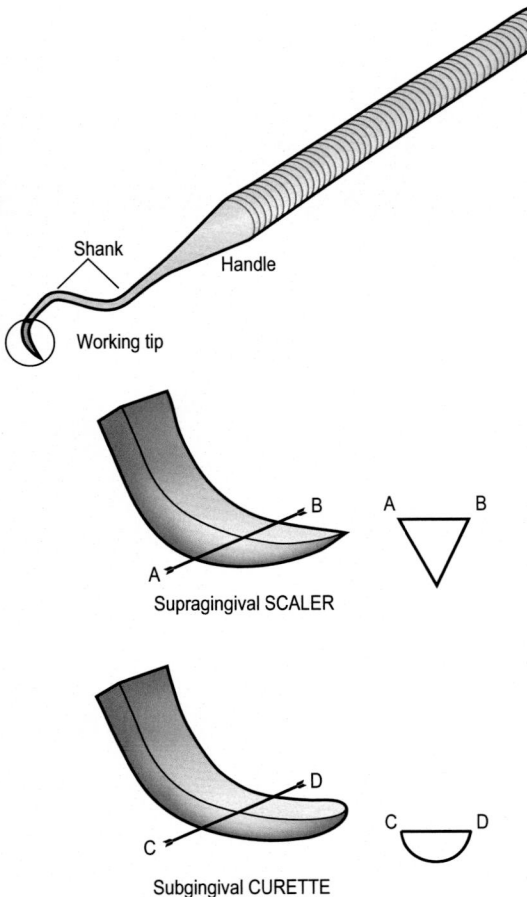

Fig. 1.6 **Scaler and curette design** Each has a handle, a shank and a working tip. The working tip of a scaler is more robust than that of a curette. Curettes are less bulky, with rounded back and tip, for use in gingival pockets. Both hand scalers and curettes require frequent sharpening to maintain their cutting edges.

instruments (scaler, curette) prior to using mechanical scaling equipment.

Sonic scalers are driven by compressed air, so they require a compressed air-driven dental unit for operation. The tip oscillates at a sonic frequency and is efficient at removing dental calculus. Sonic scalers are generally less effective than ultrasonic scalers. Depending upon the design of the tip of the scaler, these instruments may be used for supra- and subgingival scaling. A thin, pointed tip, sometimes called a perio, sickle or universal insert, is the recommended insert.

Ultrasonic scalers are most commonly used in veterinary practice. The tip oscillates at ultrasonic frequencies. They are driven by a micromotor, so do not require a

compressed air-driven unit for operation. The tip vibration is generated either by a magnetostrictive mechanism or by a piezoelectric mechanism in the hand piece. The ultrasonic oscillation of the tip causes cavitation of the coolant, which aids in the disruption of the calculus on the tooth surface. Ultrasonic scalers are generally designed for supragingival use, but tips designed for subgingival scaling are available. A thin, pointed insert is recommended for supragingival use. Inserts specifically designed for subgingival use are recommended for subgingival scaling. It is essential that these tips are used with the correct frequency and sufficient water, and they need replacing at regular intervals as the tips lose efficiency with wear.

Calculus forceps

Calculus forceps have been designed to aid removal of heavy calculus from the surface of teeth. It is essential to use these forceps with extreme care and in the described manner, as inappropriate use will result in fractured teeth. These forceps must not be used to extract teeth.

Polishing

Polishing removes plaque and restores the scaled tooth surfaces to smoothness, which is less plaque retentive. Scaled teeth must be polished. It is often suggested that teeth may be 'polished' by hand using a toothbrush and prophy paste. This method is inefficient and, therefore, not recommended. Efficient polishing can be performed using either prophy paste in a prophy cup or in a brush in a slow-speed contra-angle hand piece, or by means of air polishing (particle blasting).

Prophy paste in a cup/brush in a slow-speed contra-angle hand piece

The speed of rotation of the cup/brush can be regulated. To minimize the amount of heat generated, the prophy cup or brush should not rotate faster than 5000 rpm. Each patient should receive a new polishing cup or brush.

Air polishing (particle blasting)

This technique, based on the sandblasting principle, is used to polish the supragingival parts of the teeth. The particles used (e.g. bicarbonate of soda) will polish the tooth surface without causing damage to the enamel. It is essential to protect the soft tissues (gingivae and oral mucosa) during air polishing. A simple way of protecting the soft tissues is to cover them with a piece of gauze.

Prophy paste

Prophy paste is available in bulk containers and in individual patient tubs. The latter are inexpensive and should be used to prevent contamination and the iatrogenic transmission of pathogens.

EQUIPMENT AND INSTRUMENTATION FOR TOOTH EXTRACTION

The techniques for tooth extraction are detailed in Chapter 13.

Hand instruments

Luxators, elevators and Extraktors

A selection of dental luxators, elevators and Extraktors of varying sizes is required. Our preferred selection is shown in Figure 1.7.

These instruments are used to cut/break down the periodontal ligament, which holds the tooth in the alveolus. The different sizes are required so that an appropriate range for each size of root can be selected. Luxators have a very thin working end and are used to cut the ligament, but should not be used for leverage or they may break. Elevators have a more robust working end than luxators and are used to break down the periodontal ligament with a combination of apical pressure and leverage. The Accesia 'Extraktor' is a newly developed instrument (Accesia AB, Sweden) specifically designed for tooth extraction in the dog and cat (Fig. 1.8). It combines the advantages of a luxator and an elevator into one instrument. They are shaped to adapt well to the shape of the root surface and can be used in an apical cutting motion as well as inserted horizontally between tooth roots to apply leverage. Moreover, they have sharp cutting edges on the lateral aspect, which allows them to slide around the circumference of the tooth. An extraction can be started with a luxator and completed with an elevator or it can be performed using different sizes of Extraktors only.

Periosteal elevator

Periosteal elevators of different sizes (Fig. 1.9) are required for open (surgical) extractions to expose the alveolar bone by raising a mucoperiosteal flap. However, even if a closed (non-surgical) extraction technique has been used, the gingiva may be sutured over the extraction socket. In this case, a periosteal elevator is invaluable to free the gingiva, allowing suturing over of the extraction socket without tension.

Extraction forceps

Although forceps can be used to aid ligament breakdown by rotational force on the tooth, it is very easy to snap the crown off by using excessive force. There is some truth in the saying that the only extraction forceps required are your fingers. If the tooth cannot be lifted out with your fingers, then the periodontal ligament has not been adequately broken down. In short, dental forceps are not essential, but if they are to be used, then a selection of sizes, to fit the root anatomy of the tooth being extracted, is required.

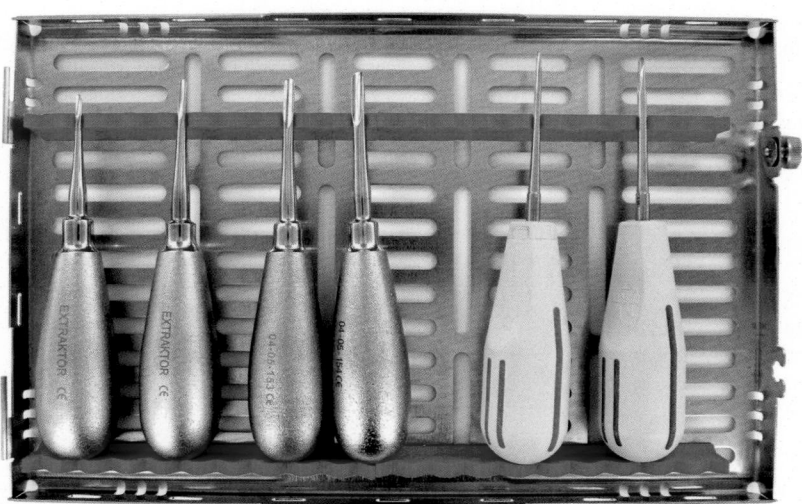

Fig. 1.7 Luxators and Extraktors The authors' favorite extraction tools are depicted. On the left are Extraktors and on the right are two luxators. Most extractions can be performed using the four different sizes (1.5, 3, 4 and 5) of Extraktors.

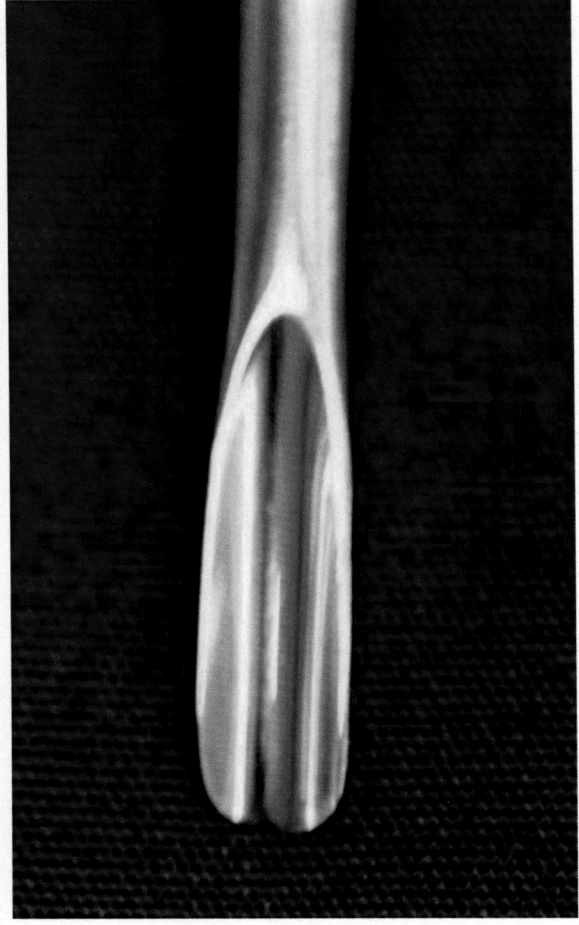

Fig. 1.8 The Extraktor This newly developed instrument combines the advantages of both a luxator and an elevator. It is designed to conform to the shape of the root and can be used in an apical cutting motion as well as inserted horizontally between roots to apply leverage. It also has lateral cutting edges, unlike the luxator or elevator, which allow the instrument to slide around the circumference of the tooth.

Power equipment

Power equipment is required to perform dentistry and oral surgery. Regular maintenance is essential to avoid problems with equipment failure.

Micromotor unit

A micromotor unit can be used for polishing teeth as well as sectioning them. For sectioning teeth, the micromotor should be set at maximum speed (20–40 000 rpm). Micromotor units do not generally include water cooling of the bur and an external source (e.g. assistant applying coolant continuously to the tissues) is required to prevent thermal damage.

Compressed air-driven unit

The basic compressed air-driven unit consists of a high-speed hand piece with water cooling, a slow-speed hand piece (with or without water cooling) and a combination air/water syringe. Most units also have a built-in ultrasonic scaler (Fig. 1.10). A high-speed hand piece, although not essential for sectioning multirooted teeth prior to extraction, facilitates the process and allows accurate application of coolant water. Investing in a high-speed hand piece with fiberoptic light is strongly recommended. The slow-speed hand piece accommodates the contra-angle hand piece used for polishing the teeth. The different hand pieces for dental units are shown in Figure 1.11. The three-way syringe can deliver either a stream of water or a spray of water and air, or air only. It is used to irrigate/lavage the mouth (water or water/air spray) and to dry the teeth (air only). Some units come with two high-speed outlets and one of these can be used with a sonic scaler and/or an air-polishing hand piece. Many units also have a pump for saline irrigation during open extractions. Suction, which is highly recommended, is also available with some units.

Investing in a compressed air-driven unit from the outset is recommended. The high-speed hand piece greatly facilitates tooth sectioning and the three-way syringe (for lavage and drying) will aid in the removal of debris and improve visibility during examination and any procedure. Suction is a real bonus. Investigate the maintenance and service options offered before making your choice.

Burs

Dental burs are made of a variety of materials including stainless steel, tungsten-carbide steel and 'diamond'. There is a wide selection of burs available to fit both the slow- and the high-speed hand piece. A selection of round, pear-shaped, tapered fissure and straight fissure burs will be required for sectioning of teeth and removal of alveolar bone (Fig. 1.12A). 'Diamond' burs abrade rather than cut and may be safer for the inexperienced user. High-speed burs (Fig. 1.12B) are used to section teeth and perform cavity preparation.

MISCELLANEOUS

Sharpening

Scalers and curettes, luxators and elevators all require regular sharpening. The basic goals of sharpening are to conserve a sharp cutting edge, and to preserve the original shape of the instrument. Dental instrument sharpening

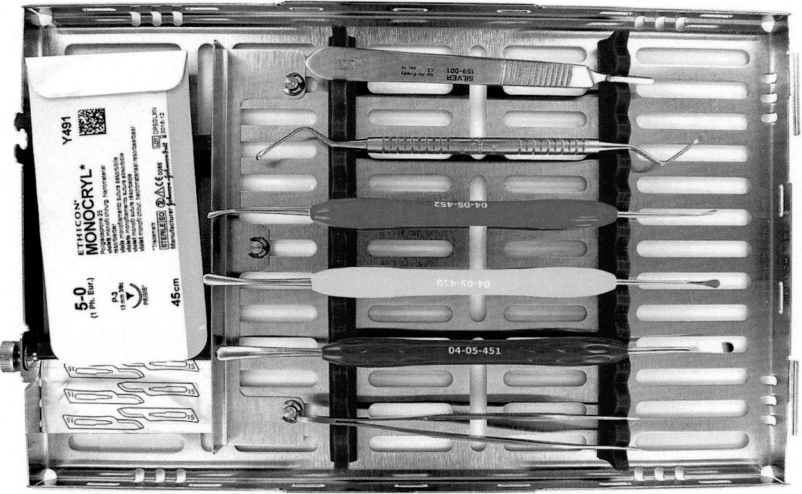

Fig. 1.9 Equipment for tooth extraction The authors' preferred periosteal elevators are shown. The size 15 blade shown (should always be used in a handle) is preferred.

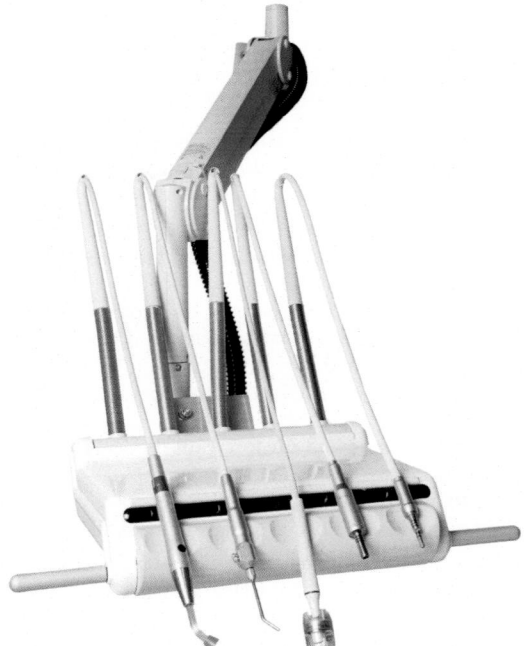

Fig. 1.10 A dental unit The depicted unit has the following components from left to right: light gun (for transilluminating teeth and curing light-cure dental materials); an air–water syringe; an ultrasonic scaler (driven by a built-in micromotor); slow-speed and high-speed outlet (will need separate compressor).

kits (stones and instructions) are available through dental and veterinary wholesalers. Attending a course to learn how to sharpen instruments is strongly recommended.

In general, a fine-grade stone, e.g. Arkansas, is recommended to avoid changing the basic shape of the instrument. A course-grade stone removes too much metal and should not be used. Instruments that are very dull should be professionally reground or replaced with new ones that are maintained.

Scalers and curettes

Instruments must be sharp if scaling is to be completed efficiently with minimal trauma to the gingival tissues. When the blade of the instrument is maintained properly, greater control of the working end occurs. Fewer repetitive strokes are required and there is thus less operator fatigue.

Scalers and curettes should be sharpened before each use, i.e. after cleaning and disinfection. Sharpening of dirty instruments will contaminate the sharpening stone. Sharpening should be performed in a light room with a bright light, so that the cutting edge(s) of the blade are clearly visualized. Acrylic testing sticks are available to check the adequacy of the sharpening procedure.

Hand-held sharpening stones are the best way to restore the cutting edge on a dull instrument while maintaining its original shape. Fine stones will maintain the cutting edge on instruments that are frequently sharpened, without removing an excessive amount of the blade. To prevent 'grooving', the whole surface of the stone should be used during sharpening.

Water (not oil) should be used on the stone. The care of stones requires wiping with a clean cloth to remove

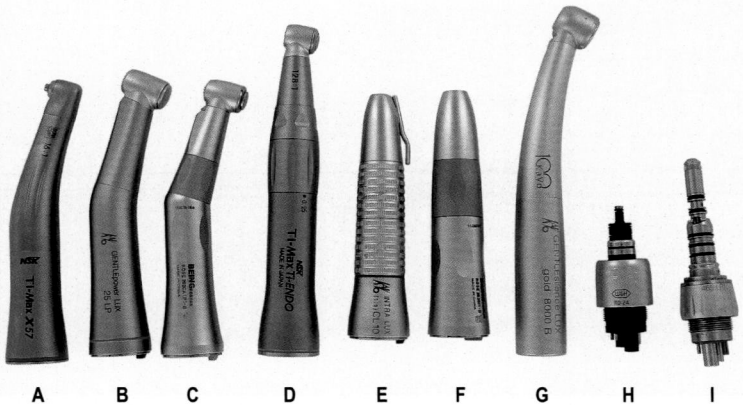

A   B   C   D   E   F   G   H   I

Fig. 1.11 The different hand pieces for dental units From the left are: three slow-speed contra-angle hand pieces; an endodontic hand piece; two straight hand pieces – one with external water/saline and the other with internal; a high-speed (30 000 rpm or more) hand piece; a rotaquick connector (for motor and turbine or blaster); and a multiflex connector (for turbine or blaster). Slow-speed hand pieces run at the speed of the micromotor, i.e. 20–40 000 rpm unless geared up or geared down. A blue ring or no color marking around the connecting end of the hand piece (C, E and F) means that the hand piece will run at the speed of the micromotor. A green ring around the connecting end of the hand piece (A) means that the hand piece is geared down, i.e. runs slower than the micromotor. The degree of speed reduction is often engraved on the hand piece. The one depicted furthest left in the picture is 16 : 1, i.e. the hand piece will run 16 times slower than the micromotor. The hand piece depicted 4th from left is an endodontic hand piece with reduction gear 128 : 1. A red ring indicates that the hand piece is geared up, i.e. runs faster than the micromotor. The one depicted in the picture (B) is 1 : 5, i.e. runs five times faster than the micromotor.

metal particles and then scrubbing or ultrasonically cleaning. Stones can be autoclaved safely.

There are several techniques for sharpening scalers and curettes detailed in the literature. A simple, but effective technique is as follows:

1. The terminal shank of the scaler (Fig. 1.13A) or curette (Fig. 1.14A) is placed on the stone in such a way that the reflection of the working end is seen on the stone.
2. The instrument is placed so that the blade engages the stone and the reflection (shadow) of the working end disappears (Fig. 1.13B for scaler and Fig. 1.14B for curette).
3. The stone is held stationary and the engaged instrument is pulled towards you (Fig. 1.15).

Make sure that you are familiar with the component parts of the scaler and curette before attempting sharpening. It may be useful to have a sharp, unused scaler and curette available for comparison during the learning phase. Also, have an acrylic stick handy to test the cutting edge.

Luxators, elevators and extraktors

Luxators, elevators and extraktors also need to be sharpened regularly, usually after each use, i.e. after cleaning and disinfecting. If the working end has been damaged, they should be professionally reground.

Luxators and elevators are easily sharpened with a cylindrical Arkansas stone. We prefer to use a 'stationary stone, moving instrument technique' to sharpen these instruments. The technique is as follows:

1. Place the cylindrical stone flat on the table.
2. Place a few drops of water on the stone.
3. Hold the handle of the luxator or elevator in the palm of the hand, with the index finger extended straight on the shank.
4. Apply the working end of the luxator or elevator to the stone.
5. Exert mild pressure and push or pull the luxator and elevator along the stone.
6. Check sharpness on an acrylic stick.
7. Repeat as necessary until the instrument is sharp.

Extraktors can be sharpened using either a flat stone or ideally a specially designed stone (Fig. 1.16). If a flat stone is used, then place the extraktor with its convex side against the stone, angle around 20° and push the instrument forward on the stone. For best results, use the specially designed stone. Place the extraktor in the correct groove and push forwards while rotating the instrument to maintain the lateral cutting edges.

Scalpel blade

The use of a scalpel blade to free the gingival attachment to the tooth is recommended for both closed and open

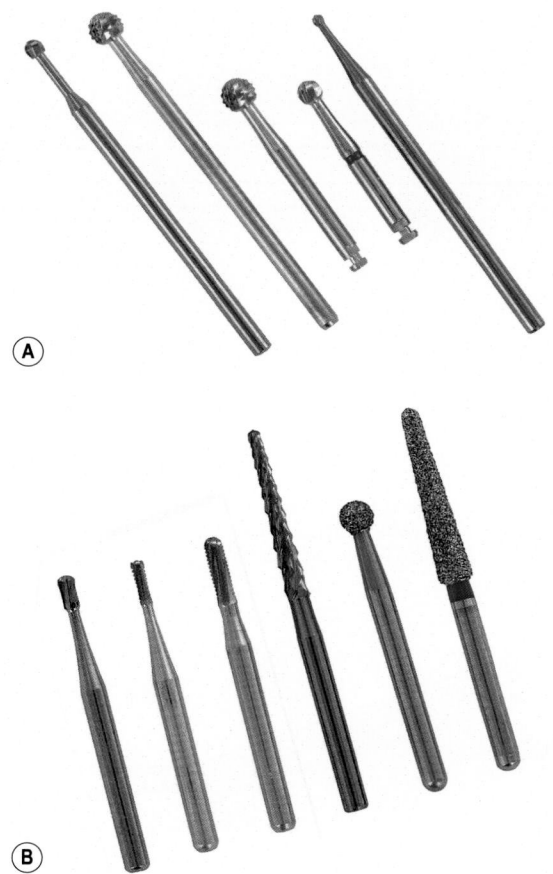

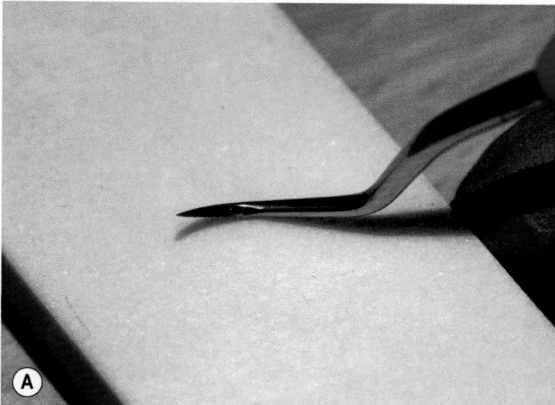

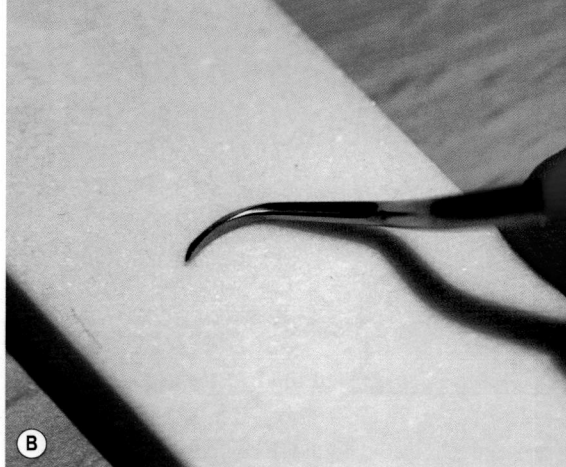

Fig. 1.12 Slow-speed and high-speed burs (A) Slow-speed burs. A selection of burs for slow-speed hand pieces. The long burs with friction grip attachment are for use in a straight hand piece; while the shorter ones with latch-key attachment are for use in a contra-angle hand piece. Slow-speed burs can be used to section teeth but are predominantly used to safely remove alveolar bone during extraction. Water cooling is essential. (B) High-speed burs. A selection of burs for high-speed hand pieces. Note that all burs are friction grip. A latch-key attachment is not possible at speeds in excess of 300 000 rpm. High-speed burs are used to section teeth and for cavity preparation. To avoid thermal injury to the tooth and bone and blunting of the bur, the water should never be turned off when using a high-speed bur.

Fig. 1.13 Sharpening a scaler The terminal shank of the scaler is placed on the stone in such a way that the reflection of the working end is seen on the stone (A). The instrument is then rotated so that the blade engages the stone and the shadow of the working end disappears (B).

cavity. Monocryl® (polyglecaprone, Ethicon) is currently our suture material of choice.

Suction

Suction is invaluable. Excess water and debris can easily be removed, improving visibility for the operator and increasing safety for the patient (reducing the risk of aspiration). In addition, blood loss can be estimated more accurately. Invest in either a compressed air-driven unit that incorporates suction or a separate suction unit.

Care of power equipment

Power equipment also requires care and maintenance. The manufacturer and/or supplier of power equipment need

extraction technique. A size 15 or 11 blade, used in the handle, is ideal (see Fig. 1.9).

Suture kit and suture material

A suture kit with small (ophthalmic) instruments should be available. An absorbable suture material with a swaged-on needle should always be used in the oral

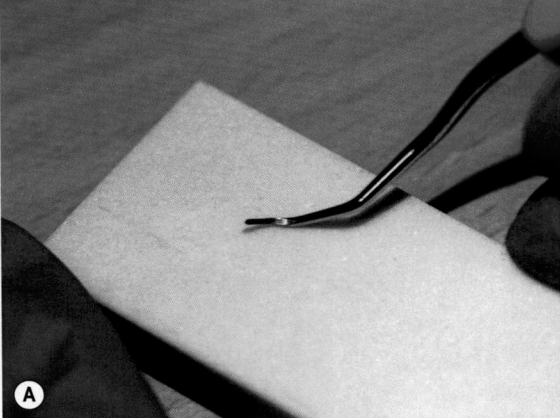

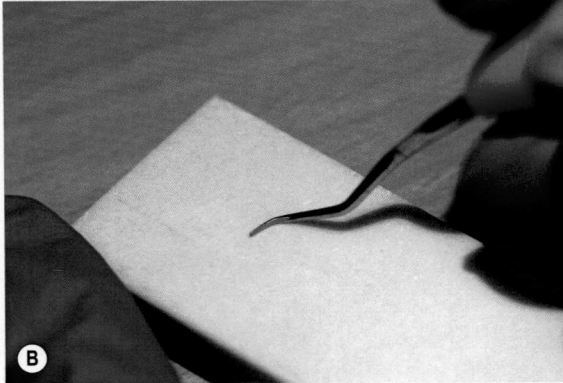

Fig. 1.14 Sharpening a curette The terminal shank of the curette is placed on the stone in such a way that the reflection of the working end is seen on the stone (A). The instrument is then rotated so that the blade engages the stone and the shadow of the working end disappears (B).

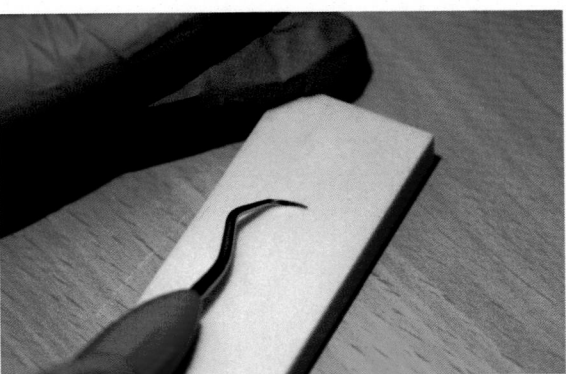

Fig. 1.15 Sharpening a scaler or curette The stone is held stationary and the engaged scaler or curette is pulled towards you. Use a few drops of water (not oil) to lubricate the stone. Use the length of the stone and avoid using the same area every time to avoid grooving in the stone. Test the cutting edge with an acrylic stick and repeat until the instrument is sharp, i.e. acrylic flakes are readily removed from the stick.

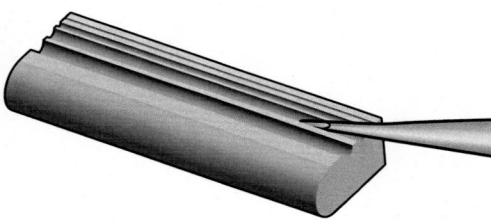

Fig. 1.16 Sharpening the Extraktor The Extraktor is placed in the correct groove for its size with its convex side against the stone. The instrument is pushed forward while rotating it to maintain the unique lateral cutting edges.

to supply you with detailed information of how to care and maintain the unit that you purchase. An annual service contract should be part of the purchase agreement.

There are similarities and differences in the care and maintenance of different units and you need to check with your supplier exactly how your unit should be looked after. The following guidelines are applicable to most air-driven units.

Unit:

- Dental lines need to be disinfected at least once a week using a 6% hydrogen peroxide solution, e.g. KaVo Oxygenal.
- External water needs to decanted and the lines left to dry at the end of each day and when the machine is not in use.
- If you have suction, then change the tip between each patient. The system should be flushed with

water and disinfected daily using a foam-free cleanser designed for dental suction systems, e.g. MD 555 (Durr Dental).

Compressor:

- The compressor needs to be positioned in an area with good ventilation, minimal moisture and no dust.
- It must be an oil-free compressor.
- Filters should be checked and changed regularly.
- Water condensation collects and should be removed.

Cleaning and sterilizing hand pieces

Each patient should receive clean and sterile hand pieces.

Hand pieces need to be lubricated after cleaning, i.e. prior to sterilization. They then need to be lubricated again after sterilization, i.e. prior to use. Hand pieces need to be lubricated before and after sterilization or the bearings will fail. They should be sterilized by means of autoclaving. Dry heat sterilization should not be used.

Important points relating to the high-speed hand piece are:

- Ensure that the water switch is in the 'On' position.
- Do not operate if there is insufficient water in the bottle.
- It should never be operated without a bur inserted.

After removing the bur, a brush is used to remove foreign particles from the hand piece. It is then wiped clean with a moist cloth. For the high-speed hand piece, a fine wire is provided for cleaning the water spray hole. Instructions should come with each unit as to how to dismantle hand pieces. Read these instructions carefully.

Lubricate the hand piece. We advise the use of a spray lubricant, which is inserted into the hand piece via a special lubricant nozzle. This is done without a bur in place. Once the oil has been inserted, the hand piece is ready for autoclaving. Follow the manufacturer's directions. After autoclaving is complete, make sure the hand piece returns to room temperature and lubricate the hand

piece again prior to use. Lack of lubrication will cause malfunction.

Caution:

- Never autoclave the hand piece with the bur in place.
- Never operate the hand piece without the bur inserted.
- Do not forget 'before and after sterilization' lubrication procedures.
- Dry heat sterilization is not allowed under any circumstances.

SUMMARY

- ◆ Dental procedures require a designated room or area designed to facilitate safe and effective clinical working practices.
- ◆ Dedicated anesthetic and radiographic facilities are ideal.
- ◆ Careful consideration should be given to the selection, maintenance and proper use of dental instruments and equipment.

FURTHER READING

Gorrel, C., Penman, S., 1995. Dental equipment. In: Crossley, D., Penman, S. (Eds.), Manual of Small Animal Dentistry. BSAVA, Cheltenham, Ch. 2, pp. 12–26.

Holmstrom, S.E., Frost-Fitch, P., Eisner, E.R., 2004. Dental equipment and care. In: Veterinary Dental Techniques for the Small Animal Practitioner, third ed. Saunders, Philadelphia, Ch. 2, pp. 39–129.

Wiggs, R.B., Lobprise, H.B., 1997. Dental equipment. In: Wiggs, R.B., Lobprise, H.B. (Eds.), Veterinary Dentistry: Principles and Practice. Lippincott-Raven, Philadelphia, Ch. 1, pp. 1–28.

Chapter 2

Anesthesia and analgesia

INTRODUCTION

This chapter deals with anesthetic and analgesic considerations specifically for the patient undergoing dental treatment and/or oral surgery. Detailed protocols will not be given, as there is wide variation in regimes worldwide and there are good textbooks on the subject available on the market.

ANESTHESIA

A full clinical examination of the oral cavity and all oral procedures require general anesthesia (GA). In rare circumstances, e.g. a brief oral examination or taking a few radiographs, sedation may be sufficient. However, as soon as any therapy needs to be performed, the animal should be placed under GA. Oral/dental procedures range from simple procedures in young healthy patients to lengthy complicated procedures in older, systemically compromised individuals.

GA can be maintained using an inhalational or injectable technique. However, if an injectable technique is used, the airways should always be secured with an endotracheal tube to prevent aspiration of saliva, debris and irrigation fluids.

Anesthesia is an unnatural state, and the induction process always carries a risk. The degree of risk varies and this should always be explained to the owner. It is essential that the owner or, in their absence, adult agents sign a consent form for anesthesia, indicating that they are giving their consent and have understood what has been explained to them. While the anesthetic mortality rate in fit and

healthy cats and dogs is 1 in 679 (0.15%), it increases to around 1 in 31 (3.2%) in animals that have a disease (Clarke and Hall 1990). In a more recent study (Dyson et al. 1998) investigating the morbidity and mortality associated with anesthesia (8087 dogs and 8702 cats), the incidences of complications were 2.1% in dogs and 0.13% in cats and the mortality rate was 0.11% in dogs and 0.1% in cats. Among other factors, continuous monitoring of anesthesia was associated with reduced mortality.

A thorough clinical examination must be performed prior to anesthesia. A full hematology and biochemistry panel is recommended for all geriatric (75–80% of the animal's anticipated life span is completed) patients. In the elderly, there is increasing likelihood of systemic disease that may have gone unnoticed by the client. Irrespective of age, the brachycephalic breeds pose an anesthetic challenge. Anesthesia for the trauma patient also requires careful management.

General principles of anesthesia for the dental patient

Airway security

During dental surgery, the airway must be secured by endotracheal intubation to prevent aspiration pneumonia, which may occur if debris (irrigation fluid, blood) from the oral cavity enters unprotected airways. This condition may be fatal and is easier to prevent than cure.

Endotracheal tubes

Endotracheal tubes must be checked for defective cuffs and obstructed lumens before use. Any defective tubes should be discarded. Lightweight circuits are recommended.

To reduce apparatus dead space and the risk of endo-bronchial intubation, the tubing should be cut to fit the patient from midneck to the level of the incisor teeth. Excessively long tubes that protrude from the oral cavity are prone to kinking, which may lead to pulmonary oedema as the patient inspires against an obstructed airway. The use of guarded endotracheal tubes should be considered for patients at high risk of tube kinking. Moreover, excessively long tubes are difficult to secure to the jaw with gauze bandage, which increases the risk of accidental extubation. Knots should be tied around the adaptor and not around the endotracheal tube itself.

The cuff should be carefully inflated to a point where there is no air leaking around it. Be careful not to inflate the cuff excessively as this can cause tracheal injury.

Pharyngeal packing

Pharyngeal packing should be used for greater airway security. Commonly used pharyngeal packs include surgical swabs, sponges and gauze bandage. A simple way to pack the pharynx is to insert a length of damp gauze bandage around the endotracheal tube with the free end left visible for easy removal. It is important not to pack too tightly as this impedes venous return and results in swelling of the tongue. Packs will become saturated with liquid during procedures and will then no longer offer adequate protection and should be replaced as required. It is imperative to remove any packing prior to extubation.

Eye protection

The eyes should be protected from desiccation by applying a lubricant eye ointment as required during the procedure.

Mouth gags

Mouth gags should be used with caution. Keeping the jaws wide open for prolonged periods may result in neuropraxia and inability to close the jaws. The condition is self-limiting but may take several weeks to resolve. Mouth gags should be released and the jaws closed every 10–15 min.

Suction

It is recommended to have suction available to protect the airways from saliva, irrigation fluids and other debris if required. In addition, blood loss can also be estimated by measuring the volume of blood in the suction jar.

Long anesthetic periods

Dental procedures are often lengthy and close attention to life support is needed:

- Oxygen should be delivered at an inspired concentration of at least 33% to compensate for the deterioration in pulmonary function that accompanies anesthesia even in healthy young patients.
- Reduced cardiac output and arterial blood pressure produced by anesthesia should be offset by intravenous fluid therapy. A catheter should be aseptically placed in an appropriate superficial vein before inducing anesthesia. Hartmann's (lactated Ringer's) solution should be given at a rate of 10 mL/kg per h. Catheters allow immediate venous access in an emergency and they ensure that irritant injectable agents are not given perivascularly. They should not be removed until the patient is fully recovered from anesthesia.
- Hypothermia is a complication of lengthy anesthesia and the use of cool irrigation fluids. Hypothermia results in anticholinergic-resistant bradycardia, reduced cardiac output and hemoconcentration. Cardiac fibrillation can occur at a body temperature of around 28 °C. Moreover, requirements for anesthetic agents are reduced during hypothermia and care should be taken to prevent relative overdose. Body temperature should be monitored during dental procedures and the development of hypothermia should be prevented by supplying external heat by blankets and warmed intravenous and irrigation fluids. Patients should be insulated with towels or bubble pack to prevent thermal injuries due to 'hot spots' that may occur with electrical heating mats. Circulating warm water mats may be safer.
- Hyperthermia can occasionally occur in large heavy-coated dogs connected to rebreathing circuits for long periods. Active cooling must then be initiated before damage occurs to vital organs.

Hemorrhage

The conditions covered in this book rarely result in extensive hemorrhage, unless the patient has an underlying disorder, e.g. coagulopathy, septicemia. A full hematologic examination and clotting profile should be performed prior to any potentially hemorrhagic procedure. The patient should also be cross-matched with a healthy donor prior to any such procedure. An alternative to cross-matching is autologous transfusion, where a week before surgery 10% of the patient's blood volume is removed and replaced with intravenous fluids. The blood is stored at 4 °C in acid citrate–dextrose or citrate–phosphate–dextrose transfusion packs until required.

During the procedure, blood loss should be estimated either by weighing blood-soaked swabs or by measuring the amount of blood collected in a suction jar. As a rough guide, a saturated 3×3 inch swab contains 7 mL of blood and a saturated 4×4 inch swab contains 10 mL of blood.

The normal patient can compensate for a blood loss of up to 20% of circulating volume. A dog's blood volume is 80–90 mL/kg and a cat's blood volume is 60–70 mL/kg. To compensate for hypotension, intravenous isotonic crystalloid fluid infusion should be increased to 30–40 mL/kg per h. Colloids can be used (up to 20 mL/kg) to maintain tissue perfusion but they are not a replacement for red blood cells. As the blood loss approaches 20% of circulating volume, fluid replacement therapy with blood should begin. Donor blood should be given at the same rate as patient blood is lost.

Hemostasis

Hemostasis is best achieved by identifying and ligating blood vessels or by using firm pressure for a few minutes. Vasoconstrictors such as topically applied adrenaline (epinephrine) or phenylephrine, owing to their arrhythmogenic properties if systemically absorbed, are best avoided.

Patient monitoring

All patients should be monitored continuously. Careful monitoring should enable the detection of problems before they become severe, so that they can be treated appropriately and crises can be avoided. Continuous anesthetic monitoring is associated with reduced mortality (Dyson et al. 1998).

Routine anesthetic monitoring includes inspection of respiratory function and the color of the mucous membranes, capillary refill time, listening to the sound of breathing and palpation of the peripheral pulse. This basic monitoring can be augmented with mechanical aids which give additional information and allow a more precise picture of the patient's status. This allows closer control over the course of the anesthetic. The disadvantage of mechanical monitoring devices is that they in turn must be monitored to ensure that the information they are giving is accurate. Unexpected readings should be verified by examination of the patient before they are acted on, i.e. monitor the patient, not the equipment (Box 2.1)!

Geriatric patients

Many of the patients that require dental procedures are geriatric. It must be remembered that even clinically healthy geriatric patients have physiologic changes in the cardiopulmonary system that can influence the course of anesthesia. Important age-related changes include:

- Decreased cardiac output
- Reduced ability to compensate for blood pressure and circulating volume changes
- Decreased lung compliance

Box 2.1 **Anesthesia and monitoring checklist**

- Endotracheal tube is correctly positioned and the cuff is not overinflated
- Endotracheal tube is securely fastened and not kinked
- Accidental extubation or circuit disconnection has not occurred (apnea alarms and capnograms are useful for detecting accidental disconnection)
- Monitor the central nervous system (ocular signs and muscle tone will indicate the depth of anesthesia)
- Monitor the cardiovascular system (pulse quality, auscultation of heart sounds, mucous membrane color and capillary refill). Monitoring devices that aid clinical assessment of cardiovascular function include esophageal stethoscopes, blood pressure monitors and ECG
- Monitor the respiratory system (tidal volume assessment by observing the rebreathing bag and chest wall excursions, respiratory rate, and mucous membrane color). Monitoring devices include apnea alarms and pulse oximeters
- Monitor and record body temperature (rectal or esophageal)
- Monitor renal function (a urinary catheter connected to an empty intravenous fluid bag via an administration set can measure urine output and thus give an indication of organ perfusion)
- Estimate blood loss and take appropriate measures
- Replace saturated pharyngeal packs
- Release mouth gags at regular intervals
- Reapply eye ointment as required.

- High small airway closing volume
- Decreased partial pressure of oxygen in arterial blood (PaO_2).

A noticeable decrease in circulation time is seen during induction, and further increments of injectable anesthetic agents should not be given too soon.

In addition to the age-related physiologic changes, elderly patients also have psychologic requirements in that they are easily distressed and confused by changes in routine and require gentle handling and constant reassurance.

Brachycephalic patients

In brachycephalic patients, upper airway obstruction should be anticipated. The degree of obstruction, assessed from clinical history and physical examination, needs to be determined prior to anesthesia and surgery. Chronic severe upper airway obstruction eventually results in cor pulmonale, and evidence for this should be checked.

Brachycephalic patients pose a challenge at both induction and recovery. Induction of anesthesia causes relaxation of pharyngeal musculature, and the degree of upper airway obstruction is increased until endotracheal intubation is performed. The ideal is rapid induction and rapid expert endotracheal intubation to shorten the period of increased upper airway obstruction. Mild sedation with low doses of acepromazine and an opioid, e.g. buprenorphine, is adequate in dogs. Boxers are prone to vasovagal syncope with acepromazine and should receive an anticholinergic if acepromazine is used. Alternatively, it should be avoided. Preoxygenation by mask for 5 min, if the animal will allow it, helps prevent hypoxia during induction, but mask induction using an inhalational agent should be avoided.

Airway obstruction during recovery can be dealt with in two ways. First, using an induction agent with a short plasma half-life, e.g. propofol, will ensure a rapid recovery and return of the patient's ability to maintain its own airway. Isoflurane or sevoflurane provides more rapid recoveries than halothane. Second, the use of an opioid with potent antitussive action, e.g. butorphanol, morphine or oxymorphone, can be used to allow tolerance of the endotracheal tube for a prolonged period. The endotracheal tube should be left in place for as long as possible. Ideally, the animal should be able to sit up or even stand before the endotracheal tube is removed.

Once the endotracheal tube is removed, there is still a risk of obstruction until the patient is fully awake. It is wise to have a small dose of an induction agent available so that reintubation can be performed rapidly if required. Continued oxygenation via a nasal catheter to prevent hypoxia following removal of the endotracheal tube is prudent. The patient's tongue should be pulled forwards to alleviate obstruction and the mouth kept open to encourage mouth breathing. Recovery in sternal recumbency is ideal as it allows more uniform expansion of the lungs and may promote a more rapid return to consciousness.

Maxillofacial trauma

Patients with traumatic injuries must be stabilized and other potential injuries dealt with prior to anesthesia. Most procedures can be managed with conventional endotracheal intubation, but occasionally passing the endotracheal tube through a pharyngotomy or tracheotomy site may be necessary.

Cats are prone to upper airway obstruction during anesthetic recovery if the nasal passages are occluded with blood and debris. They seem reluctant to mouth breathe during the critical time from extubation until they are completely recovered from the effect of the anesthetic. Anesthetic agents providing rapid recovery are therefore recommended.

ANALGESIA

Humans can express and describe the sensations of discomfort and/or pain that they experience, and these descriptions are well accepted. Assessment of pain in animals is much more difficult. One must rely on overt signs and the correct interpretation of these signs. Animals probably have no psychologic expectation of pain, so the confounding influence of anticipation is removed. Changed responsiveness to human contact is often a first indicator that the animal is in discomfort. Aggression or avoidance of human contact may occur, but some animals seek excessive human reassurance. Disturbance in the sleep pattern, with an animal sleeping less, is also an indicator of discomfort. Reduced grooming and changes in eating behaviour are often manifestations of chronic pain.

In the presence of oral/dental disease it is rare for the animal to stop eating, instead they change their food preferences (e.g. an animal will selectively only eat soft food) or change the way they chew (e.g. chew selectively on one side). A common feedback from clients after their pet has undergone a remedial dental procedure is that the animal is brighter in general, often showing more interest in exercise and games than prior to treatment. One can speculate that this commonly reported change in general behaviour is attributable to the removal of chronic discomfort and pain.

In human dentistry, there is a good understanding of which disease processes cause discomfort and pain. We also know which procedures are associated with postoperative pain. It seems reasonable to assume that dogs and cats experience discomfort and pain when afflicted by the same diseases and after receiving similar treatment. In following this line of reasoning, overtreatment with analgesics may occur, but the adverse consequences of this are minimal compared with the distress of withholding pain relief.

Common conditions that we know are likely to cause discomfort and/or pain in people, and are thus likely to cause similar sensations to an affected animal, include:

- Complications to periodontitis, e.g. lateral periodontal abscess, toxic mucous membrane ulcers, gingivostomatitis
- Pulp and periapical disease, e.g. acute pulpitis, periapical abscess, osteomyelitis
- Traumatic injuries, including soft-tissue lacerations and jaw fracture.

These conditions may be seen as emergencies in that treatment should not be delayed. They are covered in detail in Chapter 12, but analgesic considerations will be covered in this chapter.

Dental procedures that we know are likely to cause postoperative pain in humans, and are therefore likely to cause similar sensations in animals, include:

- Periodontal therapy, e.g. deep subgingival curettage
- Extraction, especially when extraction sockets are left to heal by granulation.

Mechanisms of pain processing

The 'pain pathway' can be split into three principal components:

1. Peripheral tissue nociceptors detect the stimulus and transmit the nociceptive signal via primary afferent nerve fibers to the spinal cord or cranial nerve nuclei.
2. Processing occurs in the spinal cord or brainstem before transmission to supraspinal structures.
3. After further processing at supraspinal sites, the signal induces the conscious perception of pain.

In addition, there are various intrinsic segmental, spinal and supraspinal endogenous mechanisms for inhibiting the transmission of the nociceptive signals. These are mediated by endogenous neurotransmitter systems (opioid, cholinergic, adrenergic, serotonergic).

The appreciation of pain is not just a moment-by-moment analysis of afferent noxious input relayed by a hard-wired transmission system. Instead, it is a dynamic process that is influenced by past experience. Clinical pain can be classified as inflammatory (relates to peripheral tissue damage) or neuropathic (relates to a damaged central nervous system). Clinical pain is characterized by changes in sensitivity, such that stimuli that are not normally perceived as painful become painful (allodynia) and an exaggerated response to a given noxious stimulus (hyperalgesia) develops and spreads to uninjured tissue (secondary hyperalgesia). This sensitization occurs at either or both peripheral and central levels. Peripheral sensitization occurs because of an increase in sensitivity of the nociceptors due to their exposure to high levels of inflammatory mediators and results in an increase in the firing rate of afferent nerve fibers. Central hypersensitivity develops because of changes in the spinal cord. An activity-dependent increase in excitability of dorsal horn neurons develops, which outlasts the nociceptive afferent inputs.

The clinical implications of peripheral and central hypersensitivity are that:

- Once pain is established, analgesic drugs, for a given dose, are much less effective, i.e. pain is more difficult to control.
- The pain perceived by the animal will be greater.

Thus, the evidence is overwhelming that pain should be *prevented* rather than just treated. It has been shown clinically in dogs (Lascelles et al. 1997) that pre-injury treatment with opioids prevents or markedly decreases the development of central hypersensitivity, but these treatments are far less effective if administered after the injury is initiated. Local analgesics (Bach et al. 1988) have shown similar protective effects. So, by preventing the surgical afferent stimuli from entering the spinal cord, central sensitization can be avoided. Thus, the severity of postoperative pain can be markedly decreased.

The concept of pre-emptive analgesia is the administration of analgesics preoperatively to reduce the severity of postoperative pain. It is important to distinguish between pre-emptive analgesia and alleviation of postoperative pain. In other words, pre-emptive analgesia may block sensitization, but it does not eliminate postoperative pain; additional measures are still required to ensure a comfortable recovery.

The optimum form of pain therapy is continuous pre-emptive analgesia, continuously preventing the establishment of sensitization. The administration of opioids or local anesthetic drugs blocks central sensitization and nonsteroidal anti-inflammatory drugs (NSAIDs) reduce the severity of the peripheral inflammatory response. The combined use of an opioid and an NSAID is more effective than using either drug alone. Local anesthetics (analgesics) can produce complete pain relief by blocking all sensory input from the affected area.

A basic analgesic routine, which can be modified as required, is as shown in Box 2.2.

Local anesthesia

Local anesthesia (LA) can be used to provide intra- and postoperative analgesia. In contrast to human patients, dogs and cats are not amenable to LA if conscious. So, the techniques are used when the animal is under GA. When given prior to the start of a procedure, the use of LA may reduce the requirement for GA drugs during surgery. When given at the end of a procedure, prior to GA recovery, they will provide postoperative analgesia.

Useful techniques in the oral cavity include infiltration anesthesia and regional nerve blocks. Infiltration anesthesia is where a small amount of anesthetic agent is deposited locally to diffuse into the tissue and exert effect. Regional anesthesia is where the anesthetic agent is deposited as close to the nerve as possible and its effect is thus to block

---

Box 2.2 **Basic analgesic plan for the dentistry and/or oral surgery patient**

- Include an opioid in the premedication
- Use local anesthetics prior to surgery and/or administer additional opioids intraoperatively
- Give opioids and/or NSAIDs postoperatively. LA (administered at the end of a procedure) will also provide postoperative analgesia
- Administer NSAIDs during recovery.

all sensation distally, e.g. placing local anesthetic close to the inferior alveolar branch of the mandibular nerve as it enters the mandibular foramen will desensitize the mandibular teeth and lower lip. In human dentistry infiltration anesthesia is the most commonly used technique and provides adequate analgesia for all teeth except the mandibular premolars and molars, where a mandibular block is used. In veterinary dentistry, the use of regional blocks has been advocated. In fact, infiltration techniques are often not described in veterinary textbooks. This is a shame, as infiltration anesthesia is easier and safer than regional blocks. The main risk with regional blocks is damage to the nerve as the anesthetic agent is placed. Iatrogenic nerve damage (the needle scratches or perforates the nerve) causes pain and it can take weeks to months before the tissue regenerates and the patient is pain free. In rare instances, there is permanent nerve damage. In human dentistry it is advised to never inject into a foramen because of the high risk of nerve damage. Moreover, the patient is conscious and reacts if the needle scratches or perforates the nerve. The sensation is described as an electric shock. In human dentistry, LA is generally not used in the anesthetized patient as there will be no reaction to nerve injury. In veterinary dentistry the described techniques for regional blocks involve placing a needle well into a foramen and are performed on an anesthetized animal where there will be no sensory feedback. In my opinion, regional blocks should be performed with great caution and only be used in areas where infiltration anesthesia is not possible, i.e. mandibular premolars and molars.

All clinically used local anesthetics are membrane-stabilizing agents. They prevent depolarization and thus stop or retard conduction of impulses. Sensation disappears in the following order: pain, cold, warmth, touch, joint and deep pressure. Procaine hydrochloride is the prototype of all local anesthetics. It is the standard drug for comparison of anesthetic effects. For LA in the oral cavity lidocaine, mepivacaine, bupivacaine and ropivacaine are all suitable. The local anesthetic drug chosen for postoperative pain relief should ideally have a long duration of action, and therefore bupivacaine (onset 15 min, duration 4–6 h) is the drug of choice. Lidocaine can be used during surgery for more immediate effect.

The mechanism of action of all local anesthetic drugs is similar. The salt of the anesthetic base (RNH^+Cl^-) is an ionizable quaternary amine with little or no anesthetic properties of its own because it is not lipid soluble and therefore not absorbed in the nerve membrane. After deposition in tissue that is slightly alkaline and has considerable buffering capacity, the anesthetic base is liberated as follows:

$$RNH^+Cl^- \rightleftharpoons Cl^- + RNH^+ \rightleftharpoons RN + H^+$$

The free anesthetic base (RN) is absorbed in the outer lipid nerve membrane, where anesthetic action takes place.

If sufficient local buffering capacity exists to remove the dissociated H^+, this reaction proceeds to the right, and active base is liberated which exerts an anesthetic effect. In inflamed or infected tissue, however, the pH is acidic and the result is that only small amounts of free base dissociate from the anesthetic salt, resulting in poor LA.

In human dentistry and oral surgery, vasoconstrictors (adrenaline, L-adrenaline) are routinely used in combination with the local anesthetic. The main reason is to delay systemic absorption of the local anesthetic, thus reducing the toxicity and increasing the margin of safety. Local anesthetics produce analgesia when given in small doses intravenously, but are potent proconvulsants and can induce marked myocardial depression and cardiac dysrhythmias when administered systemically. The addition of vasoconstrictors, by reducing systemic absorption of the local anesthetic, will also increase intensity and prolong anesthetic activity. However, they may increase the risk of cardiac arrhythmias and ventricular fibrillation. In veterinary dentistry and oral surgery, local anesthetics are generally used without the addition of vasoconstrictors. Safe maximum doses are: 4 mg/kg lidocaine and 1–2 mg/kg bupivacaine. I use local anesthetics with added vasoconstrictor to ensure that the anesthetic agent remains locally active for a prolonged period.

A 22–30 gauge, 1 inch needle is used for the regional blocks in dogs; a shorter needle is easier for infiltration anesthesia and for regional blocks in cats. The use of a dental local anesthetic syringe and needle (Fig. 2.1) is strongly recommended. The safe maximum dose is calculated for each animal. In general, 0.25–1.00 mL of local anesthetic agent is deposited per site. Always aspirate for blood before injecting.

Infiltration

Infiltration anesthesia involves depositing a small amount of local anesthetic (bleb technique) into the gingiva and alveolar periosteum in the region of the apex of the tooth that needs to be desensitized (Figs 2.2–2.4). The anesthetic agent diffuses into the tissue to have local effect on the nerve. The infiltrates are deposited buccally and palatally/lingually as required. This technique can be used to provide desensitization of all teeth in the upper jaw. In fact, regional blocks are not necessary in the upper jaw. Infiltration can also be used to desensitize incisors (Fig. 2.5) and rostral premolars in the lower jaw. It is only for the distal premolars and molars in the mandible that a regional block is required.

Regional blocks

Regional anesthesia is where the anesthetic agent is deposited as close to the nerve as possible and its effect is thus to block all sensation distally. Figures 2.6 and 2.7 describe the pathways of innervation. Nerve blocks that have been described for use in dentistry and oral surgery are:

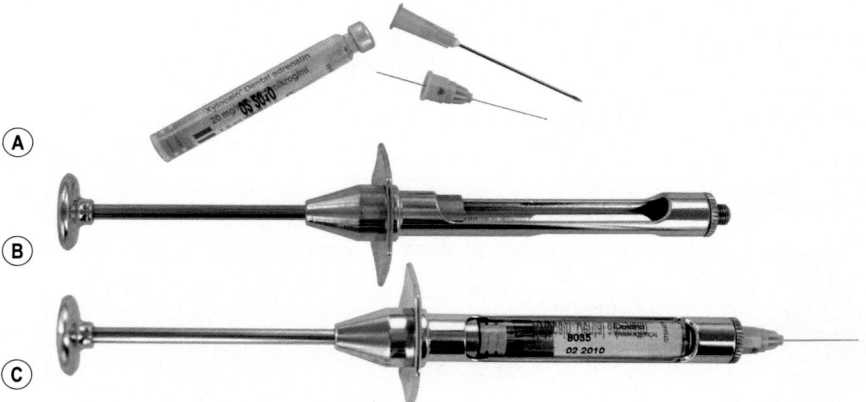

Fig. 2.1 **A dental local anesthetic needle and syringe** (A) The ampoule with local anesthetic agent and the needle. An 18-gauge needle is depicted as well to highlight how fine the dental needle is. (B) The metal syringe case. (C) The device assembled and ready for use.

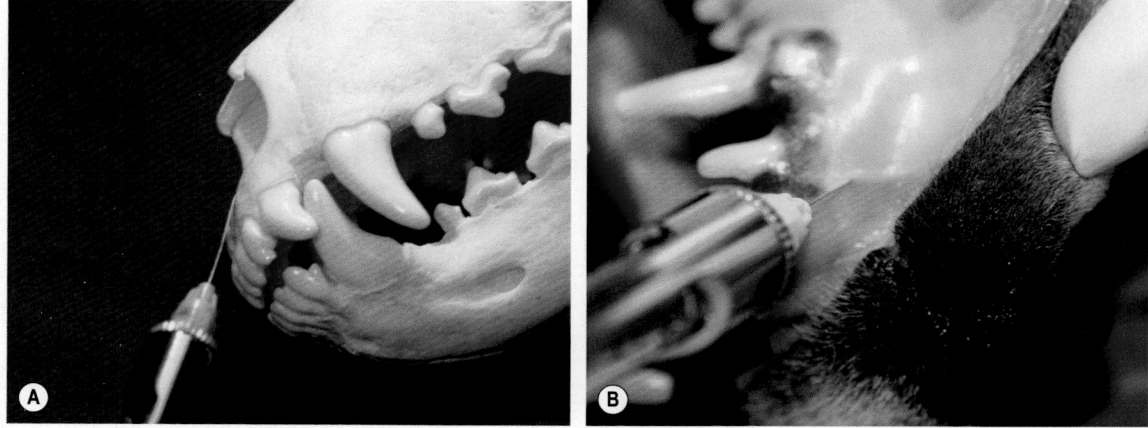

Fig. 2.2 **Technique for infiltration anesthesia for desensitization of the buccal aspect of an upper incisor** A small amount of local anesthetic is deposited into the gingiva and alveolar periosteum in the region of the tooth that needs to be desensitized. The anesthetic agent diffuses into the tissue to have local effect on the nerve. The location for buccal desensitization of an upper incisor is shown on a skull (A) and on a cadaver (B).

- Infraorbital
- Mandibular
- Mental.

All four quadrants of the jaws can be blocked at the same session if required, e.g. extraction of most or all teeth.

In the following, the three blocks will be described but, in my opinion, the only block that is required for veterinary dentistry is the mandibular block. Infiltration techniques can be used at all locations of the oral cavity except the lower distal premolars and molars and is a far safer technique.

Infraorbital nerve block. Blocking the infraorbital nerve will desensitize the upper lip and nose, roof of the nasal cavity, skin ventral to the infraorbital foramen and the maxillary teeth. An extraoral approach is possible, but the intraoral approach is much easier. The procedure (Fig. 2.8) is as follows.

The lip is lifted and the infraorbital foramen is located by palpation. The needle is inserted a short distance into the canal. Remember that the infraorbital canal is much shorter than normal in brachycephalic dogs and cats and it is not recommended to insert the needle into the pterygopalatine fossa. A suggested guideline is to insert

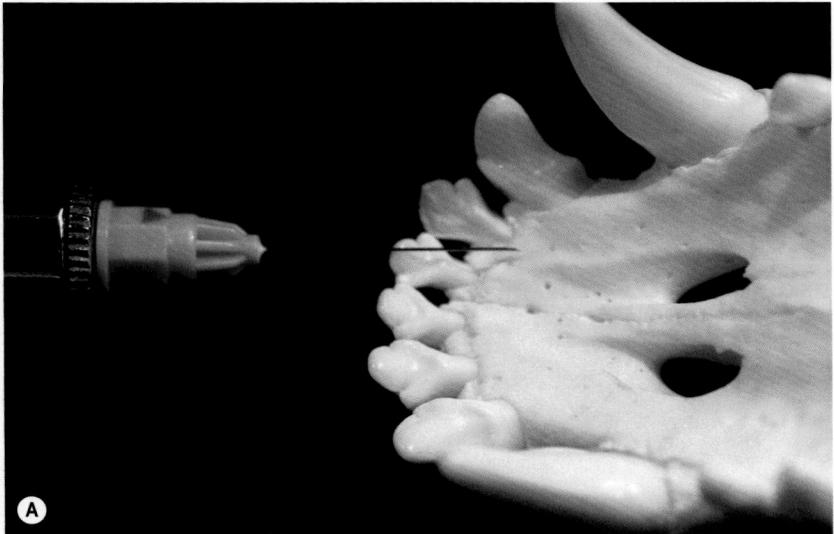

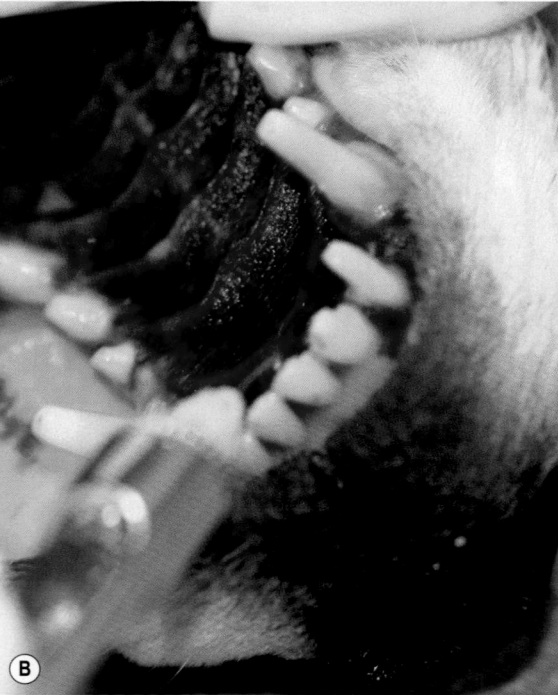

Fig. 2.3 Technique for infiltration anesthesia for desensitization of the palatal aspect of an upper incisor
It is often necessary to place anesthetic agent palatally as well. The location for palatal desensitization of an upper incisor is shown on a skull (A) and on a cadaver (B).

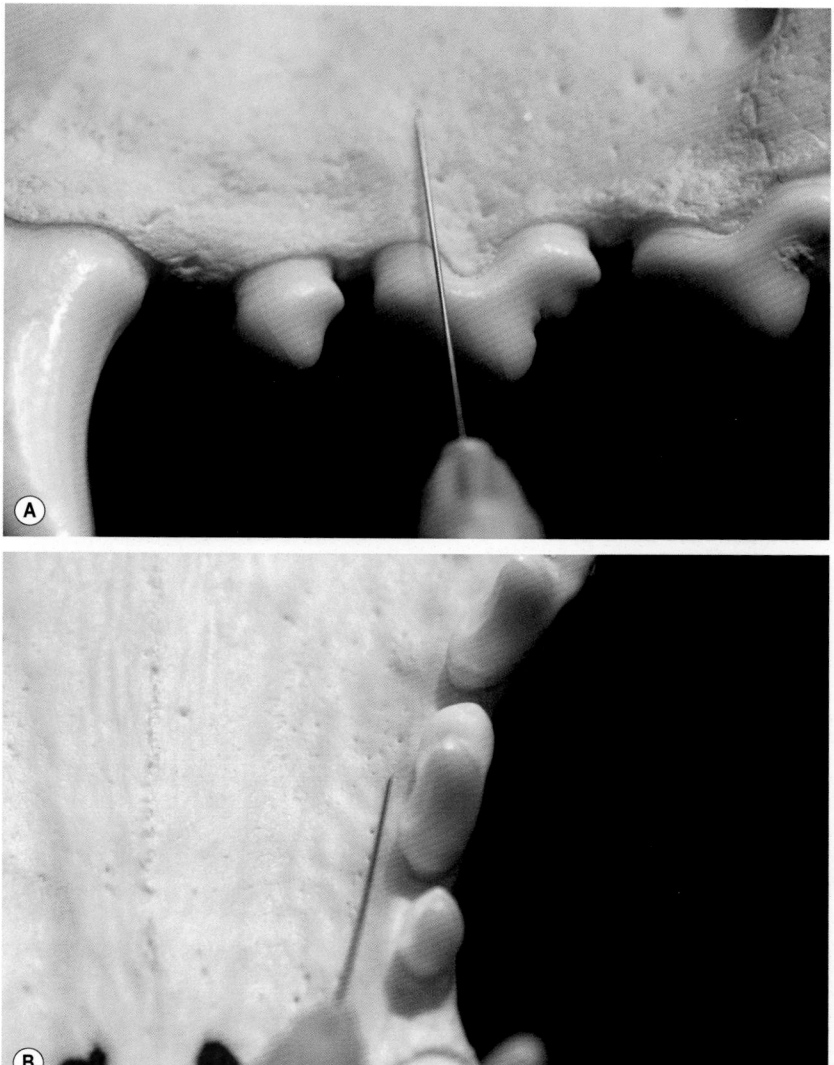

Fig. 2.4 Technique for infiltration anesthesia for desensitization of an upper premolar The buccal (A) and palatal (B) locations where local anesthetic agent is deposited are depicted on a skull.

the needle into the canal no further than a distance that is less than the width of the upper 4th premolar. Following aspiration to ensure that the needle is not into the blood vessels, the calculated amount of local anesthetic is deposited. Place a finger over the infraorbital foramen for 20–30 s after withdrawing the needle to encourage the local anesthetic to track back in the canal and block the middle superior alveolar branches that supply the cheek teeth, and also to prevent hematoma formation at the injection site.

I never use this technique owing to the high risk of nerve damage when inserting a needle in the foramen and into the canal.

Mandibular block. Blocking the inferior alveolar branch of the mandibular nerve will desensitize the mandibular teeth and lower lip. In the mandibular block the inferior alveolar nerve is blocked prior to its entering the mandibular canal. This block can be performed using either an extraoral or an intraoral approach.

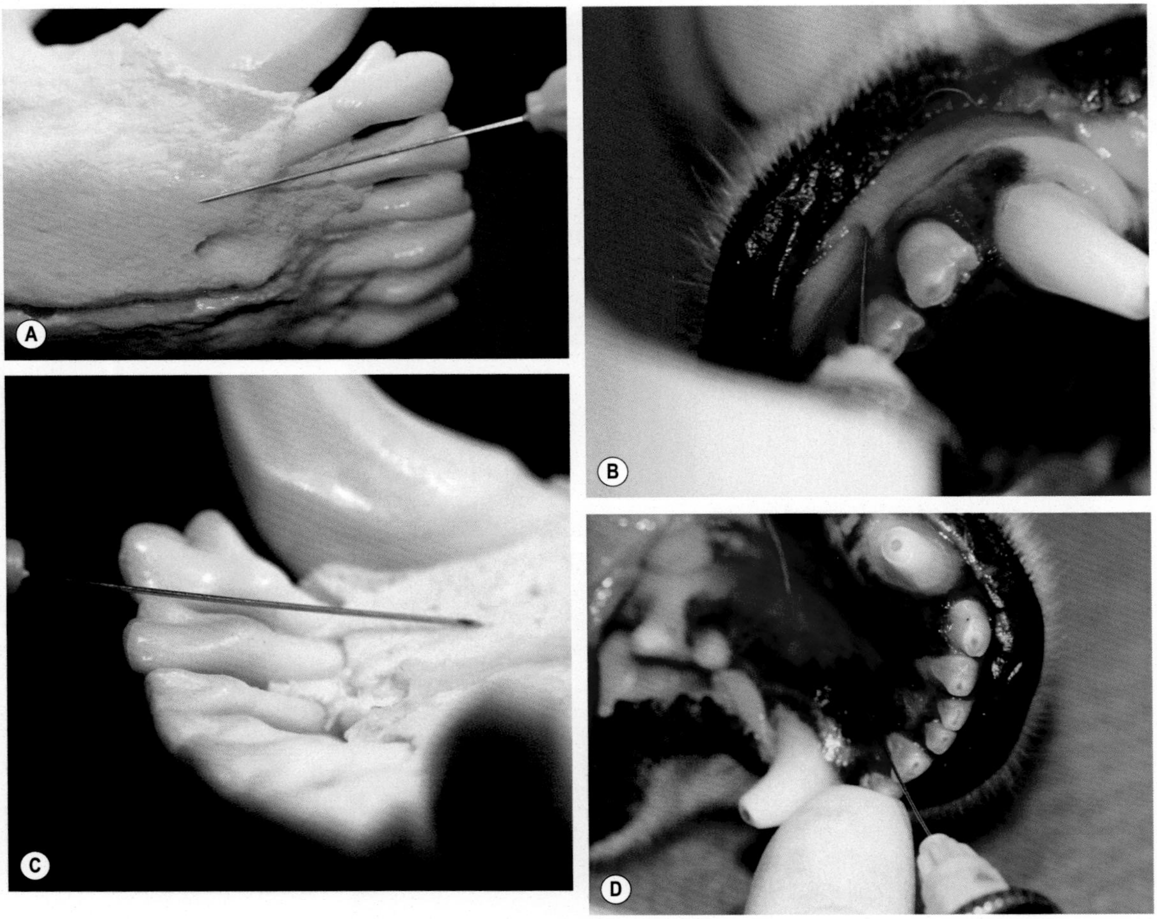

Fig. 2.5 Technique for infiltration anesthesia for desensitization of a lower incisor The buccal and palatal locations where local anesthetic agent is deposited are depicted on a skull (A,C) and on a cadaver (B,D).

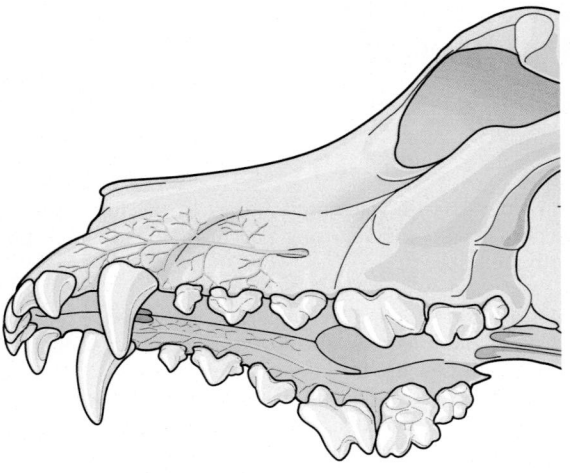

Fig. 2.6 Sensory innervation of the upper jaw The *infraorbital nerve* is the continuation of the maxillary nerve in the pterygopalatine fossa. Before entering the infraorbital canal (at the maxillary foramen), the nerve gives off *caudal superior alveolar branches*, which supply the posterior cheek teeth. Within the canal, the infraorbital nerve gives off *middle superior alveolar branches* to the cheek teeth. Just before it emerges from the infraorbital foramen (at the infraorbital foramen), it gives off the *rostral superior alveolar branches*, which supply the upper canine and incisor teeth. The infraorbital nerve divides into a number of large fascicules upon emerging from the infraorbital foramen. These are distributed to the skin and sinus or tactile hair of the upper lip and muzzle. There are external and internal *nasal branches* and *superior labial branches*. The *palatine nerves* (derived from the sphenopalatine branches of the maxillary nerve) provide the sensory innervation to the roof of the mouth, soft palate, tonsil and lining membrane of the nasal cavity.

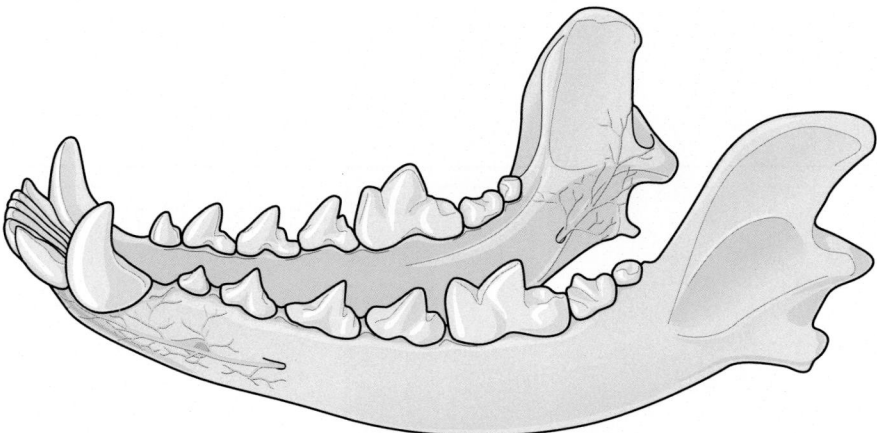

Fig. 2.7 Sensory innervation of the lower jaw The *inferior alveolar nerve* leaves the ventral lateral trunk of the mandibular division of the trigeminal nerve and enters the mandibular canal at the mandibular foramen. The *inferior alveolar nerve* accompanies the inferior alveolar artery and gives off sensory branches to the mandibular teeth. Several branches (*mental nerves*) leave the nerve rostrally and pass out through the mental foramina. The *mental nerves* are distributed to the incisor teeth and skin ventral to the incisor teeth.

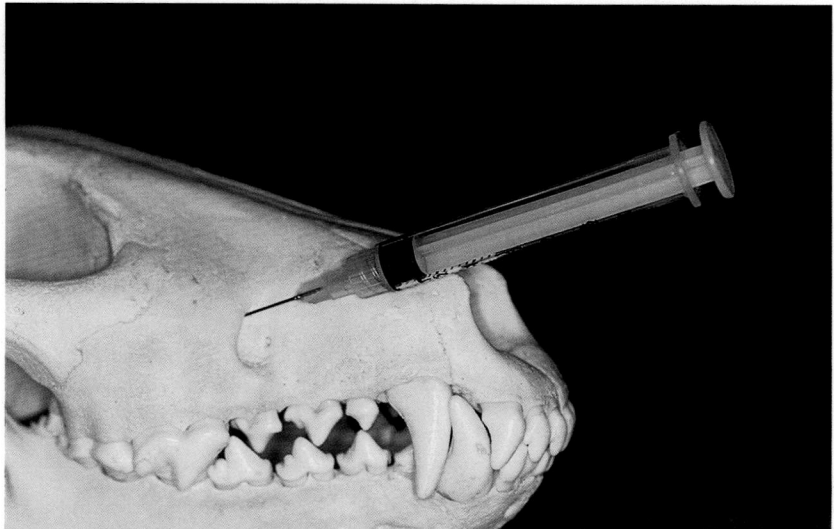

Fig. 2.8 The infraorbital block

For the extraoral approach (Fig. 2.9), the needle is inserted into the skin at the lower angle of the jaw, approximately 1.5 cm rostral to the angular process. The needle is passed dorsally along the medial surface of the mandibular ramus, staying close to the bone to avoid inadvertently blocking the lingual nerve. The mandibular foramen can be palpated intraorally and the needle point guided accurately to the nerve. The calculated dose of local anesthetic is deposited in and around the nerve as it enters the mandibular foramen.

The intraoral approach (Fig. 2.10) involves palpating the mandibular foramen intraorally and directing the needle to that area using an oral approach. The easiest way is to slide the needle along the medial aspect of the ventral mandible, with the syringe held parallel to the hemimandible to be blocked (Fig. 2.10A). When the point of the needle is close to the foramen, move the syringe barrel over to the premolar region of the contralateral side (Fig. 2.10B) to give better access to the area around the foramen. The needle should be close to the bone of the

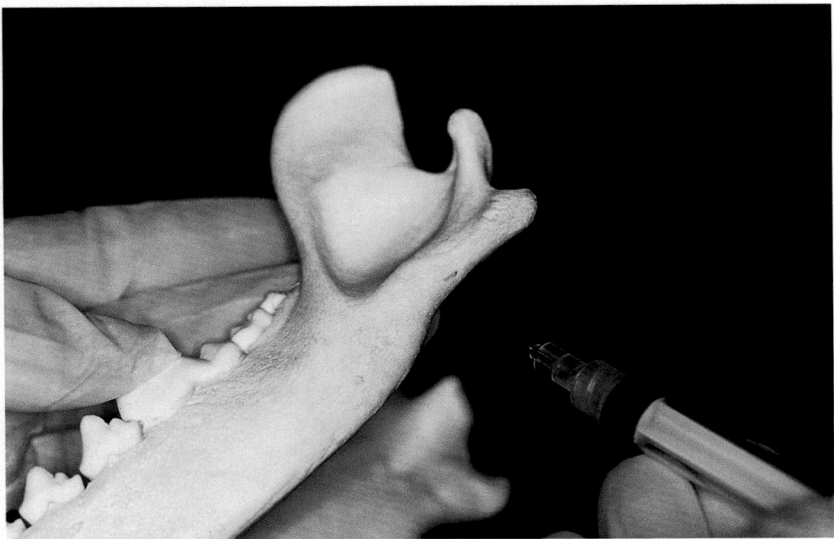

Fig. 2.9 **The mandibular block** Mandibular block (extraoral approach).

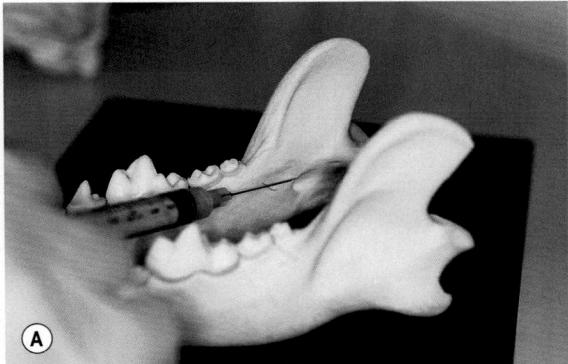
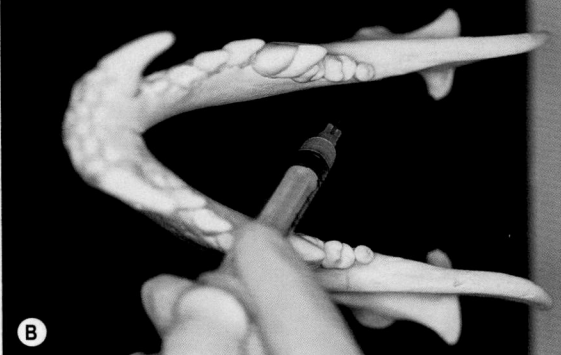

Fig. 2.10 **The mandibular block** Mandibular block (intraoral approach).

ventral mandible to avoid inadvertently blocking the lingual nerve. The calculated dose is deposited.

Mental block. Blocking the mental nerve branches will desensitize the lower lip and the teeth rostral to the mental foramina. The needle is inserted into the middle mental foramen at the level of the 2nd premolar tooth (Fig. 2.11) and the calculated dose of local anesthetic is deposited. It is not practically possible to perform a mental block in cats and small dogs as the middle mental foramen may not be palpable and/or may be too small a diameter to successfully insert even a fine needle.

In my opinion, this block should never be performed. There is absolutely no need to enter into the foramen. A much less traumatic and safer option is to deposit a bleb of anesthetic in the region of the foramen and allow the agent to diffuse into the nerves. Another option is to perform infiltration anesthesia of individual teeth. A third option is to use the mandibular block.

Complications with local anesthesia

Infiltration anesthesia is rarely associated with complications other than the rare hematoma at the injection site.

Regional anesthesia may result in tongue biting and/or cheek chewing in the postoperative period, hematoma, nerve damage resulting in pain (often also with paresthesia) and trismus. As already mentioned, nerve damage occurs when the injection needle scrapes or perforates the nerve (likely if the needle is inserted into the foramen or canal). The injury causes pain and often also paresthesia

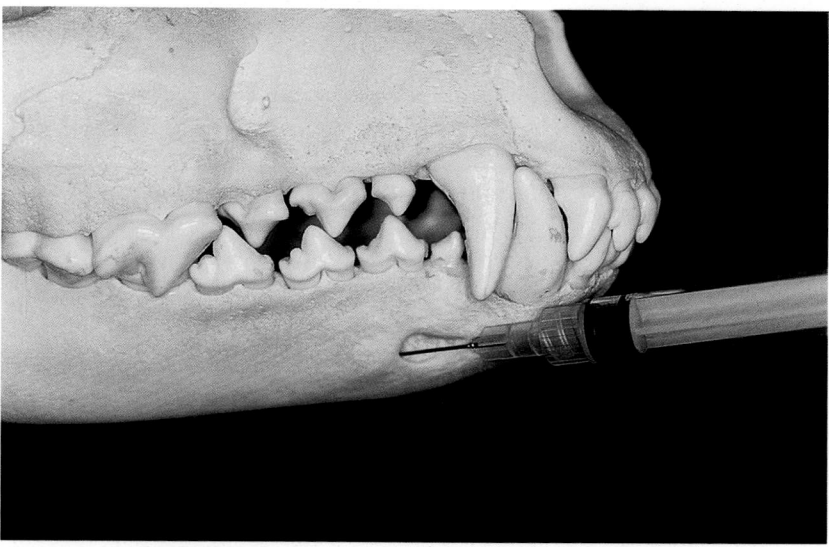

Fig. 2.11 The mental block

and can take weeks to months to resolve. Permanent injury is possible. Trismus may occur if the needle causes trauma to or if local anesthetic is placed in the medial pterygoid muscle. The patient loses the ability to fully open the mouth. The condition is self-limiting but may take weeks to resolve.

Indications for local anesthesia

This is a controversial topic. Some authors advocate routine use of LA for all dental/oral surgery. I am more restrictive and use it more selectively. Situations where I feel that LA is useful include open extraction of several teeth, jaw fracture repair, and bone resection, e.g. mandibulectomy, maxillectomy procedures.

Guidelines for LA:

- Inject slowly
- Aspirate
- Avoid injecting into inflamed/infected tissue
- Avoid injecting into the foramina
- Avoid injecting below the periosteum.

Non-pharmacologic methods of pain relief

Sound nursing measures also have a profound impact on reducing the level of postoperative discomfort and pain. A quiet environment allowing the animal to sleep is most important. The intensity of acute postoperative pain generally diminishes quickly. Sleeping it off is beneficial! Cats, in particular, appreciate a quiet environment postoperatively; a barking dog in the same room is not conducive

to a stress-free recovery! Giving a low dose of a sedative if the patient is particularly agitated should be considered.

Giving the animal some attention at regular intervals helps reduce the distress associated with pain and the unfamiliar environment, otherwise a cycle of pain/distress/sleeplessness can develop.

The provision of a comfortable bed in a warm, but not too hot, environment is beneficial. Food and water should be offered as early as possible in the postoperative period. Pain and inflammation increase the basic metabolic rate and a high level of nutrition is required to promote healing. Offering food as early as possible not only speeds recovery, but can also have a soothing effect.

SPECIAL TECHNIQUES

There are certain situations where special techniques for intubation and feeding are required and the clinician needs to be familiar with these.

Intubation

In some circumstances, pharyngotomy or tracheotomy intubation is required.

Pharyngotomy

Occasionally, it may be required to pass the endotracheal tube from the trachea through a temporary pharyngotomy to connect to the breathing circuit. This allows access to the oral cavity without the hindrance of an endotracheal tube. Pharyngotomy intubation is essential in situations where occlusion needs to be maintained, e.g. fracture repair.

Orotracheal intubation, using a wire-reinforced endotracheal tube, is performed. The skin at the cervical area and over the angle of the mandible is clipped and surgically prepared. An index finger is inserted into the oral cavity to locate the pyriform sinus rostral to the epihyoid bone. The skin is incised and tissue dissected through to the oral cavity. The adaptor is removed from the endotracheal tube and forceps are thrust through the pharyngotomy incision and used to grasp and pull the proximal end of the endotracheal tube laterally. Be careful not to push the endotracheal tube in too far and accidentally perform an endobronchial intubation! The adaptor is reconnected and anesthesia using an inhalational technique is continued. Injectable anesthetic drugs may be required to maintain anesthesia during movement of the endotracheal tube. Propofol is ideal for this purpose, as it does not accumulate with repeated boluses.

Elective tracheotomy

This may be required for an animal that cannot open its mouth sufficiently to allow orotracheal intubation (e.g. chronic masseteric muscle myositis), or as an emergency procedure in animals with acute upper airway obstruction. Anesthesia can be induced and maintained with incremental boluses of a non-cumulative anesthetic agent such as propofol until the tracheotomy is performed. The skin over the ventral surface of the neck is clipped and surgically prepared. The ventral surface of the trachea at the level of the 2nd, 3rd and 4th tracheal rings is exposed by a midline incision and retraction of the sternohyoideus muscles. Tracheal incision can be performed in two ways. In either method, two stabilizing sutures are placed around the tracheal rings at the site of the tracheal incision to facilitate later apposition. Access to the trachea is gained by means of a transverse incision through the annular ligament and mucosa between two tracheal rings. The incision should extend to up to 65% of the circumference of the trachea. This method is useful for short-term intubation.

Alternatively, a U-shaped ventral tracheal flap is created based on the 2nd tracheal ring and extending two rings distally. The flap is raised as a hinge to allow placement of the endotracheal tube. This method is suitable for long-term intubation as it prevents excessive pressure of the tube on surrounding tissues. Ideally, the incision should be left to heal by granulation. This does require intensive care to allow cleaning of the tracheotomy site and constant observation of the patient. Some clinicians therefore prefer to close the site, but there is risk of subcutaneous emphysema, localized swelling and subsequent airway obstruction.

Feeding tubes

In patients that cannot eat or drink normally, placement of a feeding tube offers an alternative method of providing nutrition and fluids.

Indwelling nasogastric intubation

This technique is limited to short periods of feeding with liquidized foods. It is useful following full mouth extraction in cats with chronic gingivostomatitis and is rarely required for more than 1–2 days.

A nasogastric tube can be placed in either the conscious or the anesthetized animal. The easiest and safest way of doing it is to place the feeding tube while the animal is under GA with an endotracheal tube in place.

A lubricated 5 or 6 French gauge polyvinyl infant feeding tube is passed into the ventral nasal meatus. In the conscious patient, the nasal mucosa should be desensitized with a local anesthetic agent and the head should be held with the nose pointing down while the tube is being advanced, as this position helps prevent accidental insertion into the trachea. The tube should be advanced until the distal end is positioned in the distal esophagus. Placement should be verified by radiography or by auscultation of bubbles when air or sterile saline is instilled through the tube. The tube should then be capped and sutured in place with butterflies made from sticky tape. An Elizabethan collar will be necessary in some animals to prevent them from removing the tube.

Esophagostomy tube

This site is currently the preferred position for placement of a feeding tube. It prevents potential complications such as aspiration and damage to the mucosa, which can be associated with pharyngotomy intubation, and avoids the complication of peritonitis from gastrostomy tubes.

With the animal under GA, the left lateral cervical region is clipped and prepared for surgery. Curved forceps are inserted into the proximal cervical esophagus, caudal to the hyoid bone, via the pharynx. The tips of the forceps are turned laterally and pressure applied so the tips can be palpated. A skin incision large enough to accommodate the feeding tube is made over the tips of the forceps. The forceps are then pushed through the esophagus or, in large dogs, an incision is made. The distal end of the premeasured feeding tube (marked from stomach or distal esophagus to incision site) is grasped by the forceps and pulled through the esophagus out of the mouth. With the aid of forceps, the distal end is then turned back on itself and fed back into the esophagus until the loop disappears. The distal tip is correctly positioned using the mark on the tube. Placement should be verified by radiography.

SUMMARY

◆ Most dental treatment requires general anesthesia, and standard good clinical practice should be followed.

◆ Specific considerations in the dental patient include airway protection, surgical access, the advanced age of many dental patients and prolonged anesthetic times. Attention should be given to maintaining body temperature and fluid balance.

◆ Pre-emptive and postoperative analgesia using opioids and/or non-steroidal anti-inflammatory drugs should be considered for all patients.

◆ Local anesthesia, administered intraoperatively, can also be a useful part of the analgesic regime.

◆ Short-term feeding tubes should be used in patients unwilling or unable to eat despite receiving appropriate analgesia.

REFERENCES

Bach, S., Norveng, M.F., Tijellden, N.U., 1988. Phantom limb pain in amputees during the first twelve months following amputation after preoperative lumbar epidural blockade. Pain 33, 297–330.

Clarke, K.W., Hall, L.W., 1990. A survey of anesthesia in small animal practice: AVA/BSAVA report. Journal of the Association for Veterinary Anesthesia 17, 4–10.

Dyson, D.H., Maxie, M.G., Schnurr, D., 1998. Morbidity and mortality associated with anesthetic management in small animal veterinary practice in Ontario. Journal of the American Animal Hospital Association 34 (4), 325–335.

Lascelles, B.D., Cripps, P.J., Jones, A., et al., 1997. Postoperative central hypersensitivity and pain: the pre-emptive value of pethidine for ovariohysterectomy. Pain 73, 461–471.

FURTHER READING

Crowe, D.T., 1986. Enteral nutrition for critically ill or injured patients. Parts I, II and III. Compendium of Continuing Education (Small Animal) 8, 603–826.

Crowe, D.T., Devey, J.J., 1997. Esophagostomy tubes for feeding and decompression: clinical experience in 29 small animal patients. Journal of the American Animal Hospital Association 33, 393–403.

Duke, T., 1999. Anaesthetic management: dental and maxillofacial surgery. In: Seymour, C., Gleed, R. (Eds.), Manual of Small Animal Anaesthesia and Analgesia. BSAVA, Cheltenham, pp. 147–153.

Hartsfield, S.M., 1990. Anaesthetic problems of the geriatric dental patient. Problems in Veterinary Medicine 2, 24–45.

Moon, P.F., 1999. Fluid therapy and blood transfusion. In: Seymour, C., Gleed, R. (Eds.), Manual of Small Animal Anaesthesia and Analgesia. BSAVA, Cheltenham, pp. 119–137.

Muir, W.W. III., Hubbell, J.A.E., 1995. Handbook of Veterinary Anesthesia, second ed. Mosby, St Louis.

Waterman-Pearson, A.E., 1999. Analgesia. In: Seymour, C., Gleed, R. (Eds.), Manual of Small Animal Anaesthesia and Analgesia. BSAVA, Cheltenham, pp. 59–70.

Chapter | **3** |

Antibiotics and antiseptics

INTRODUCTION

In the late 1930s and early 1940s, the appearance of potent chemotherapeutic agents selectively active against bacteria revolutionized the treatment of bacterial infections. The discovery of such drugs led many to believe that bacterial infections were about to vanish! Antimicrobial agents have been extensively used (in both human and veterinary medicine) for more than half a century and the potential and limitations of this therapy are now better understood. Problems, resulting from the widespread use of antibiotics, have modified the general perception of the capabilities of antimicrobial agents. Over the years, bacteria have developed a marked ability to withstand or repel many antibiotic agents. Bacteria are increasingly resistant to many formerly potent agents. The use of antibiotics may disturb the delicate ecologic equilibrium of the body, allowing the proliferation of resistant bacteria and/or non-bacterial organisms. Sometimes this may initiate new infections that are worse than the ones originally treated. In addition, no antibacterial drug is completely non-toxic and the use of any antimicrobial agent will have accompanying risks. It must also be remembered that resistant bacteria can cross the species barrier. Antibiotics and antiseptics have a role to play in the management of oral diseases, but their use should be limited and selective. Dosing regimens and strategies that lead to optimal efficacy of antimicrobial agents must be implemented.

ANTIBIOTICS

Antibiotics can be used for prevention and for therapy.

Preventive use of antibiotics

The main objective of preventive (prophylactic) antibiotics is *to prevent treatment-induced bacteremia*. Periodontal therapy, tooth extraction and surgical treatment of oral trauma cause a considerable bacteremia, which typically clears in around 20 min. The preventive or prophylactic use of antibiotics should only be necessary in patients that cannot cope with the treatment-induced bacteremia.

Animals that *should receive* preventive antibiotic administration are:

- Geriatric or debilitated animals
- Patients with pre-existing heart and/or systemic diseases
- Immunocompromised patients.

In addition to preventing treatment-induced bacteremia, preventive antibiotic administration helps control wound infection. Consequently, animals that *may benefit* from receiving preventive antibiotic administration are those affected by:

- Gross infection
- Chronic stomatitis.

The choice of prophylactic antibiotic and protocol remains controversial. A wide variety of microorganisms is found in the flora of the mouth and saliva. Antibiotic prophylaxis requires a drug with antimicrobial activity against Gram-positive and Gram-negative aerobes and anaerobes. The timing of administration of antibiotics is critical. It is generally accepted that antibiotics should be administered within 2 h of the surgery and not continued for more than 4 h after the procedure (Peterson 1994; Callender 1999). In addition, antibiotics must be given at a high enough dose to reach a tissue level four times higher than the minimal inhibitory concentration

© 2013 Elsevier Ltd.

31

of the causative organisms. A number of studies have shown that ampicillin, amoxicillin–clavulanic acid, certain cephalosporins and clindamycin meet the above requirements in dogs, cats and humans (Harvey et al. 1995a,b; Johnson et al. 1997; Callender 1999; Mueller et al. 1999).

The standard protocol used by the Dentistry and Oral Surgery Service, Veterinary Medical Teaching Hospital, University of California Davis, is 20 mg/kg i.v. of ampicillin prior to surgery (at the time of catheter placement for anesthesia). This dose is repeated after 6 h if the catheter is still in place. Metronidazole is given intravenously in addition to ampicillin in the presence of severe infection to ensure a wider anaerobic spectrum.

The protocol used in my referral practice in the UK is to give twice the therapeutic dose of amoxicillin or amoxicillin–clavulanic acid by intramuscular injection at the time of premedication for anesthesia. This gives 20–30 min for the drug to disperse before the animal is anesthetized and the surgical procedure is started. In fractious animals, who are unlikely to tolerate an intramuscular injection while conscious, we may choose to administer the antibiotic immediately after induction of anesthesia. Examination and patient preparation will ensure that at least 20 min has elapsed before the surgical procedure is started.

Therapeutic use of antibiotics

The therapeutic use of antibiotics is *indicated in patients with* local and systemic signs of *established infection*, i.e. marked swelling, pus formation, fever, lymphadenopathy and an elevated white blood cell count. Clinical judgment is important in making the diagnosis of infection and deciding on antibiotic therapy. Antibiotic administration 'just to be on the safe side' is not prudent use of antimicrobials!

Principles for prudent use of therapeutic antibiotics

The causative agent should be identified and the antibiotic sensitivity determined. In the oral cavity, the organisms involved have been well defined and are known to include a mixed flora of aerobic and anaerobic, Gram-positive and Gram-negative bacteria (Peterson 1994). Empirical antibiotic treatment based on previous susceptibility studies is, therefore, acceptable. Amoxicillin–clavulanic acid and clindamycin, and to a lesser extent cephalosporins, provide broad antibacterial activity against oral infections in dogs and cats (Harvey et al. 1995a,b). *Culture is indicated for infection not responding to the initial treatment, recurrent infection, postoperative wound infection and osteomyelitis.*

The antibiotic with the narrowest antibacterial spectrum should be used. This will minimize the risk of development of resistant bacteria (Peterson 1994).

Combinations of antibiotics are discouraged. The exception to this rule is the combination of amoxicillin or cephalosporins with metronidazole in severe mixed infections in which anaerobes are believed to play a major role.

A bactericidal antibiotic is preferable to a bacteriostatic agent. A bactericidal antibiotic (amoxicillin, cephalosporins and metronidazole) is preferred over a bacteriostatic antibiotic (clindamycin), mainly because there is less reliance on host inflammatory and immune reactions. Other considerations include the toxicity of the antibiotic and the patient's history of previous allergic reactions to a particular antibiotic.

The antibiotic of choice must be administered at the proper dose and correct time interval. Refer to a current compendium of data sheets for veterinary products for correct dosing and time interval. A 7-day course of antibiotics is generally recommended. Osteomyelitis generally requires a longer period of treatment (Rosin et al. 1993). Suboptimal dosing and/or pulse therapy is not recommended.

The patient must be monitored for response to treatment and the potential development of adverse reactions. Re-evaluation of the diagnosis is required if there is no response to treatment. Culture and antibiogram may well be indicated.

Minor adverse reactions, e.g. mild gastrointestinal side-effects and inappetance, due to changes in the gut flora as a result of systemic treatment with amoxicillin and clindamycin, occasionally occur.

Antibiotics and periodontal disease

In veterinary practice, antibiotics are often used indiscriminately (incomplete diagnostic work-up, incorrect dose and time intervals, inadequate monitoring of response to treatment) for patients with periodontal disease.

The indication for preventive (prophylactic) use of antibiotics in animals with gingivitis and/or periodontitis is well defined (indicated for individuals that cannot cope with treatment-induced bacteremia). In contrast, the indication for therapeutic use of antibiotics in the management of periodontal disease is not well defined. A thorough understanding of the etiology and pathogenesis of periodontal disease is required (see Ch. 9) for discriminate (limited and selective) therapeutic use of antibiotics. Periodontal disease is a clinical descriptive term for inflammation of the periodontium caused by the accumulation of dental plaque (a bacterial biofilm) on the tooth surfaces. It is essential to differentiate between gingivitis (inflammation limited to the gingiva) and periodontitis (inflammation involves periodontal ligament and alveolar bone) prior to instituting any treatment.

Gingivitis

In gingivitis, daily mechanical removal of dental plaque (toothbrushing) will restore inflamed gingivae to health and continued regular plaque removal will maintain gingival health. *Antibiotics* are *thus not indicated for the treatment of gingivitis.* Adjunctive use of antiseptics (covered later in this chapter) may be indicated in some patients.

Periodontitis

The role of antibiotics for treatment of periodontitis is not clear and requires further investigation. The two main questions that need to be answered before any general recommendation can be made are whether antimicrobial agents can enhance the effect of mechanical plaque removal, and whether these agents can be a substitute for such treatment.

Can antimicrobial agents enhance the effect of mechanical plaque removal? There are many similarities between human and canine periodontal disease. Consequently, data from human studies do have relevance to canine periodontal disease.

In human dentistry, it is recognized that antimicrobial treatment is of secondary importance in the treatment of periodontitis, compared to conservative periodontal therapy. Conservative periodontal therapy involves professional cleaning (supragingival scaling and polishing, subgingival scaling and root planing) in combination with meticulous daily plaque removal by the patient. Where follow-up mechanical plaque control is successfully instituted (after professional cleaning), no benefit can be shown by including antimicrobial therapy with professional mechanical debridement as compared to mechanical debridement alone (Loesche 1979). No similar study has been performed in dogs or cats.

Various antibiotic regimens have been tested for the treatment of human patients not responding to conservative periodontal therapy. Although favorable short-term effects have been reported; a great variability in treatment response among patients has been noted. Re-emergence of putative pathogens has been observed and has been considered the reason for recurrence of disease. In dogs where no post-scaling homecare is provided, a demonstrable long-term retardation effect following short-term antimicrobial therapy has been reported in one study (Sarkiala et al. 1993). The ultimate evidence for the efficacy of systemic antibiotics must be obtained from longer-term treatment studies in animals with periodontitis. At present, no such data are available.

To summarize, reducing the bacterial load postoperatively can be achieved by mechanical plaque control. The use of systemic antibiotics in combination with conservative periodontal therapy will at best achieve a retardation of the disease process.

Can periodontitis be treated with antimicrobial agents alone? There are some specific features of periodontal disease which suggest that treatment by antimicrobial agents alone, i.e. in the absence of professional periodontal therapy and homecare, will not be sufficient. First, there is generally a lack of bacterial invasion of the tissues in periodontal disease. Bacteria in the subgingival plaque interact with host tissues even without direct tissue penetration. Thus, for any microbial agent to have an effect there is the requirement that the agent is available at a sufficiently high concentration not only within, but also in the subgingival environment outside the periodontal tissues. Second, periodontal pockets contain a large number of different bacteria. This may cause problems for antimicrobial agents to work properly because they may be inhibited, inactivated or degraded by non-target microorganisms. Third, subgingival plaque is a biofilm and it is known that biofilms effectively protect the bacteria from antimicrobial agents. Finally, the majority of microorganisms associated with periodontal disease can frequently be detected at low numbers in the absence of disease. In the therapy of opportunistic infections, elimination is not a realistic goal. Successfully suppressed putative pathogens are likely to grow back if favorable ecologic conditions (e.g. deep periodontal pockets) persist. Therefore, continuous control of ecologic factors will be necessary after initial treatment.

It is important to understand that *in vitro* tests cannot be directly correlated to clinical efficacy, as they do not reflect the true conditions found in periodontal pockets. In particular, they do not account for the biofilm effect. Demonstration of *in vitro* susceptibility is therefore no proof that an agent will work in the treatment of periodontal disease.

At our present level of understanding, systemic antimicrobial therapy cannot be recommended as prevention and/or first-line treatment of periodontal disease for any species, and definitely not in the absence of mechanical periodontal therapy. Professional periodontal therapy followed by meticulous mechanical plaque control by the patient (owner) remains the way to treat periodontitis. *In some very specific situations*, e.g. severe local infection, or a systemically ill or immunocompromised individual, *antibiotics may be a useful adjunctive modality.* However, *the adjunctive use of antiseptics rather than antibiotics is likely to achieve the same result and is associated with fewer hazards*, e.g. resistance development. In short, antibiotics have not been shown to prevent periodontitis; neither have they been shown to have any significant role in the treatment of periodontitis.

Antibiotic delivery

In the few specific situations where antibiotics may be a useful adjunctive modality, the method of delivery needs to be determined. Antibiotic agents may be delivered by direct placement into the periodontal pocket (local route) or via the systemic route. Each method of delivery has specific advantages and disadvantages.

Local therapy may allow application of an agent at a concentration that cannot be achieved by the systemic route. Local application may thus be particularly successful if the treatment of target microorganisms is confined to the clinically visible lesions.

On the other hand, systemically administered agents may reach widely distributed microorganisms. Studies in humans have shown that periodontal bacteria may be distributed throughout the whole mouth in some patients, including non-dental sites such as the dorsum of the tongue and/or the tonsillary crypts (van Winkelhoff et al. 1988; Mombelli et al. 1991, 1994; Muller et al. 1995). Disadvantages of systemic antibiotic therapy relate to the fact that the drug is dispersed over the whole body and only a small portion of the dose actually reaches the subgingival flora. In addition, adverse drug reactions, e.g. resistance, are more likely to occur if drugs are distributed via the systemic route.

ANTISEPTICS

Antiseptics have two major roles in veterinary dentistry and oral surgery:

1. To reduce the number of bacteria in the oral cavity prior to and during a procedure
2. To supplement mechanical plaque control.

It is good practice to rinse the oral cavity with a suitable antiseptic prior to and during dentistry and oral surgery (Summers et al. 2000). This reduces the number of potential pathogens, providing a cleaner environment to work in and thus reducing the bacteremia induced by dental procedures. It also reduces the number of bacteria in the aerosol generated by dental equipment, e.g. ultrasonic scalers. This is beneficial to the operator and assistant.

Chlorhexidine gluconate, an aqueous, non-alcohol-containing solution, is generally regarded to be the oral antiseptic of choice in animals. The correct concentration should be used. A 0.2% solution is generally recommended as being safe, but a 0.05% solution may be indicated if the oral mucosa is exposed to the solution throughout the procedure. Care should be taken to avoid the eyes (Morgan et al. 1996).

Numerous chemical agents have been evaluated for the supplementation of mechanical plaque control. Clinically effective antiplaque agents are characterized by a combination of intrinsic antibacterial activity and good oral retention properties. Agents that have been evaluated include

chlorhexidine, essential oils, triclosan, sanguinarine, fluorides, oxygenating agents, quaternary ammonium compounds, substituted amino-alcohols and enzymes. Of these, the greatest effect on the reduction of plaque and gingivitis can be expected from chlorhexidine. Chlorhexidine is the gold standard and the agent against which all antiplaque agents are tested.

Antiplaque agents delivered from toothpastes, gels or mouth rinses can augment mechanical oral hygiene to control the formation of supragingival plaque and the development of early periodontal disease. It must be emphasized that none of these agents will prevent gingivitis on their own, i.e. in the absence of mechanical plaque removal. Moreover, all these agents are associated with adverse side-effects. These effects vary according to the chemical agent and include poor taste, a burning and/or numbing of oral mucous membranes, staining of teeth and soft tissues, and allergic reactions. The use of chemical antiplaque agents should be seen as adjunctive to the mechanical removal of plaque.

Some examples of situations where adjunctive use of topical chlorhexidine is useful are:

- Immediately postoperatively when discomfort from treatment (deep subgingival debridement, multiple extractions) may prevent mechanical plaque removal with a toothbrush
- Intermittent use when an inflammatory process flares up, e.g. cats with chronic gingivostomatitis
- Adjunct to toothbrushing when toothbrushing is performed suboptimally, e.g. animal will not allow proper brushing, or owner is not technically capable of efficient brushing.

Chlorhexidine gluconate is available as an aqueous solution and as a semi-fluid gel. It can be applied with a syringe, a piece of gauze or a toothbrush.

SUMMARY

- Antibiotics should be employed rationally based on accepted principles of preventive or therapeutic use. Indiscriminate and inappropriate use should be avoided.
- Empirical drug choice based on published studies of the nature of oral infections is usual, with culture and sensitivity being reserved for problem cases.
- Antibiotics are not indicated in the treatment of gingivitis. Their role in periodontitis is doubtful and is definitely secondary to conservative periodontal therapy.
- The oral antiseptic of choice is chlorhexidine.

REFERENCES

Callender, D.L., 1999. Antibiotic prophylaxis in head and neck oncologic surgery: the role of Gram-negative coverage. International Journal of Antimicrobial Agents 12 (Suppl. 1), S21–S25.

Harvey, C.E., Thornsberry, C., Miller, B.R., Shafer, F.S., 1995a. Antimicrobial susceptibility of subgingival bacterial flora in dogs with gingivitis. Journal of Veterinary Dentistry 12(4), 151–155.

Harvey, C.E., Thornsberry, C., Miller, B.R., Shafer, F.S., 1995b. Antimicrobial susceptibility of subgingival bacterial flora in cats with gingivitis. Journal of Veterinary Dentistry 12(4), 157–160.

Johnson, J.T., Kachman, K., Wagner, R.L., et al., 1997. Comparison of ampicillin/sulbactam versus clindamycin in the prevention of infection in patients undergoing head and neck surgery. Head and Neck 19, 367–371.

Loesche, W.J., 1979. Clinical and microbiological aspects of chemotherapeutic agents used according to the specific plaque hypothesis. Journal of Dental Research 58, 2404–2414.

Mombelli, A., McNabb, H., Land, N.P., 1991. Black pigmenting Gram-negative bacteria in periodontal disease. 1. Topographic distribution in the human dentition. Journal of Periodontal Research 26, 301–307.

Mombelli, A., Gmur, R., Gobbi, C., et al., 1994. Actinobacillus actinomycetemcomitans in adult periodontitis. 1. Topographic distribution before and after treatment. Journal of Periodontology 65, 820–826.

Morgan, J.P., Haug, R.H., Kosman, J.W., 1996. Antimicrobial skin preparations for the maxillofacial region. Journal of Oral and Maxillofacial Surgery 54, 89–94.

Mueller, S.C., Henkel, K.O., Neumann, J., et al., 1999. Perioperative antibiotic prophylaxis in maxillofacial surgery: penetration of clindamycin into various tissues. Journal of Craniomaxillofacial Surgery 27, 172–176.

Muller, H.P., Eickholz, P., Heinecke, A., et al., 1995. Simultaneous isolation of Actinobacillus actinomycetemcomitans from subgingival and extracrevicular locations of the mouth. Journal of Clinical Periodontology 22, 413–419.

Peterson, L.J., 1994. Principles of antibiotic therapy. In: Topazian, R.G., Goldberg, M.H. (Eds.), Oral and Maxillofacial Infections, third ed. W.B. Saunders, Philadelphia, pp. 160–197.

Rosin, E., Dow, S.W., Daly, W.R., et al., 1993. Surgical wound infection and use of antibiotics. In: Slatter, D.H. (Ed.), Textbook of Small Animal Surgery, second ed. W.B. Saunders, Philadelphia, pp. 84–95.

Sarkiala, E., Asikainen, S.E.A., Kanervo, A., et al., 1993. The efficacy of tinidazole in naturally occurring periodontitis in dogs: Bacteriological and chemical results. Veterinary Microbiology 36, 273–288.

Summers, A.N., Larson, D.L., Edmiston, C.E., et al., 2000. Efficacy of preoperative decontamination of the oral cavity. Plastic and Reconstructive Surgery 106, 895–900.

van Winkelhoff, A.J., Van der Velden, U., Clement, M., et al., 1988. Intra-oral distribution of black-pigmented Bacteroides species in periodontitis patients. Oral Microbiology and Immunology 3, 83–85.

Chapter 4

Anatomy of the teeth and periodontium

INTRODUCTION

The dentition of dogs and cats resembles that of man. There are differences in tooth number and shape, but the basic anatomy is similar. The dentition of rodents and lagomorphs is covered in Chapter 14.

Each tooth has a crown (above the gum) and one or more roots (below the gum). The bulk of the mature tooth is composed of dentine, which is covered by enamel on the crown and by cementum on the roots. The centre of the tooth contains the pulp or endodontic system. Figure 4.1 depicts the basic structure of a tooth.

The crowns of dog and cat teeth have a more tapered shape with sharp cutting edges and fewer chewing surfaces than human teeth. Also, the teeth are spaced further apart and, where there is contact between teeth, the contact area is smaller and not as tight. Humans, dogs and cats are *diphyodont*, i.e. primary (deciduous) teeth are followed by a permanent dentition. Dental formulae describe the type and number of teeth in each quadrant of the oral cavity. 'I' represents incisor teeth, 'C' represents canine teeth, 'P' represents premolars and 'M' represents molars. The respective dental formulae of the primary and permanent dentitions of dog and cat are shown in Box 4.1.

The formation of the crown of both primary and permanent teeth occurs within the alveolar bone. Enamel formation is completed before the tooth erupts into the oral cavity. Once the enamel has formed, the ameloblasts (the cells which produce the enamel matrix) are lost and further development of enamel does not occur. The only natural form of repair that can occur to enamel after eruption is surface mineralization, through deposition of minerals, mainly from saliva, into the superficial enamel layer.

Although enamel formation is completed by the time the tooth erupts, dentine production is just beginning. Moreover, root development, i.e. growth in length and formation of a root apex, is by no means complete at the time of eruption. Figure 4.2 depicts maturation of a permanent tooth following eruption.

The primary teeth start forming *in utero* and erupt between 3 and 12 weeks of age. The permanent crowns start forming at or shortly after birth and mineralization of the crowns is complete by around 11 weeks of age. Resorption and exfoliation of the primary teeth and replacement by the permanent dentition occurs between 3 and 7 months of age in the dog and between 3 and 5 months of age in the cat. Once the crowns of the permanent teeth have erupted, root development continues for several months. The approximate ages when teeth erupt in dogs and cats are shown in Table 4.1.

ANATOMY OF THE TEETH

As already mentioned, the teeth consist of enamel, dentine, cementum and pulp. The detailed structure of these tissues will be discussed below.

Enamel

Enamel is the hardest and most mineralized tissue in the body. It does not have a nerve or a blood supply. The inorganic content of mature enamel amounts to 96–97% of the weight, the remainder being organic material and water (Fejerskov and Thylstrup 1979). The inorganic material consists of calcium hydroxyapatite crystals arranged in an orderly fashion at right angles to the tooth surface. The

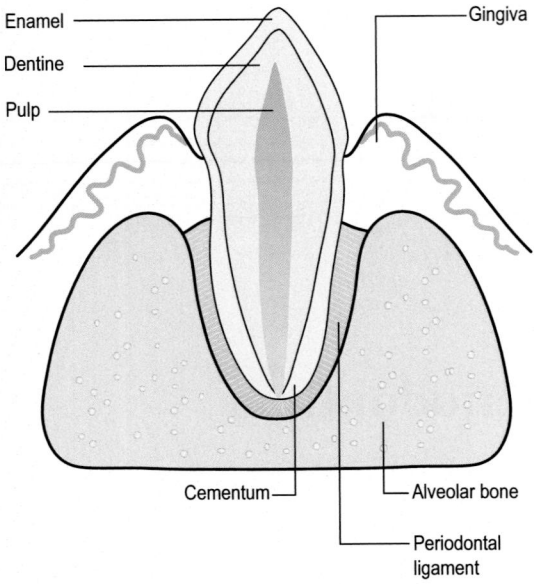

Fig. 4.1 Basic anatomy of the tooth and periodontium

Table 4.1 Approximate ages (in weeks) when teeth erupt in dogs and cats

Teeth	Primary		Permanent	
	Puppy	Kitten	Dog	Cat
Incisors	4–6	3–4	12–16	11–16
Canines	3–5	3–4	12–16	12–20
Premolars	5–6	5–6	16–20	16–20
Molars	–	–	16–24	20–24

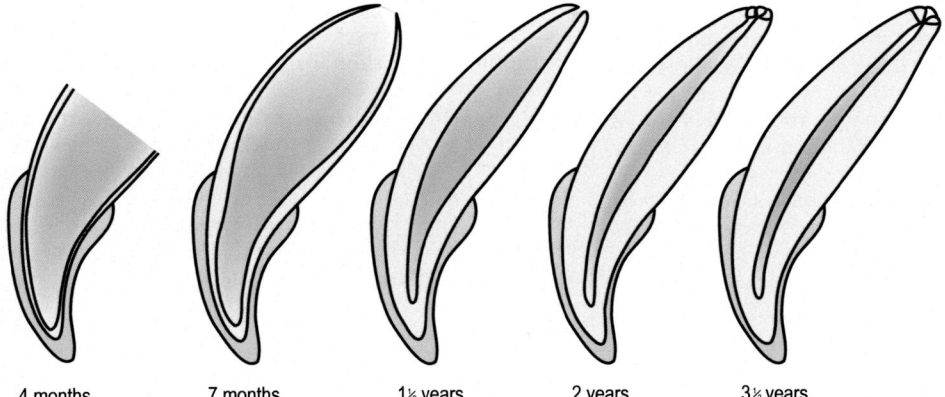

| 4 months | 7 months | 1½ years | 2 years | 3½ years |

Fig. 4.2 **Maturation of a permanent canine tooth after eruption** Enamel formation is complete at the time of eruption, while dentine production and root development (root elongation and formation of an apex) are just beginning. The apical foramen of an immature tooth is a single wide opening. As the individual ages, closure of the apex (apexogenesis) occurs by continuous deposition of dentine and cementum until, in mature teeth, the root apex consists of numerous small openings or foramina allowing the passage of blood vessels, lymphatics and nerves.

organic content is made up of soluble and insoluble proteins and peptides.

The enamel of dog and cat teeth is thinner than that of human teeth, generally being 0.2 mm thick in the cat and 0.5 mm in dogs, rarely exceeding 1 mm even at the tips of the teeth (Crossley 1995). This compares with a thickness of up to 2.5 mm in humans (Schroeder 1991).

Dentine

The bulk of the mature tooth is made up of dentine, which is continuously deposited throughout life by odontoblasts lining the pulp system. The primary dentine is the first layer that forms. It is the dentine that is present at the time of tooth eruption. Throughout life, there is a slow continuous physiologic deposition of dentine, which is called secondary dentine. In response to trauma, dentine is laid down rapidly and in a less organized fashion. This type of dentine is called reparative or tertiary dentine.

The composition of dentine on a wet weight basis is 70% inorganic material, 18% organic material and 12% water (Mjör 1979). The inorganic portion of dentine consists mainly of calcium hydroxyapatite crystals that are similar to those seen in cementum and bone, but smaller than the hydroxyapatite crystals seen in enamel. The organic portion consists mainly of collagen.

Dentine has a tubular structure. Dentinal tubules make up 20–30% of the volume of dentine. The tubules traverse the entire width of the dentine, from the pulpal tissue to the dentino-enamel junction in the crown or the dentino-cementum junction in the root. They contain the cytoplasmic processes of the odontoblasts and dentinal fluid. The dentine tubules are more numerous and have a wider diameter closer to the pulp than towards the enamel or cementum surface. The number of dentine tubules $(20\,000–40\,000/mm^2)$ and diameter (tapering from 3–4 μm near the pulp to under 1 μm in the outer layer of dentine) is similar in cats, dogs, monkeys and humans (Forssell-Ahlberg et al. 1975).

Cementum

Cementum, although part of the tooth, is classified as part of the periodontium and is discussed later in this chapter.

Pulp

The pulp is composed of connective tissue liberally interspersed with tiny blood vessels, lymphatics, myelinated and unmyelinated nerves and undifferentiated mesenchymal cells. As already mentioned, the pulp system is lined by odontoblasts, which produce dentine.

In the crown, the section containing the pulp is called the pulp chamber, and in the root(s) it is called the root canal(s). The root canal opens into the periapical tissues at the root apex. The apical foramen of immature teeth is a single wide opening. As the individual ages, closure of the apex (apexogenesis) occurs by continuous deposition of dentine and cementum (Fig. 4.2) until, in mature teeth, the root apex consists of numerous small openings or foramina allowing the passage of blood vessels, lymphatics and nerves.

ANATOMY OF THE PERIODONTIUM

The periodontium is an anatomic unit which functions to attach the tooth to the jaw and provide a suspensory apparatus resilient to normal functional forces. It is made up

of gingiva, periodontal ligament, cementum and alveolar bone (Fig. 4.1).

The gingiva

The gingiva surrounds the teeth and the marginal parts of the alveolar bone, forming a cuff around each tooth. It can be divided into the free gingiva, which is closely adapted to the tooth surface, and the attached gingiva, which is firmly attached to the underlying periosteum of the alveolar bone (Figs 4.3, 4.4). The attached gingiva is delineated from the oral mucosa by the mucogingival line, except in the palate where no such delineation exists. An interdental papilla is formed by the gingival tissues in the spaces between the teeth (the interproximal spaces).

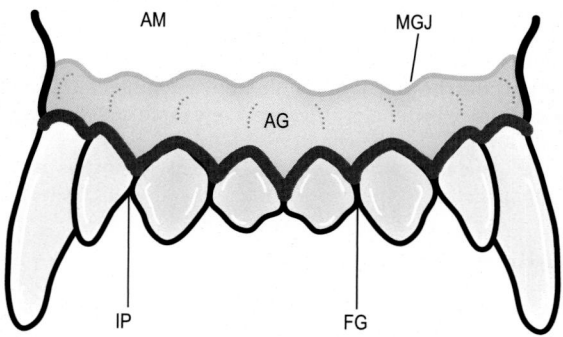

Fig. 4.3 The visible landmarks of clinically normal gingiva MGJ, mucogingival junction or line; AM, alveolar mucosa; AG, attached gingiva; FG, free gingiva; IP, interdental papilla.

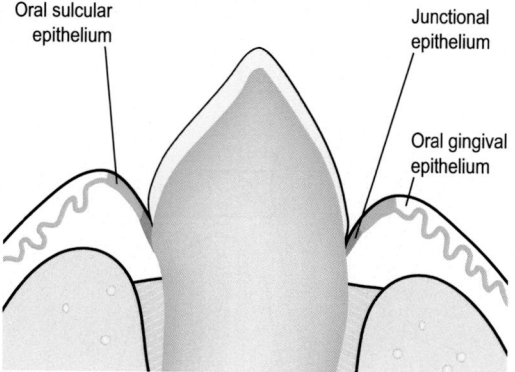

Fig. 4.4 The gingival cuff The oral surface is lined by a parakeratinized squamous cell epithelium: the oral gingival epithelium. The gingival sulcus is lined by the oral sulcular epithelium, which is closely apposed but not adherent to the tooth. The junctional epithelium or epithelial attachment is adherent to the tooth surface. Both the sulcular epithelium and the junctional epithelium are non-keratinized squamous cell epithelia.

The margin of the free gingiva is rounded in such a way that a small invagination or sulcus is formed between the tooth and the gingiva. Therefore, the gingival sulcus is a shallow groove surrounding each tooth. The depth of the sulcus can be assessed by gently inserting a graduated periodontal probe until resistance is encountered. This resistance is taken to be the base of the sulcus. The depth from the free gingival margin to the base of the sulcus can thus be measured (Fig. 4.5). In the periodontally healthy individual, the sulcus is 1–3 mm deep in humans and dogs and 0.5–1.0 mm in cats.

The oral surface of the gingiva is lined by a parakeratinized squamous cell epithelium: the oral gingival epithelium. The gingival sulcus is lined by the oral sulcular epithelium. In addition to the sulcular epithelium, which is closely apposed to the tooth surface but not attached, there is a thin layer of highly permeable epithelium which is adherent to the tooth surface called the epithelial attachment or junctional epithelium. Both the oral sulcular epithelium and the junctional epithelium are non-keratinized squamous cell epithelia and have a very rapid cell turnover (5–8 days).

The gingival connective tissue is densely fibrous and firmly attached to the periosteum of the alveolar bone.

Periodontal ligament

The periodontal ligament is the connective tissue that attaches the root cementum to the alveolar bone. It acts as a suspensory ligament for the tooth, and is in a continual stage of physiologic activity.

The collagen fibers within the ligament are arranged in functional groups. Individual fibers do not span the entire distance between bone and cementum; they branch and reunite in an interwoven pattern. All fibers follow a wavy course that allows for slight movement of the tooth and will absorb mild impact to the tooth.

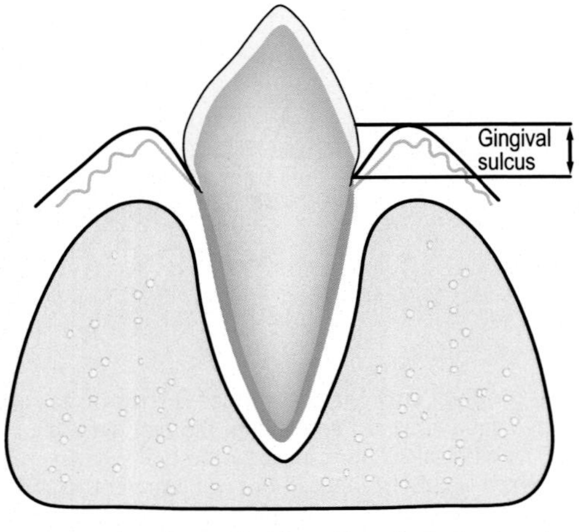

Cementum

The cementum is an avascular bone-like tissue that covers the root surface. It does not contain Haversian canals and is therefore denser than bone. It is less calcified than enamel or dentine, but, like dentine, cementum deposition is continuous throughout life. Cementum is a very important component involved in tooth support, as it is capable of both resorptive and reparative processes. Resorption and apposition are, however, slower than in bone.

Alveolar bone

The alveolar bone is composed of the ridges of the jaw that support the teeth. The roots of the teeth are contained in deep depressions, the alveolar sockets in the bone. The alveolar bone develops during tooth eruption and undergoes atrophy with tooth loss. It responds readily to external and systemic influences. The usual response to stimuli results in resorption, but this may be accompanied by deposition in some situations.

Alveolar bone consists of four layers. In addition to the three layers found in all bones, namely periosteum, dense compact bone and cancellous bone, there is a fourth layer called the cribriform plate, which lines the alveolar sockets. Radiographically, this appears as a fine radiodense line called the lamina dura. The crest of the alveolar bone is normally located around 1 mm below the cemento-enamel junction. Blood vessels and nerves run through the alveolar bone and perforate the cribriform plate. The majority of these blood vessels and nerves supply the periodontal ligament.

Fig. 4.5 The gingival sulcus The gingival sulcus is measured from the free gingival margin to the base of the sulcus.

SUMMARY

- Cats and dogs (like humans) are diphyodont, i.e. primary (deciduous) teeth are shed to make way for the permanent dentition.
- The bulk of the mature tooth is composed of dentine, covered by enamel on the crown and cementum on the roots.
- Enamel is the hardest tissue in the body, consisting mainly of calcium hydroxyapatite. Its formation is complete by the time of tooth eruption. Regeneration is not possible, only repair by surface mineralization.
- The endodontic system (pulp) makes up the center of the tooth and contains odontoblasts, which produce dentine throughout the life of the animal.
- The periodontium serves to support the tooth and absorb functional forces. It consists of the gingiva, periodontal ligament, cementum and alveolar bone.

REFERENCES

Crossley, D.A., 1995. Results of a preliminary study of enamel thickness in the mature dentition of domestic dogs and cats. Journal of Veterinary Dentistry 12 (3), 111–113.

Fejerskov, O., Thylstrup, A., 1979. Dental enamel. In: Mjör, I.A., Fejerskov, O. (Eds.), Histology of the Human Tooth, second ed. Munksgaard, Copenhagen, pp. 75–103.

Forssell-Ahlberg, K., Brännström, M., Edwall, L., 1975. The diameter and number of dentinal tubules in rat, cat, dog and monkey. A comparative scanning electron microscope study. Acta Odontologica Scandinavica 33, 234–250.

Mjör, I.A., 1979. Dentin and pulp. In: Mjör, I.A., Fejerskov, O. (Eds.), Histology of the Human Tooth, second ed. Munksgaard, Copenhagen, pp. 43–74.

Schroeder, H.E., 1991. Oral Structural Biology. Thieme, New York.

Chapter | 5 |

Occlusion and malocclusion

INTRODUCTION

Occlusion is the term used to describe the 'bite', i.e. the relationship of teeth in the same jaw as well as the relationship of teeth in opposing jaws. Occlusion is determined by the shape of the head, jaw length and width and the position of the teeth. By definition, malocclusion is an abnormality in the position of the teeth. Malocclusion is common in dogs, but it also occurs in cats. The clinical significance of malocclusion is that it may cause discomfort and sometimes pain to the affected animal. In some cases, it may be the direct cause of severe oral pathology. It is consequently important to diagnose malocclusion early in the life of the animal so that preventative measures can be taken.

Malocclusion can result from jaw length and/or width discrepancy (skeletal malocclusion), from tooth malpositioning (dental malocclusion), or a combination of both. The development of the occlusion is determined by both genetic and environmental factors. It is known that jaw length, tooth bud position and tooth size are inherited (Stockard 1941). It is also known that the development of the upper jaw, mandible and teeth are independently regulated genetically (Stockard 1941). Disharmony in the regulation of these structures results in malocclusion. Alteration of jaw growth by hormonal disorder, trauma or functional modification may result in skeletal malocclusion (Hennet and Harvey 1992a). Although tooth bud position is inherited, various events during development and growth may alter the definitive tooth position.

It is claimed that at least 50% of malocclusions are acquired and have no genetic cause (Beard 1989; Shipp and Fahrenkrug 1992). There are no data to support such a claim in dogs or cats. Not much research has been done and there are no large epidemiologic studies available.

Specific genetic mechanisms regulating malocclusion are unknown. A polygenic mechanism, however, is likely and explains why not all siblings in successive generations are affected by malocclusion to the same degree, if affected at all. With a polygenic mechanism, the severity of clinical signs is linked to the number of defective genes.

The most reasonable approach suggested (Hennet and Harvey 1992b; Hennet 1995) to evaluate whether malocclusion is hereditary or acquired is as follows:

- Skeletal malocclusion is considered inherited unless a developmental cause can be reliably identified.
- Pure dental malocclusion, unless known to have breed or family predisposition, should be given the benefit of doubt and not be considered inherited.

NORMAL OCCLUSION

When evaluating occlusion it is important to look at all parameters and not to base judgment solely on the positioning of the incisor teeth. In fact, the canine and premolar relationships often give a better guide to the occlusion.

The shape of the head affects the positioning of the teeth. Malocclusion occurs in any of the three head shapes (dolichocephalic, mesocephalic and brachycephalic), but is more common in brachycephalic breeds. The normal head type in the feral dog and cat is the mesocephalic head. We breed for brachycephalic or dolichocephalic, which leads to abnormal occlusion.

Dog

In the mesocephalic dog, the mandible is shorter and less wide than the upper jaw. Consequently, the mandibular

43

incisors and molars occlude with the palatal surfaces of their upper jaw counterparts. The normal bite of the adult mesocephalic dog is characterized by the following:

Scissor bite of the incisor teeth (Fig. 5.1)

- The upper incisors are rostral to the lower incisors.
- The incisal tips of the mandibular incisors contact the cingulae of the upper incisors.

Interdigitation of the canine teeth (Fig. 5.2)

- The mandibular canine fits into the diastema (space) between the upper 3rd incisor and the upper canine,

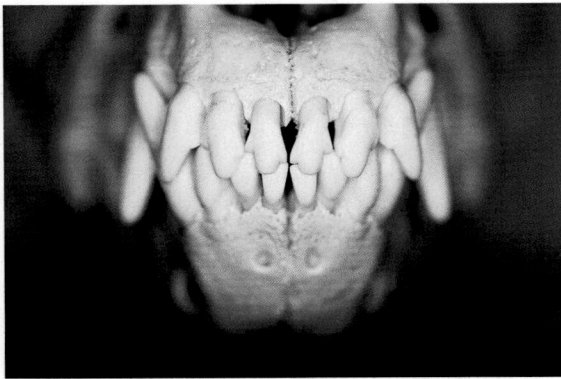

Fig. 5.1 Scissor bite of the incisor teeth The upper incisors are rostral to the lower with the incisal tips of the mandibular incisors contacting the cingulae of the upper incisors.

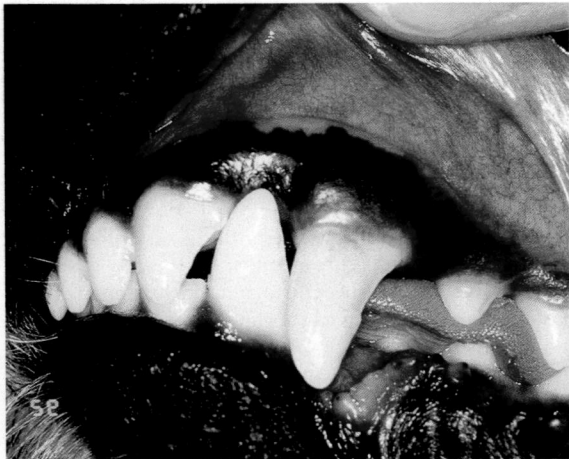

Fig. 5.2 Interdigitation of the canine teeth There should be equal space on either side of the mandibular canine crown.

touching neither. In other words, there should be equal space on either side of the mandibular canine crown.

The incisor scissor bite and canine interdigitation form the dental interlock, which coordinates rostral growth of the upper jaw and mandible.

Interdigitation of the premolars (Fig. 5.3)

- The cusps (tips) of the premolars oppose the interdental spaces of the opposite arcade, with the mandibular 1st premolar being the most rostral. This interdigitation is called the 'pinking shear' effect.

Premolar and molar relationships (Fig. 5.4)

- The mesiobuccal surface of the 1st mandibular molar occludes with the palatal surface of the maxillary 4th premolar.
- The distal occlusal surface of the mandibular 1st molar occludes with the palatal occlusal surface of the maxillary 1st molar.

Cat

The incisor and canine occlusion of the adult meso-cephalic cat is the same as in the dog. The premolar and molar occlusion differs (Fig. 5.5) from the dog as follows:

- The most rostral premolar is the maxillary 2nd premolar (the cat lacks the 1st maxillary premolar and the first two mandibular premolars).
- The buccal surface of the 1st mandibular molar occludes with the palatal surface of the maxillary 4th premolar.
- The maxillary 1st molar is located distopalatal to the maxillary 4th premolar and does not occlude with any other tooth.

The cat does not have any teeth with occlusal (chewing) surfaces.

SKELETAL MALOCCLUSION

Brachycephalic dogs have a shorter than normal upper jaw (Fig. 5.6) and dolichocephalic dogs have a longer than normal upper jaw (Fig. 5.7); in both cases the mandible is not responsible for any rostrocaudal discrepancy.

Mandibular prognathic bite

In the mandibular prognathic bite, often called 'under-shot' (Fig. 5.8), the mandible is longer than the upper jaw and some or all of the mandibular teeth are rostral to their normal position. The degree of malocclusion varies as follows:

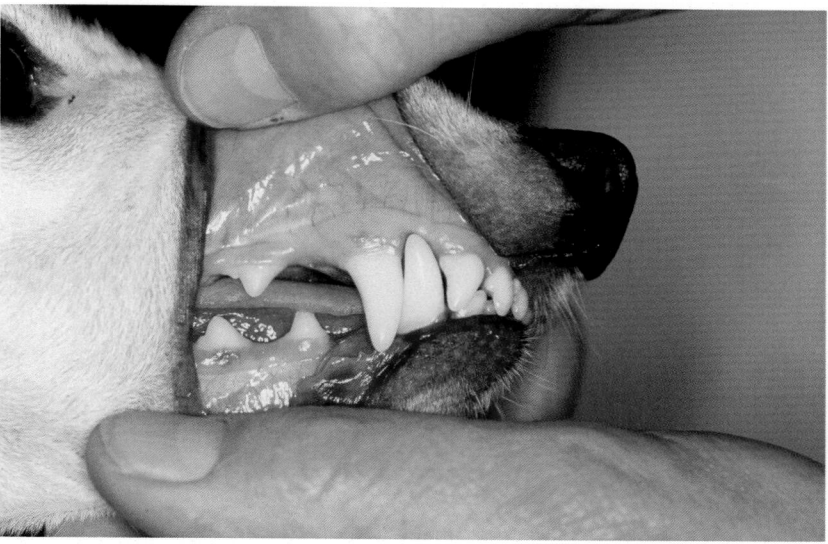

Fig. 5.3 Interdigitation of the premolars The mandibular 1st premolar should be the most rostral of the premolars.

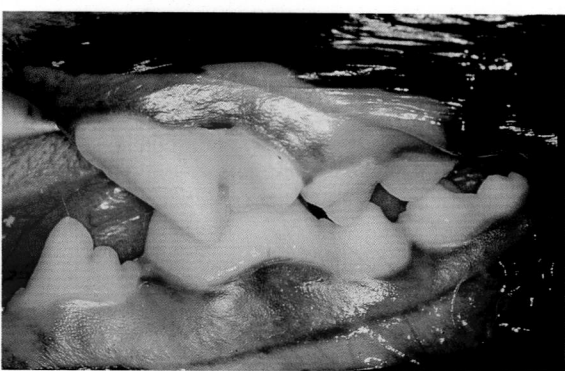

Fig. 5.4 Premolar and molar relationships in the dog The mesiobuccal surface of the 1st mandibular molar occludes with the palatal surface of the maxillary 4th premolar, and the distal occlusal surface of the mandibular 1st molar occludes with the palatal occlusal surface of the maxillary 1st molar.

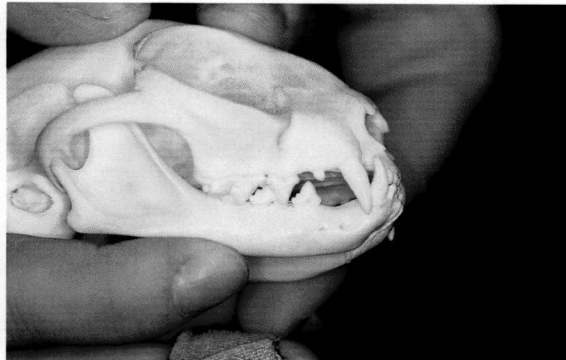

Fig. 5.5 Premolar and molar relationships in the cat The most rostral premolar is the maxillary 2nd premolar. The buccal surface of the 1st mandibular molar occludes with the palatal surface of the maxillary 4th premolar. The maxillary 1st molar is located distopalatal to the maxillary 4th premolar and does not occlude with any other tooth.

- Normal incisor occlusion, but the mandibular canines touch the upper 3rd incisors and the mandibular premolars are rostrally displaced, which disrupts the 'pinking shear' effect.
- Level bite: the upper and lower incisors meet at their incisal edges; the lower canines touch the upper 3rd incisors and the mandibular premolars are rostrally displaced.
- Reverse scissor bite: the lower incisors are rostral to the upper incisors by 0.5 mm to 5 cm or more; the lower canines may be caudal to but touching the

upper 3rd incisors, or may be rostral to the upper 3rd incisors; the mandibular premolars are rostrally displaced to a similar degree.

If the dental interlock prevents the mandible from growing rostrally to its genetic potential, lateral or ventral bowing of the mandible may occur to accommodate the length. This results in an open bite and is characterized by increased space between the premolar cusp. In addition, the caudal angle of the mandible is caudal to the temporomandibular joint to accommodate the extra length of the mandible.

45

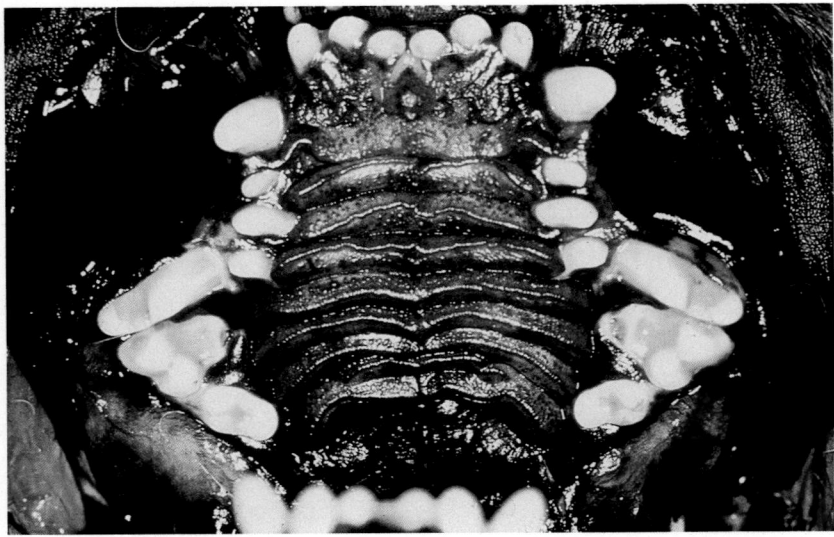

Fig. 5.6 **Brachycephalic** Brachycephalic dogs have a shorter than normal upper jaw. A short jaw results in reduced interdental spaces with rotation and/or overlap of teeth.

Mandibular brachygnathic bite

A mandibular brachygnathic bite, often called 'overshot', occurs when the mandible is shorter than normal (Fig. 5.9). The degree of malocclusion varies as follows:

- The upper incisors are rostral to the lower incisors by 0.5 mm to 5 cm or more.
- The upper canines are caudal to but touching the mandibular canines, level with the lower canines or rostral to the mandibular canines.
- The mandibular premolars are caudally displaced relative to the maxillary premolars, disrupting the 'pinking shear' effect. The degree of displacement is similar to that of the incisors and canines.

Wry bite

A wry bite (Fig. 5.10) occurs if one side of the head grows more than the other side. In its mildest form, a one-sided prognathic or brachygnathic bite develops. In more severe cases, a crooked head and bite develop with a deviated midline. An open bite may also develop in the incisor region so that the affected teeth are displaced vertically and do not occlude. The space between the upper and lower incisors can vary from 0.5 mm to 2 cm.

Narrow mandible

In some animals, the mandible is too narrow with respect to the upper jaw. The result is that the lower canines impinge on the maxillary gingivae or the hard palate instead of fitting into the diastema between the upper 3rd incisor and upper canine on either side. The animal may not be able to close its mouth and injury to the gingivae or palatal mucosa commonly occurs (Fig. 5.11). In untreated severe cases, an oronasal communication may develop over time.

This condition is seen in both the primary (deciduous) and permanent dentition. Persistent primary canines will further exacerbate the condition as the permanent canines erupt medially to their primary counterparts in the mandible. The incorrect dental interlock will interfere with the normal growth in width and length of the developing mandible. The condition can also be caused by persistent primary mandibular canines in a mandible of normal width.

DENTAL MALOCCLUSION

Dental malocclusion is malpositioning of teeth where there is no obvious skeletal abnormality, i.e. there is no jaw length or width discrepancy. Dental malocclusion may also occur in association with skeletal malocclusion.

Anterior crossbite

This is a clinical term used to describe a reverse scissor occlusion of one, several or all of the incisors (Fig. 5.12).

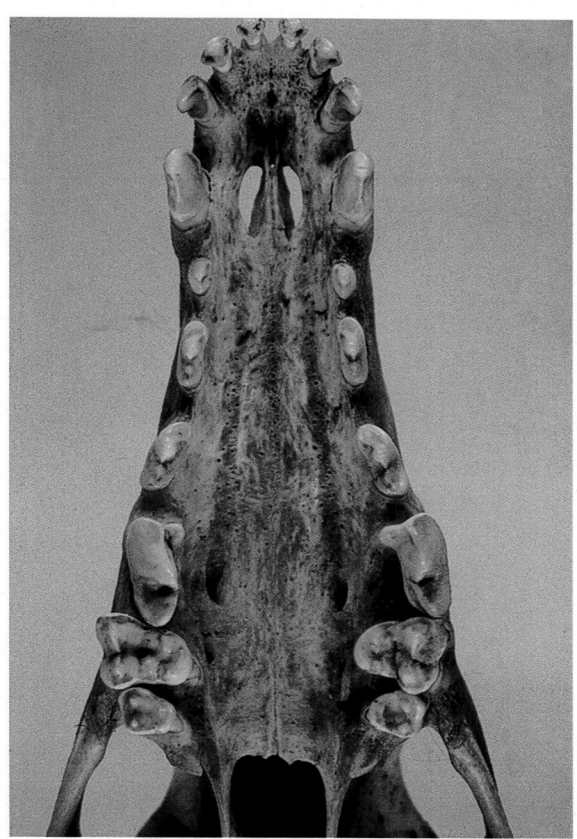

Fig. 5.7 Dolichocephalic Dolichocephalic dogs have a longer than normal upper jaw. The increased jaw length results in interdental spaces that are wider than normal.

The condition is thought to be secondary to persistent primary incisors. However, there is probably a skeletal origin as well since affected animals often develop a mandibular prognathic bite. In other words, an anterior crossbite in an immature animal may be the first sign of a developing mandibular prognathism.

Anterior crossbite is common in medium and large breed dogs where persistent primary teeth are less common. The cause can be either a dental malocclusion (i.e. linguoversion of the upper incisors) or a skeletal malocclusion (i.e. mandibular prognathism or maxillary brachygnathism). Anterior crossbite in humans usually has a skeletal origin.

Malocclusion of the canine teeth

The two most common abnormalities in canine tooth position are as follows.

Rostral displacement of the maxillary canines

Persistent primary canines may be responsible for this condition. A breed predisposition has been reported in the Shetland sheepdog.

Medial displacement of the lower canines

Persistent primary mandibular canines are thought to be the cause of this condition. Yet, the condition is not frequent in toy breeds, where persistent primary teeth are common. This malocclusion is frequent in dolichocephalic breeds, where it is of skeletal origin in that the mandible is too small for the long maxilla.

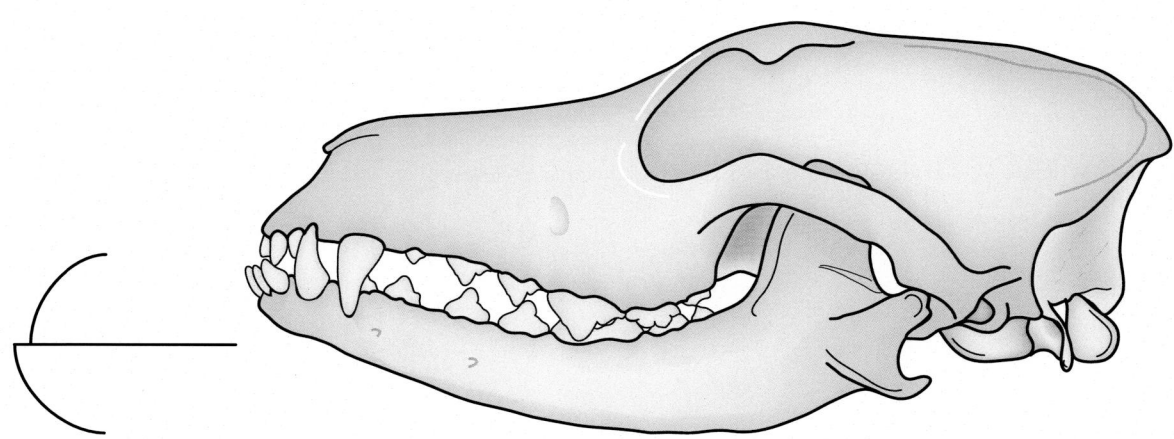

Fig. 5.8 Mandibular prognathic bite The mandible is longer than the upper jaw. This is normal for brachycephalic breeds.

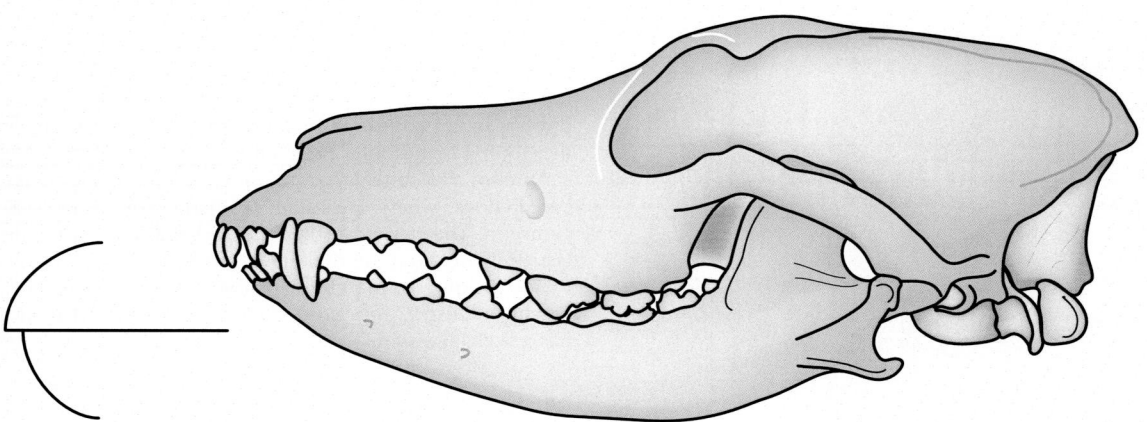

Fig. 5.9 Mandibular brachygnathic bite The mandible is too short in relation to the upper jaw. This is normal for dolichocephalic breeds.

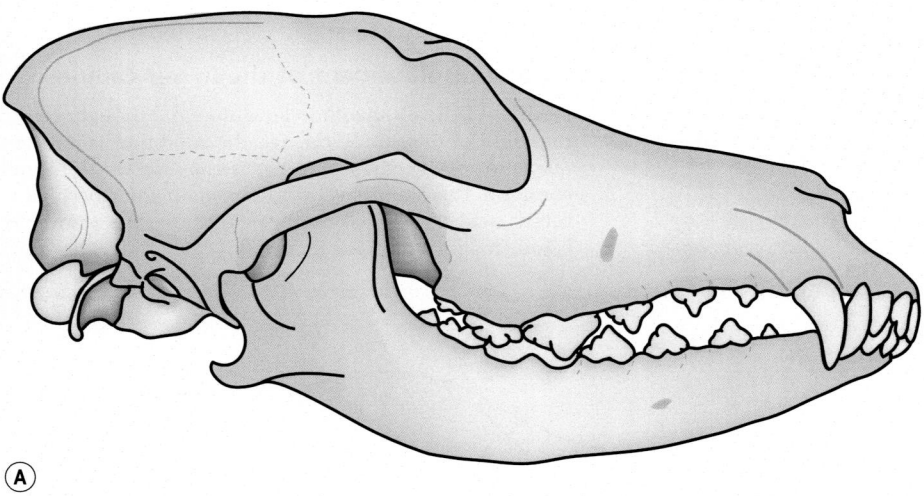

(A)

Fig. 5.10 Wry bite (A) Right lateral view of the skull showing normal occlusion.

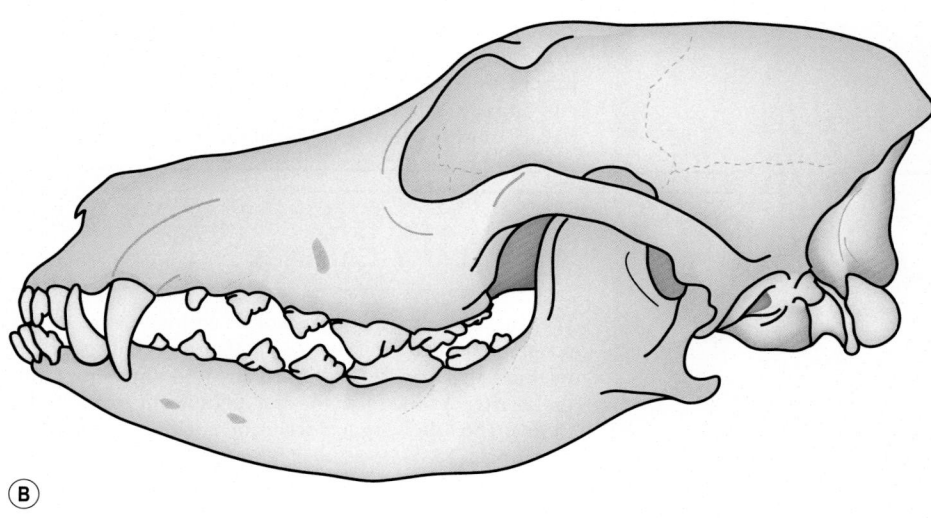

Fig. 5.10, cont'd
(B) Left lateral view of the skull showing a mandibular prognathic bite. (C) Rostral view of the skull showing a midline deviation and an open bite. Note that the left side of the skull is more developed than the right.

Ⓑ

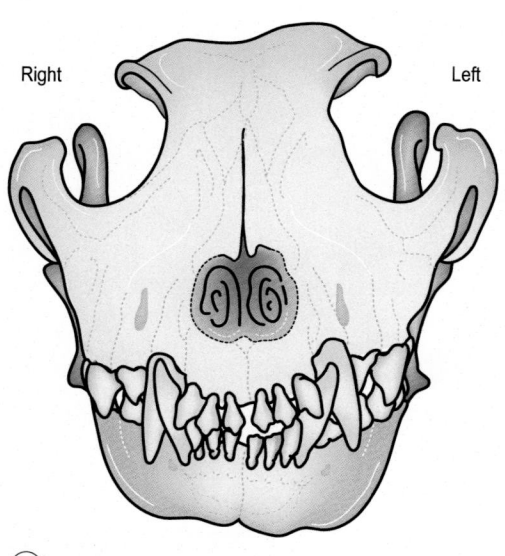

Right   Left

Ⓒ

Malocclusion of the premolars and molars

Posterior crossbite (Fig. 5.13) is used to describe an abnormal relationship of the carnassial teeth, seen commonly in the dolichocephalic breeds, where the normal buccolingual relationship is reversed.

MALOCCLUSION ASSOCIATED WITH PERSISTENT PRIMARY TEETH

Persistent primary teeth, i.e. primary teeth that are still in place when the permanent counterpart starts erupting,

may interfere with the normal eruption pathway of the permanent counterparts. The smaller breeds are more often affected by this condition. The mode of inheritance is not known but it seems to be familial. The three most commonly affected areas are the lower canines, the upper canines and the incisors.

MANDIBULAR CANINES

The mandibular permanent canine begins eruption medial to its primary counterpart. Once the primary tooth is lost, the permanent canine flares out laterally to occupy the

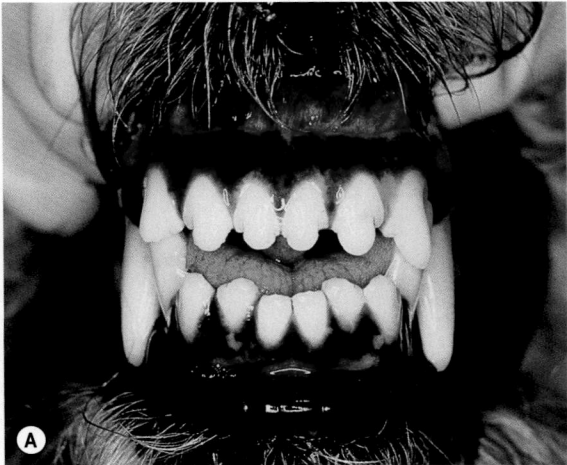

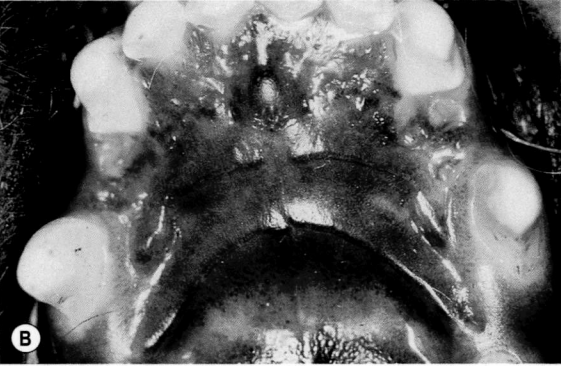

Fig. 5.11 Narrow mandible (A) The mandibular canines do not fit into the diastema between the upper 3rd incisor and upper canine on either side. Instead, they impinge on the maxillary gingivae and hard palate. The dog is unable to close its mouth. (B) Note the injury to the maxillary gingivae and palatal mucosa.

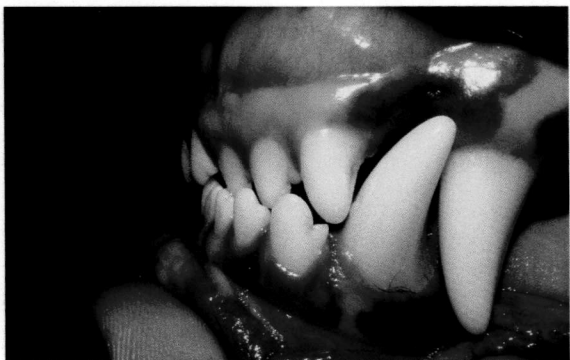

Fig. 5.12 Left anterior crossbite The left incisors have a reverse scissor occlusion.

diastema between the upper 3rd incisor and upper canine. If the primary canine is not lost, the permanent canine may be forced to continue erupting medial to the persistent primary counterpart and will impinge on the hard palate causing pain, inflammation and possibly, with time, an oronasal communication.

MAXILLARY CANINES

The maxillary permanent canine erupts rostral to its primary counterpart (Fig. 5.14). If the primary tooth is retained, this may force the permanent tooth to erupt into the diastema intended for the permanent mandibular canine. The following malocclusion situations could then develop:

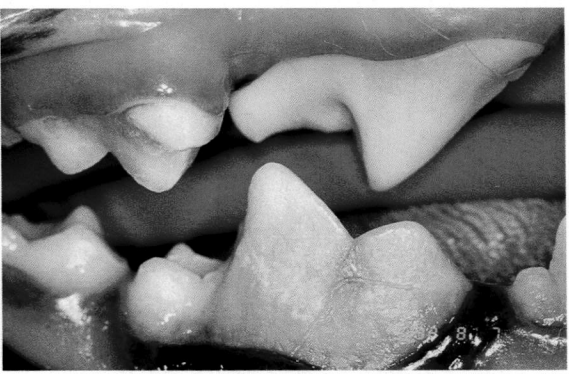

Fig. 5.13 Posterior crossbite The normal buccolingual relationship of the carnassial teeth is reversed.

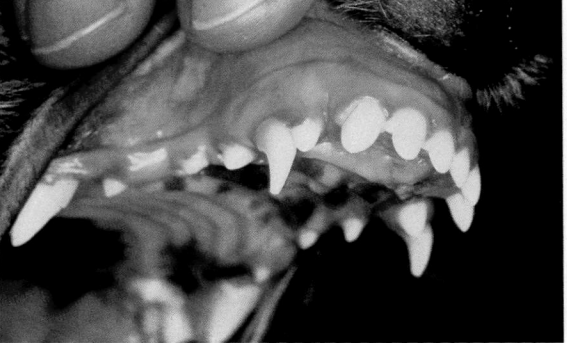

Fig. 5.14 Persistent primary maxillary canine Owing to the persistent primary maxillary canine, the permanent maxillary canine is being forced to erupt in the diastema that the permanent mandibular incisor normally occupies. Malocclusion will develop.

- The maxillary or mandibular canine may become impacted, i.e. does not erupt fully.
- The mandibular canine may push the upper 3rd incisor or the upper canine in a labial/buccal direction.
- The mandibular canine may be forced to erupt medial to the maxillary canine, thus impinging on the hard palate with possible formation of an oronasal communication, if left untreated.

Incisors

The permanent incisors erupt caudal to their primary counterparts. Retention of one or more of the primary teeth may interfere with scissor occlusion of the permanent teeth, with upper incisors occluding behind the mandibular incisors, i.e. an anterior crossbite, which may result in localized soft-tissue trauma.

Dental interlock-induced abnormalities

A maloccluding dental interlock may form when a growth spurt of either the maxilla or mandible coincides with the eruption of primary or permanent canines and incisors that interact to form the dental interlock. Once this interlock has been established, the maxilla and mandible are forced to grow rostrally at the same rate, irrespective of the genetic information. For example, mandibular canines that are locked rostral to the upper 3rd incisors will cause a non-hereditary mandibular prognathic bite; mandibular canines that are locked medial and more caudal than normal will cause a narrow mandible and a mandibular brachygnathic bite.

OCCLUSAL EVALUATION

Occlusal evaluation should ideally be performed in the conscious animal and involves the following steps:

1. Assessment of symmetry of the head, face and dentition.
   The midpoints of the mandibular and maxillary arches should be in alignment with the midsagittal plane of the head (Fig. 5.15).
2. Count teeth.
   All should be present (Fig. 5.16).
3. Evaluate incisor occlusion.
   The large cusps of the lower incisors should occlude near the cingulum on the palatal side of the upper incisors (Fig. 5.17).
4. Evaluate canine occlusion.
   The mandibular canine teeth should occlude buccal to the gingiva of the maxilla and should be

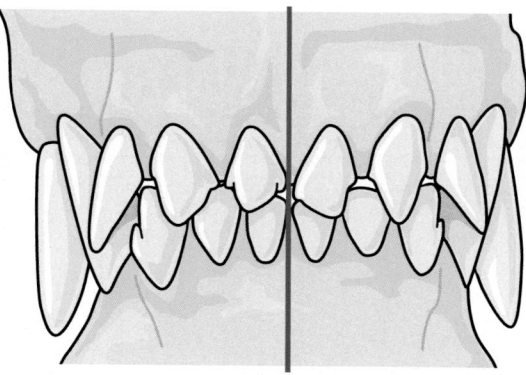

Fig. 5.15 Symmetry of head, face and dentition

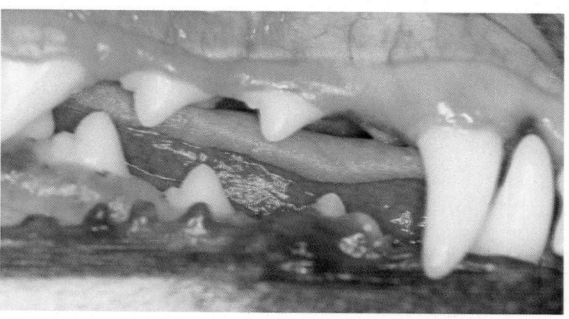

Fig. 5.16 Count teeth The upper 1st premolar is missing in this dog. Teeth that are missing on clinical examination require radiographic confirmation.

equidistant between the maxillary canine tooth and the maxillary 3rd incisor. This relationship is called the 'dental interlock' and is the most reliable reference point in the mouth (Figs 5.2, 5.18).

5. Evaluate premolar occlusion.
   The large cusp of the lower 4th premolar should divide the space between the upper 3rd and upper 4th premolars, the central cusp pointing interproximally between the two teeth (Fig. 5.19).
6. Evaluate occlusal plane of upper and lower arches.
   The premolars should interdigitate from the 2nd premolars back to the cusps of the upper 4th premolars, and there should be no overlapping of cusp tips (Fig. 5.20).

The molars should occlude to allow cusps to function in crushing.

The premolars and molars should be aligned mesial to distal in a smooth curve, with none of the teeth rotated.

A checklist for occlusal evaluation is shown in Box 5.1.

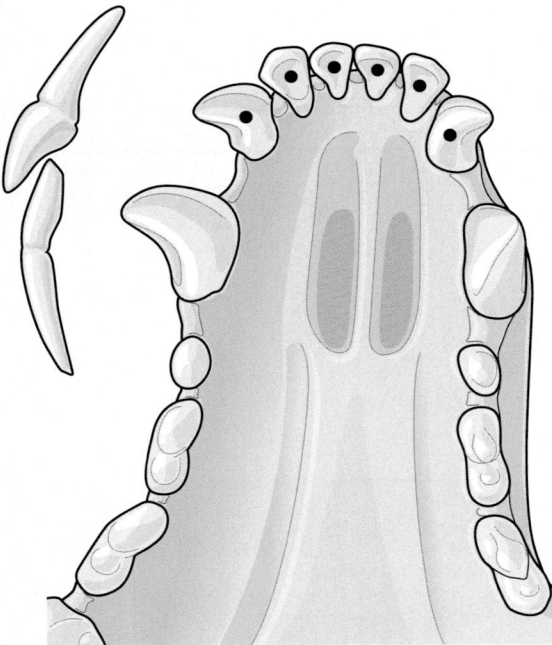

Fig. 5.17 Incisor occlusion The large cusps of the lower incisors should occlude near the cingulum on the palatal side of the upper incisors.

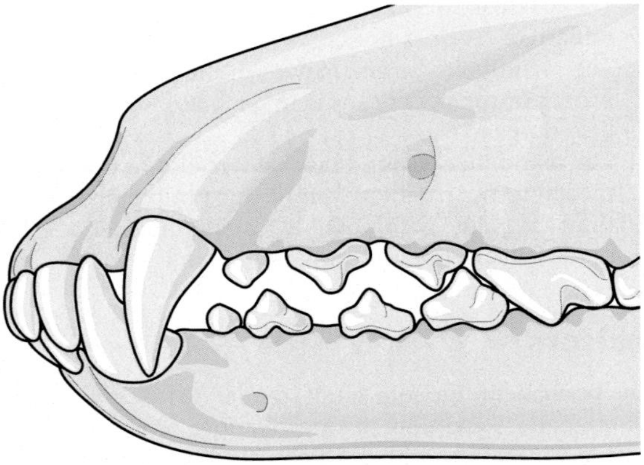

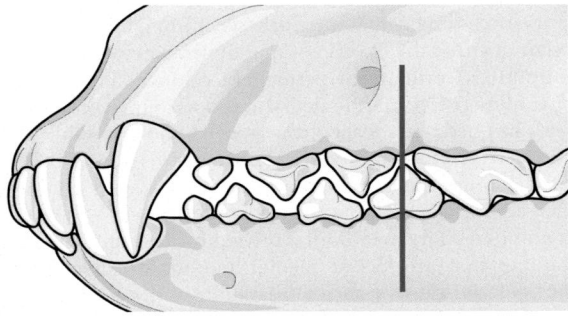

Fig. 5.18 The dental interlock The mandibular canine teeth should occlude buccal to the gingiva of the maxilla and should be equidistant between the maxillary canine and the maxillary 3rd incisor.

Fig. 5.19 Premolar occlusion The large cusp of the lower 4th premolar should divide the space between the upper third and upper 4th premolar, the central cusp pointing interproximally between the two teeth.

CLASSIFICATION OF OCCLUSION

There are numerous classification systems for occlusion. The one described below is the one currently advised by both the American Veterinary Dental College and the European Veterinary Dental College.

Normal occlusion is as described above and summarized in Figure 5.21. There are then three classes of abnormal occlusion and an, as yet, unclassified group.

Abnormal occlusion

Class I

A Class I abnormal occlusion is a bite which is generally normal with one or more teeth out of alignment or rotated. The following abnormalities qualify as a Class I malocclusion:

- A shift in interdigitation between maxillary and mandibular premolars
- An anterior crossbite (Fig. 5.12)
- A posterior crossbite (Fig. 5.13)
- Lingually displaced mandibular canines (Fig. 5.11)
- Rostrally angled maxillary canines.

Class II

A Class II abnormal occlusion is defined by the fact that the mandibular premolars and molars are positioned distal to the normal relationship. This is a skeletal malocclusion and is 'normal' for dolichocephalic breeds (Fig. 5.9).

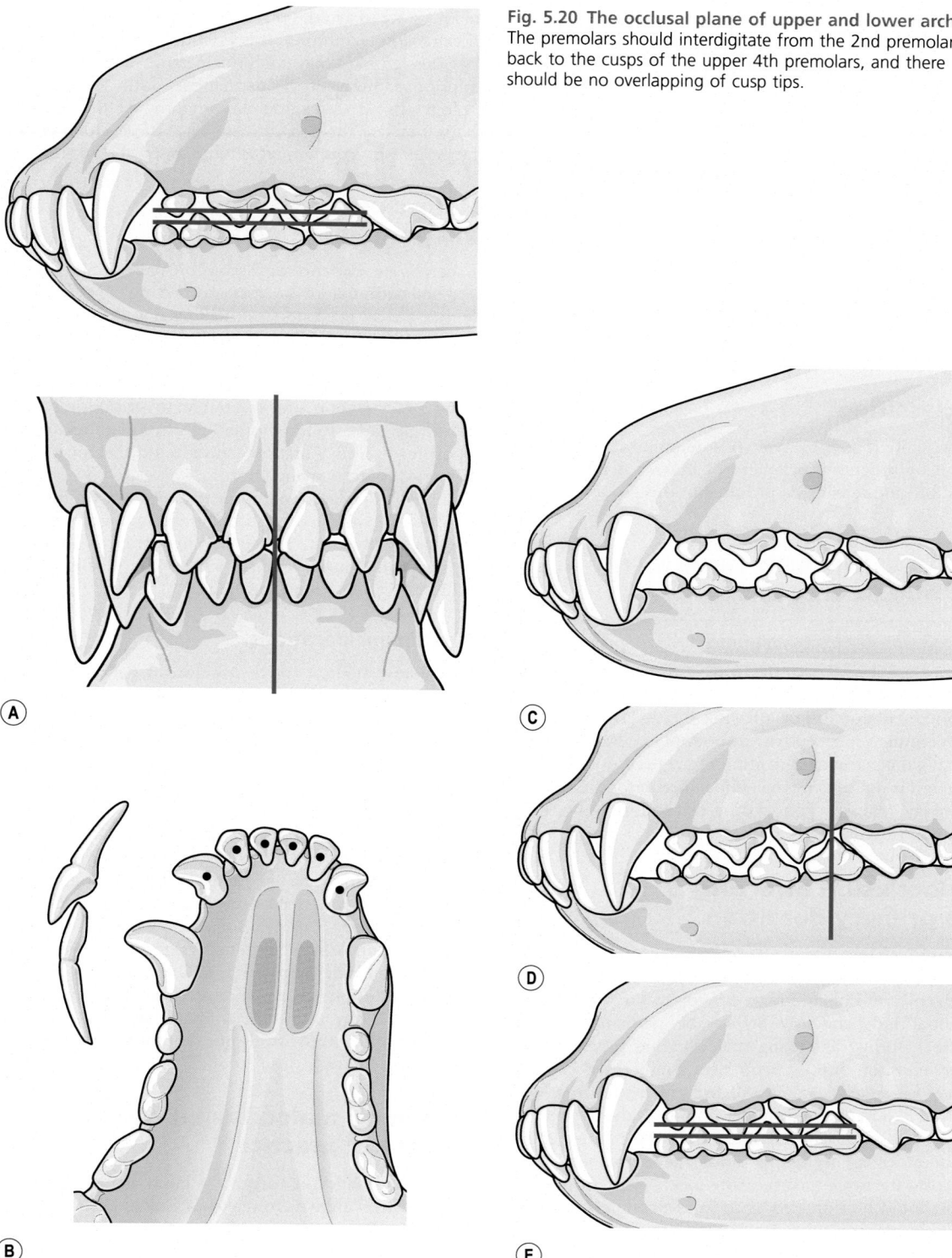

Fig. 5.20 The occlusal plane of upper and lower arches The premolars should interdigitate from the 2nd premolars back to the cusps of the upper 4th premolars, and there should be no overlapping of cusp tips.

Ⓐ

Ⓑ

Ⓒ

Ⓓ

Ⓔ

Fig. 5.21 Summary of the five features of normal occlusion

Many different terms are used to describe a Class II malocclusion. The more common are mandibular brachygnathism, retrusive mandible, distal mandibular excursion, overjet, overshot, overbite, distoclusion.

Class III

A Class III abnormal occlusion is defined by the fact that the mandibular premolars and molars are positioned rostral to the normal relationship. This is a skeletal malocclusion and is 'normal' for brachycephalic breeds (Fig. 5.8).

Many different terms are used to describe a Class III malocclusion. The more common are mandibular prognathism, protrusive mandible, mesial mandibular excursion, underjet, undershot, underbite, mesioclusion.

Unclassified

The wry bite (Fig. 5.10), which is an abnormal occlusion caused by difference in length of the two halves of the mandible and maxilla, is included in this group.

PREVENTION AND TREATMENT OF MALOCCLUSION

Prevention is always better than treatment. Early recognition of a problem is essential to avoid discomfort and pain to the animal and prevent the development of severe pathology. Malocclusion affecting the primary dentition may require interceptive orthodontics. Malocclusion affecting the permanent dentition may need no treatment at all, if it is not causing the animal discomfort or any oral pathology. Malocclusion causing discomfort and pathology always needs treating.

Malocclusion affecting the primary dentition

Primary teeth involved in malocclusion should be extracted as early as possible, i.e. at 6–8 weeks of age. This will allow the maxilla and mandible to develop to their full genetic potential independently before the permanent dental interlock forms. Extracting maloccluding primary teeth before eruption of their permanent counterparts is called *interceptive orthodontics*. It will prevent dental interlock-induced malocclusion from developing. If the developing malocclusion is of skeletal origin, the value of interceptive orthodontics is negligible, since the permanent teeth will form the same incorrect interlock. Persistent primary teeth should be extracted as soon as possible to prevent malocclusion.

The roots of primary teeth are longer and narrower than the roots of the permanent teeth. Extraction requires care

and patience to avoid tooth fracture (see Ch. 13 for details of extraction technique). It is essential not to fracture the root as a remnant may continue to cause deviation of the eruption pathway of the permanent tooth. Preoperative radiographs to determine the anatomy of the primary tooth, but also the position and stage of development of the permanent counterpart, should always be taken.

Malocclusion affecting the permanent dentition

If there is no evidence of discomfort/pain or any associated oral pathology, malocclusion affecting the permanent dentition may need no treatment. Malocclusion causing discomfort and pathology, however, always needs treating. The treatment options available are orthodontics, tooth shortening or extraction. In many instances, tooth shortening or extraction are preferable to orthodontics on ethical grounds. Tooth shortening often requires pulpal exposure. In this situation, endodontic therapy of the shortened tooth is mandatory.

Lingually displaced mandibular canines in young dogs can often be corrected by stimulating the dogs to play, as often as possible, with specific rubber toys of an appropriate size and shape (Verhaert 1999). The details of this technique can be found in Chapter 10.

Ethical considerations

In humans, medical (predisposition to periodontal diseases), functional (alteration of mastication or speech) and psychological (alteration of esthetics) problems relating to malocclusion are the primary reason for orthodontic treatment. In human orthodontics, whether malocclusion is hereditary or acquired is not a consideration when planning treatment. This is in contrast to veterinary orthodontics where esthetics and ethical concerns are linked, and treatment for the sole purpose of showing dogs or cats cannot be encouraged. The aim of any treatment is primarily to make the animal comfortable; esthetics is a secondary consideration.

It is essential to determine whether the presenting malocclusion is hereditary or not. Orthodontic correction of a malocclusion is contraindicated where the malocclusion is hereditary, unless the animal is also neutered. The rationale for this is to avoid spread of inherited malocclusion within a breed.

Managing malocclusion cases in general practice

Occlusal evaluation is part of the basic oral examination of a conscious animal. To make an evaluation, the practitioner needs to be able to identify normal occlusion for the species and breed and have an understanding of the etiology and pathogenesis of malocclusion as detailed earlier in this chapter. It is essential to determine whether the malocclusion is of skeletal, dental or combination origin. Preventive measures (such as controlled playing with an appropriate rubber toy, interceptive orthodontics or extraction of persistent primary teeth) should be carried out early in the animal's life. In most instances, treatment other than prevention is best left to a veterinarian with special skills in dentistry, namely expertise in endodontics and orthodontics.

Principles of orthodontic movement

Orthodontic movement of teeth can be described as prolonged application of pressure to the tooth, resulting in movement of the tooth as the bone around it remodels. Bone on the compression side undergoes lysis allowing the tooth to move and bone formation on the tension side ensures that the tooth stays in the new position. In the ideal situation bone lysis and bone formation should be in equilibrium. In most practical situations, there is an imbalance and lysis occurs more rapidly. A retention phase maintaining the tooth in the new position while allowing time for bone formation is, therefore, necessary in many cases.

The optimal orthodontic force is one that moves teeth rapidly without resulting in structural damage, while causing the least amount of discomfort or pain. Factors that need to be considered for any orthodontic appliance are the magnitude of the force, the distribution of the force and the duration of the force. The ideal force is a light continuous force. Heavy continuous forces are most damaging and should be avoided. Apart from the orthodontic forces applied, normal growth processes and forces from the lips, cheeks and tongue resting on the teeth will determine the outcome of the treatment. Possible complications to orthodontic movement of teeth include pulpal disease, external root resorption, tooth mobility and pain. In short, the outcome of an orthodontic procedure is rarely predictable and needs frequent monitoring based on clinical signs and radiography.

SUMMARY

- Malocclusion is common and may cause pain/discomfort and severe oral pathology.
- It is essential to diagnose malocclusion early in the life of the animal.
- Prevention is the best strategy.
- Skeletal malocclusions and persistent primary teeth are hereditary.
- Orthodontic treatment of an inheritable malocclusion should only be considered in the neutered animal.
- In most instances, treatment, other than prevention, is best left to a veterinarian with special skills in dentistry.
- The aim of any treatment is to make the animal comfortable with a functional bite; esthetic considerations are of secondary importance.

REFERENCES

Beard, G., 1989. Anterior crossbite: interceptive orthodontics for prevention, Maryland bridges for correction. Journal of Veterinary Dentistry 6 (2), 14.

Hennet, P.R., 1995. Orthodontics in small carnivores. In: Crossley, D.A., Penman, S. (Eds.), Manual of Small Animal Dentistry. BSAVA, Cheltenham, pp. 182–192.

Hennet, P.R., Harvey, C.E., 1992a. Craniofacial development and growth in the dog. Journal of Veterinary Dentistry 9 (2), 11–18.

Hennet, P.R., Harvey, C.E., 1992b. Diagnostic approach to malocclusions in dogs. Journal of Veterinary Dentistry 9 (2), 23–26.

Shipp, A.D., Fahrenkrug, P., 1992. Practitioner's Guide to Veterinary Dentistry. Dr Shipp's Laboratories, Beverley Hills, pp. 117–147.

Stockard, C.R., 1941. The Genetic and Endocrinic Basis for Differences in Form and Behaviour. The American Anatomical Memoirs No. 19. The Wistar Institute of Anatomy and Biology, Philadelphia.

Verhaert, L., 1999. A removable orthodontic device for the treatment of lingually displaced mandibular canine teeth in young dogs. Journal of Veterinary Dentistry 16 (2), 69–75.

FURTHER READING

Gorrel, C., 2008. Malocclusion. In: Saunders Solutions in Veterinary Practice – Small Animal Dentistry. Saunders/Elsevier, Philadelphia, pp. 129–167.

Holmstrom, S.E., Frost, P., Eisner, E.R., 2004. Dental equipment and care. In: Veterinary Dental Techniques for the Small Animal Practitioner, third ed. Saunders, Philadelphia, pp. 499–558.

Chapter | 6 |

Oral examination and recording

INTRODUCTION

Optimal treatment relies on a good diagnostic work-up. Oral diagnosis is based on the results of clinical examination and radiography, with guidance from the case history. Additional diagnostic tests are used when indicated. *A permanent record should be made of relevant medical and dental history, diagnostic data and details of all treatment performed.*

ORAL EXAMINATION

Examination of the oral cavity is part of every physical examination; however, oral examination in a conscious animal will only give limited information. Definitive oral examination can only be performed under general anesthesia. *All detected abnormalities should be recorded.* It saves time if one person performs the examination and another individual takes the notes and enters the findings on the dental record.

Conscious examination

Oral examination of a conscious animal is limited to visual inspection and some digital palpation. Gentle technique is essential.

Examination involves assessing not only the oral cavity proper, but also palpation of:

- The face (facial bones and zygomatic arch)
- Temporomandibular joint
- Salivary glands (mandibular/sublingual; the parotids are usually only palpable if enlarged)
- Lymph nodes (mandibular, cervical chain).

Having looked at the entire face, the mouth is first examined by gently holding the jaws closed and retracting the lips (do not pull on the fur to retract lips) to look at the soft tissues and buccal aspects of the teeth. This is the optimal time to evaluate occlusion. Chapter 5 details the normal occlusal relationships in the dog and cat.

A checklist for evaluation of dental occlusion is shown in Box 6.1.

Finally, the animal is encouraged to open its mouth. One method of achieving this in the dog is to place a thumb and finger on the margin of the alveolar bone caudal to the canine teeth of the upper and lower jaws on one side and with gentle pressure encouraging the animal to open its jaws. Another method, useful for both dogs and cats, is to approach the animal from lateral, one hand is placed over the muzzle and the lips are gently pressed into the oral cavity, while tilting the head slightly upwards. A finger from the other hand is placed on the lower incisors and gentle pressure is exerted. Do not use the fur under the mandible to try to pull the jaw down.

Most animals allow at least a cursory inspection of the oral cavity once the jaws have been opened. The mucous membranes of the oral cavity should be examined as well as the teeth. Apart from color and texture of the mucous membranes, look for evidence of a potential bleeding problem (petechiation, purpura, ecchymoses). In addition, look for vesicle formation and ulceration, which could indicate a vesiculo-bullous disorder, e.g. pemphigus, pemphigoid. Obvious pathology (tooth fracture, gingival recession, advanced furcation exposure) relating to the teeth can be identified. Assess the oropharynx (soft palate, palatoglossal arch, tonsillary crypts, tonsils and fauces) if possible. It is useful to identify any potential problems with endotracheal intubation prior to inducing anesthesia.

Examination under general anesthesia

The oropharynx should be examined prior to endotracheal intubation. Normal anatomic features of the oral cavity need to be identified and inspected. Refreshing your memory on these features from an anatomy textbook is highly recommended. It is only with knowledge of the normal that abnormalities can be identified. A checklist for the oral examination under anesthetic is summarized in Box 6.2.

Periodontium

The periodontium of each tooth needs to be assessed. Examination of the periodontium is not routinely performed in veterinary practice. It is essential to perform a thorough periodontal examination in order to correctly diagnose disease and plan treatment. The procedure for examination of the periodontium is detailed below. Instruments required include:

1. Periodontal probe
2. Dental explorer
3. Dental mirror.

The following indices and criteria should be evaluated for each tooth:

1. Gingivitis and gingival index
2. Periodontal probing depth
3. Gingival recession
4. Furcation involvement
5. Mobility
6. Periodontal (clinical) attachment level.

In animals with large accumulations of dental deposits (plaque and calculus) on the teeth, it may be necessary to remove these to assess periodontal status accurately (Fig. 6.1).

The full clinical significance of measuring and recording the periodontal parameters detailed in the following is discussed in Chapter 9.

In outline, the purpose of the meticulous periodontal examination is to:

- Identify the presence of periodontal disease (gingivitis and periodontitis)

- Differentiate between gingivitis (inflammation of the gingiva) and periodontitis (inflammation of the periodontal tissues resulting in loss of attachment and eventually tooth loss)
- Identify the precise location of disease processes

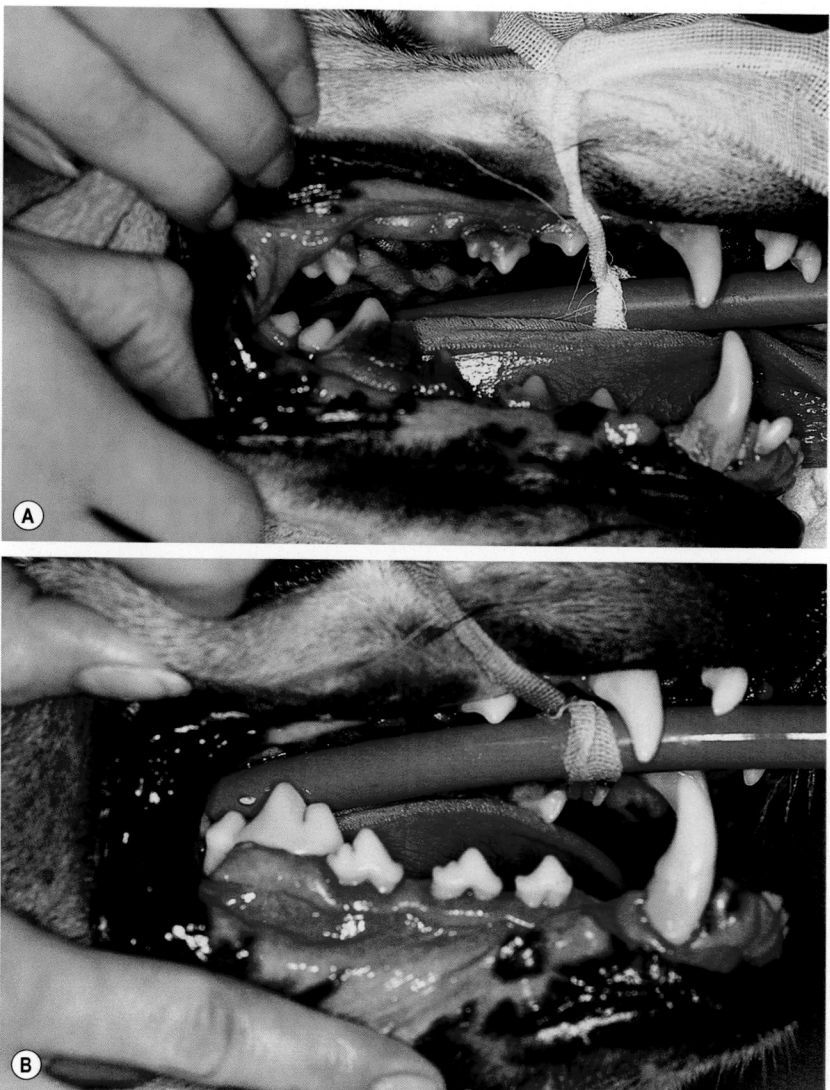

Fig. 6.1 Dental deposits and periodontal examination (A) Large amounts of plaque and calculus make it impossible to assess the severity of periodontitis. (B) The periodontal destruction is evident once the dental deposits have been removed.

• Assess the extent of tissue destruction where there is periodontitis.

Periodontal probing depth, gingival recession, furcation involvement and mobility quantify the tissue destruction in periodontitis. Radiography to visualize the extent and type of alveolar bone destruction is mandatory. Radiography of the jaws and teeth is detailed in Chapter 7. In many cases, measuring or calculating the periodontal or clinical attachment level (PAL/CAL) is also useful.

Gingivitis and gingival index

The presence and degree of gingivitis (inflammation of the gingiva) is assessed based on a combination of redness and swelling, as well as the presence or absence of bleeding on gentle probing of the gingival sulcus. Various indices can be used to give a numerical value to the degree of gingival inflammation present. In the clinical situation, a simple bleeding index is the most useful. Using this method, a periodontal probe is gently inserted into the

Table 6.1 The *modified* Löe and Silness gingival index

Gingival index 0	Clinically healthy gingiva
Gingival index 1	Mild gingivitis: slight reddening and swelling of the gingival margin; no bleeding on gentle probing of the gingival sulcus
Gingival index 2	Moderate gingivitis: the gingival margin is red and swollen; gentle probing of the gingival sulcus results in bleeding
Gingival index 3	Severe gingivitis: the gingival margin is very swollen with a red or bluish-red color; there is spontaneous hemorrhage and/or ulceration of the gingival margin

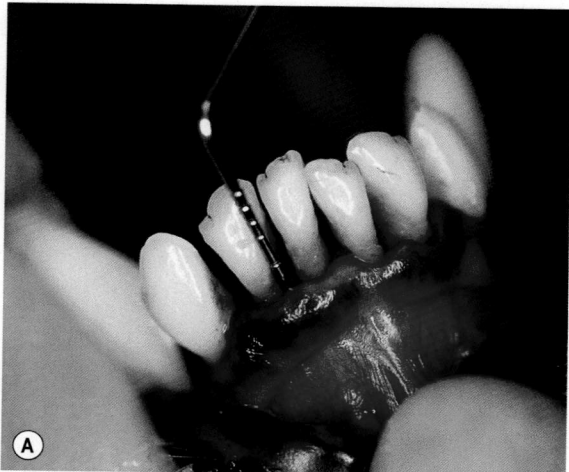

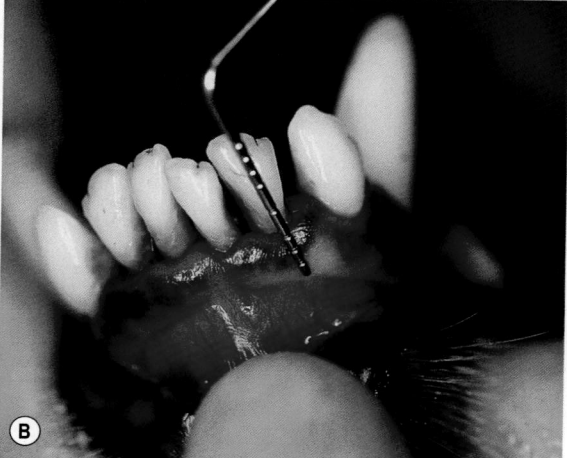

Fig. 6.2 Periodontal probing depth (PPD) (A) The PPD is measured by inserting a periodontal probe into the gingival sulcus until firm resistance is felt. The distance from the free gingival margin to the depth of the sulcus or pocket is the periodontal probing depth. It should be measured and recorded at several sites around the circumference of each tooth. (B) The probe has been placed on the surface of the gingiva to depict the depth to which it had been inserted.

gingival sulcus at several locations around the whole circumference of each tooth. A score of 0 is given if there is no bleeding and a score of 1 if the probing elicits bleeding.

An index, which relies on both visual inspection and bleeding, namely the *modified* Löe and Silness gingival index (Löe 1967), can also be used (Table 6.1). In research, this is the most commonly used method of assessing and quantifying gingivitis.

Periodontal probing depth (PPD)

The depth of the sulcus can be assessed by gently inserting a graduated periodontal probe until resistance is encountered at the base of the sulcus. The depth from the free gingival margin to the base of the sulcus is measured in millimeters at several locations around the whole circumference of the tooth (Fig. 6.2). The probe is moved gently horizontally, walking along the floor of the sulcus. The gingival sulcus is 1–3 mm deep in the dog and 0.5–1.0 mm in the cat. Measurements in excess of these values usually indicate the presence of periodontitis when the periodontal ligament has been destroyed and alveolar bone resorbed, thus allowing the probe to be inserted to a greater depth. The term used to describe this situation is periodontal pocketing.

All sites with periodontal pocketing should be accurately recorded. Gingival inflammation resulting in swelling or hyperplasia of the free gingiva will, of course, also result in measuring sulcus depths in excess of normal values. In these situations, the term 'pseudopocketing' is used, as the periodontal ligament and bone are intact (i.e. there is no evidence of periodontitis) and the increase in PPD is due to swelling or hyperplasia of the gingiva.

Gingival recession

Gingival recession (Fig. 6.3) is also measured using a periodontal probe. It is the distance (in mm) from the cemento-enamel junction to the free gingival margin. At sites with gingival recession, the PPD may be within normal values despite loss of alveolar bone due to periodontitis.

Furcation involvement

Furcation involvement refers to the situation where the bone between the roots of multirooted teeth is destroyed

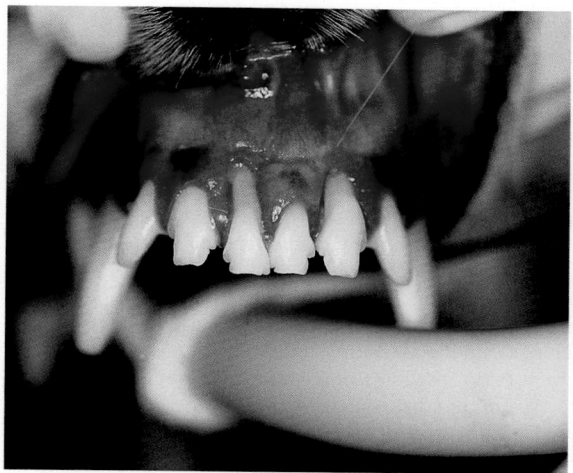

Fig. 6.3 Gingival recession Gingival recession is measured from the cemento-enamel junction to the free gingival margin using a graded periodontal probe. The right upper 1st incisor and the left upper 2nd incisor have extensive gingival recession affecting their buccal aspects, most of the root surfaces are exposed.

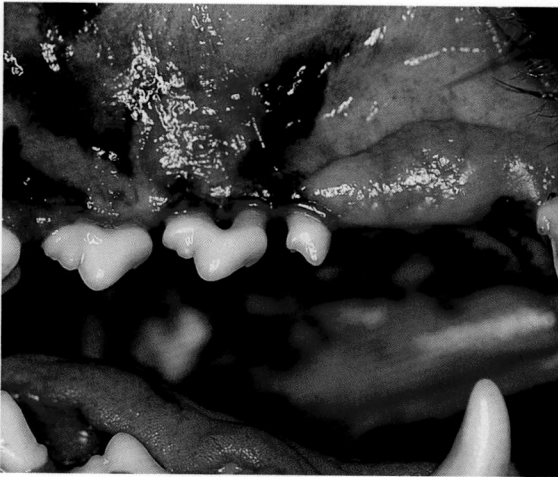

Fig. 6.4 Furcation involvement The furcation sites of multirooted teeth should be examined with either a periodontal probe or a dental explorer so that the degree of furcation involvement can be graded. The right maxillary 2nd premolar has a grade 3 furcation, i.e. the explorer or probe can be passed through it.

by periodontitis (Fig. 6.4). The furcation sites of multi-rooted teeth should be examined with either a periodontal probe or a dental explorer. The grading of furcation involvement is listed in Table 6.2.

Tooth mobility

The extent of tooth mobility should be assessed using a suitable instrument, e.g. the blunt end of the handle of a dental mirror or probe. It should not be assessed using fingers directly, since the yield of the soft tissues of the fingers will mask the extent of tooth mobility. The grading of mobility is listed in Table 6.3.

Periodontal/clinical attachment level (PAL/CAL)

Periodontal probing depth is not necessarily correlated with severity of attachment loss. As already mentioned, gingival hyperplasia may contribute to a deep pocket (or pseudopocket if there is no attachment loss), while gingival recession may result in the absence of a pocket but also minimal remaining attachment. PAL records the distance from the cemento-enamel junction (or from a fixed point on the tooth) to the base or apical extension of the pathologic pocket. It is thus a more accurate assessment of tissue loss in periodontitis. PAL is either directly measured with a periodontal probe or it is calculated (e.g. PPD + gingival recession).

Table 6.2 Grading of furcation involvement

Grade 0	No furcation involvement
Grade 1	Initial furcation involvement: the furcation can be felt with the probe/explorer, but horizontal tissue destruction is less than one-third of the horizontal width of the furcation
Grade 2	Partial furcation involvement: it is possible to explore the furcation but the probe/explorer cannot be passed through it; horizontal tissue destruction is more than one-third of the horizontal width of the furcation
Grade 3	Total furcation involvement: the probe/explorer can be passed through the furcation from buccal to palatal/lingual

RECORDING

The information resulting from the examination and any treatment performed needs to be recorded. A basic dental record consists of written notes and a completed dental chart. Additional diagnostic tests and radiographs are included as indicated.

A completed dental record is a legal document that can be referred to:

- During treatment – to ensure that all treatment is performed
- At post-treatment discharge – to inform the owner of the condition of the teeth and of treatment performed

Table 6.3 Grading of tooth mobility

Grade 0	No mobility
Grade 1	Horizontal movement of ≤1 mm
Grade 2	Horizontal movement of >1 mm. Note that multirooted teeth are scored more severely and a horizontal mobility in excess of 1 mm is usually considered a Grade 3 even in the absence of vertical movement
Grade 3	Vertical as well as horizontal movement is possible

- At any time or by any person in the practice – for information related to the mouth at a specific date.

The dental chart is a diagrammatic representation of the dentition, where information (findings and, respectively treatment) can be entered in a pictorial and/or notational form. It provides a simple way of recording most of your findings and treatments. However, it is only a chart and needs to be supplemented by clinical notes, radiographs, etc. to make a complete dental record.

Copy of the dog and cat dental record sheets used in our clinic are depicted in Figures 6.5 and 6.6. The front is used to record clinical findings and the back is used to enter diagnosis, draw up a treatment plan and record treatment performed. Figure 6.7 shows a completed form.

We number the teeth using the modified Triadan system, which is a three-digit numbering system. The first digit denotes the quadrant of the mouth and whether the tooth is part of the permanent or primary dentition (Table 6.4).

The second and third digits together denote the tooth. In dogs, the teeth are numbered consecutively from the

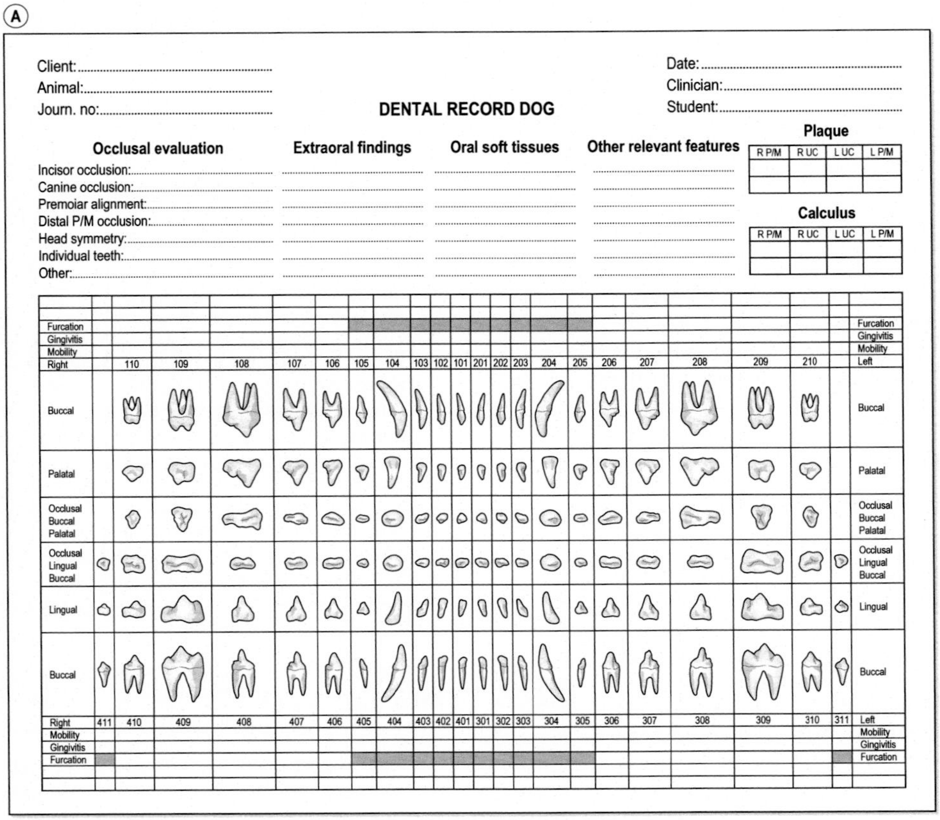

Fig. 6.5 Dental record sheets for the dog Front (A) for recording findings and back (B) for treatment planning and procedures performed.

B

Oral problem list

....

....

....

Periodontics

- ☐ Sonic scaling
- ☐ Subgingival curettage
- ☐ Pumice-polishing
- ☐ Periodontal surgery:.....................

- ☐ Ultrasonic scaling
- ☐ Peridontal debridement
- ☐ Air-polishing

Therapeutic plan

....

....

....

....

Oral surgery (Note sites on graph - X)

- ☐ Simple extraction(s):.....................
- ☐ Surgical extraction(s):.....................
- ☐ Incisional biopsy   ☐ Excisional biopsy
- ☐ Other/comments:.....................

....

....

Other dental procedures

....

....

....

....

Complications/comments

....

....

....

....

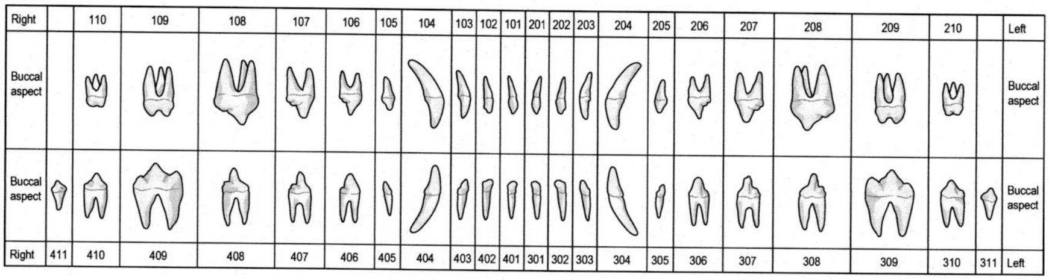

Right	110	109	108	107	106	105	104	103	102	101	201	202	203	204	205	206	207	208	209	210		Left
Buccal aspect																						Buccal aspect
Buccal aspect																						Buccal aspect
Right	411	410	409	408	407	406	405	404	403	402	401	301	302	303	304	305	306	307	308	309	310	311	Left

Fig. 6.5, cont'd

A

Client:...

Animal:...

Journ. no:...

DENTAL RECORD CAT

Date:...

Clinician:...

Student:...

	Occlusal evaluation	Extraoral findings	Oral soft tissues	Other relevant features
Incisor occlusion:................				
Canine occlusion:................				
Premoiar alignment:................				
Distal P/M occlusion:................				
Head symmetry:................				
Individual teeth:................				
Other:................				

Plaque

R P/M	R UC	L UC	L P/M

Calculus

R P/M	R UC	L UC	L P/M

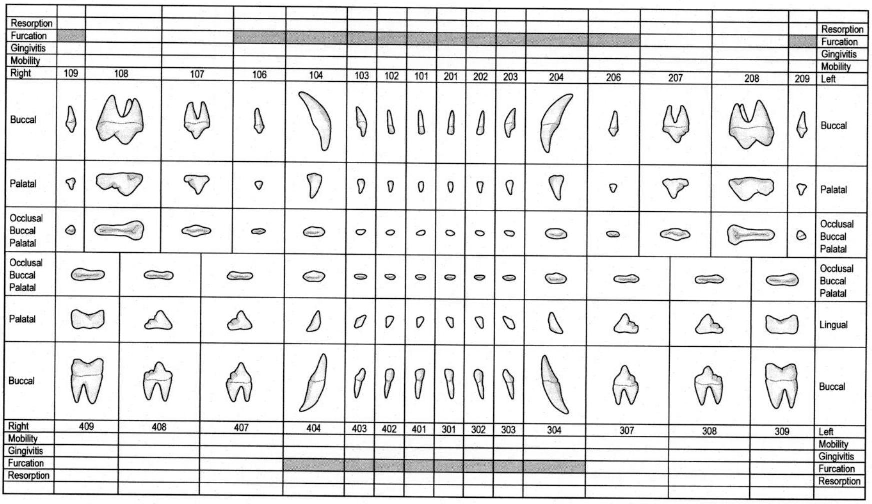

Resorption																			Resorption
Furcation																			Furcation
Gingivitis																			Gingivitis
Mobility																			Mobility
Right	109	108	107	106	104	103	102	101	201	202	203	204	206	207	208	209			Left
Buccal																			Buccal
Palatal																			Palatal
Occlusal Buccal Palatal																			Occlusal Buccal Palatal
Occlusal Buccal Palatal																			Occlusal Buccal Palatal
Palatal																			Lingual
Buccal																			Buccal
Right	409	408	407	404	403	402	401	301	302	303	304	307	308	309					Left
Mobility																			Mobility
Gingivitis																			Gingivitis
Furcation																			Furcation
Resorption																			Resorption

Fig. 6.6 Dental record sheets for the cat Front (A) for recording findings and back (B) for treatment planning and procedures performed.

Continued

(B)

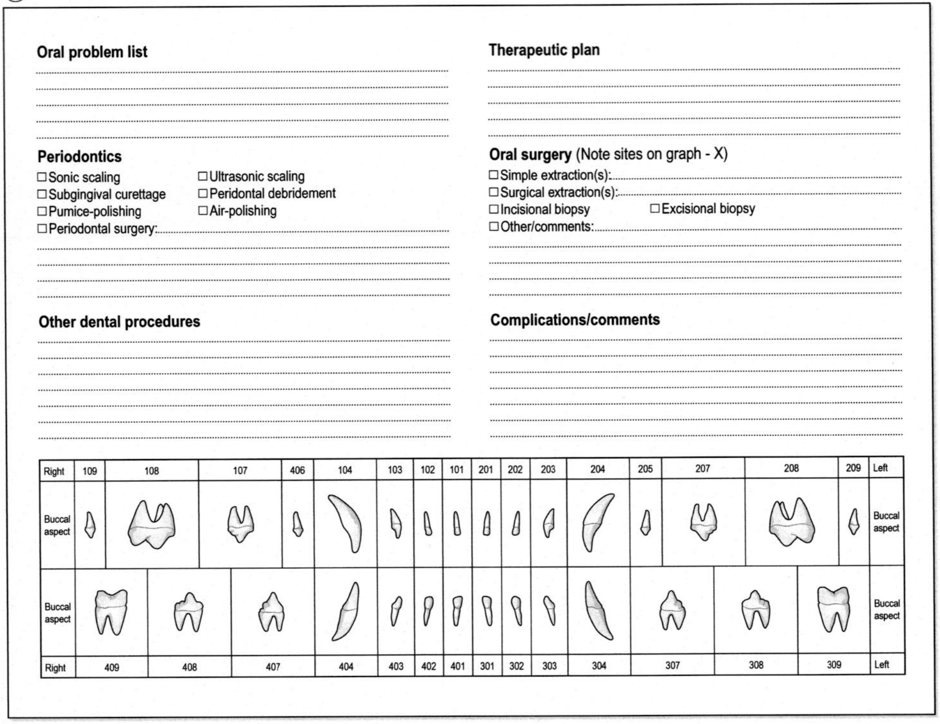

Oral problem list

Therapeutic plan

Periodontics
- ☐ Sonic scaling
- ☐ Subgingival curettage
- ☐ Pumice-polishing
- ☐ Periodontal surgery:
- ☐ Ultrasonic scaling
- ☐ Peridontal debridement
- ☐ Air-polishing

Oral surgery (Note sites on graph - X)
- ☐ Simple extraction(s):
- ☐ Surgical extraction(s):
- ☐ Incisional biopsy   ☐ Excisional biopsy
- ☐ Other/comments:

Other dental procedures

Complications/comments

Right	109	108	107	406	104	103	102	101	201	202	203	204	205	207	208	209	Left
Buccal aspect																	Buccal aspect
Buccal aspect																	Buccal aspect
Right	409	408	407	404	403	402	401	301	302	303	304	307	308	309			Left

Fig. 6.6, cont'd

(A)

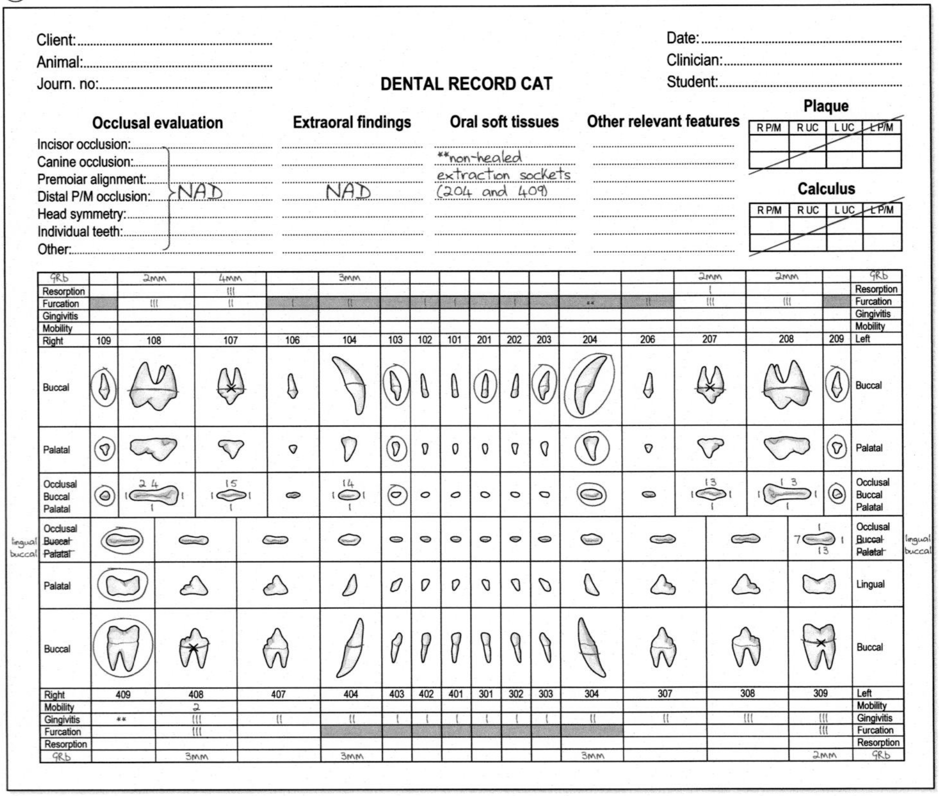

Client: _____ Date: _____
Animal: _____ Clinician: _____
Journ. no: _____ **DENTAL RECORD CAT** Student: _____

Occlusal evaluation	Extraoral findings	Oral soft tissues	Other relevant features
Incisor occlusion:		**non-healed extraction sockets (204 and 409)**	
Canine occlusion:			
Premoiar alignment:			
Distal P/M occlusion: NAD	NAD		
Head symmetry:			
Individual teeth:			
Other:			

Plaque

R P/M	R UC	L UC	L P/M

Calculus

R P/M	R UC	L UC	L P/M

9Rb	2mm	4mm	3mm									2mm	2mm		9Rb
Resorption															Resorption
Furcation											**				Furcation
Gingivitis															Gingivitis
Mobility															Mobility
Right	109	108	107	106	104	103	102	101	201	202	203	204	206	207	208	209	Left

Buccal																Buccal
Palatal																Palatal
Occlusal Buccal Palatal																Occlusal Buccal Palatal
Occlusal Buccal Palatal																Occlusal Buccal Palatal
Palatal																Lingual
Buccal																Buccal

Right	409	408	407	404	403	402	401	301	302	303	304	307	308	309			Left
Mobility		2													Mobility
Gingivitis	**														Gingivitis
Furcation															Furcation
Resorption															Resorption
9Rb	3mm	3mm				3mm						2mm			9Rb

Fig. 6.7 Completed dental record sheet for a cat Front (A) shows all findings and back (B) details treatment planning and procedures performed.

Ⓑ

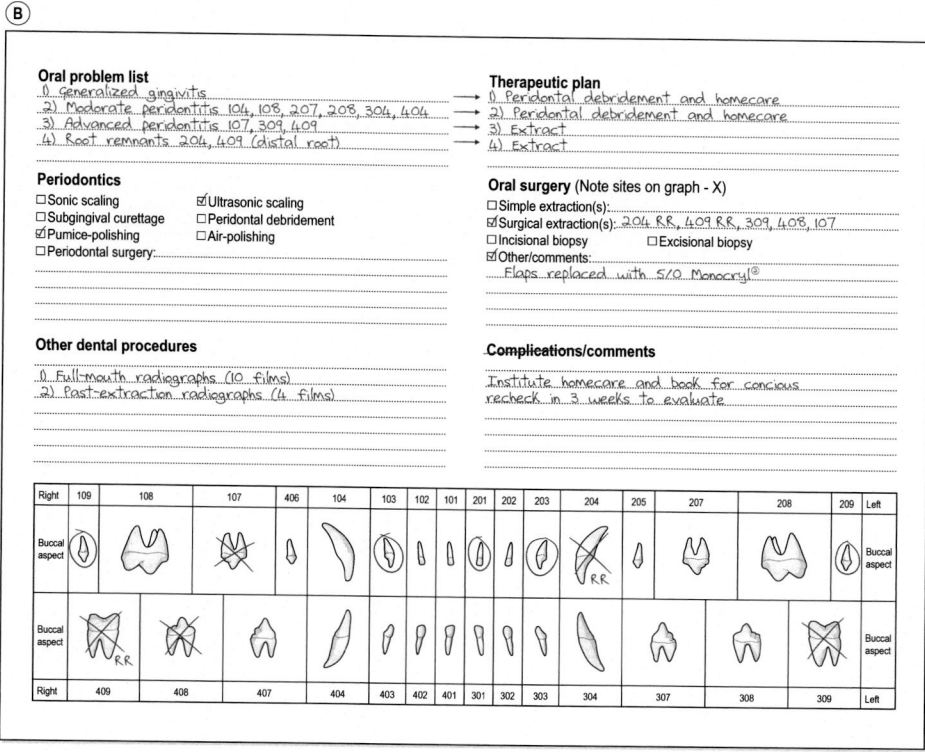

Oral problem list			**Therapeutic plan**	

Oral problem list
1) Generalized gingivitis
2) Moderate peridontitis 104, 108, 207, 208, 304, 404
3) Advanced peridontitis 107, 309, 409
4) Root remnants 204, 409 (distal root)

Therapeutic plan
→ 1) Peridontal debridement and homecare
→ 2) Peridontal debridement and homecare
→ 3) Extract
→ 4) Extract

Periodontics
☐ Sonic scaling   ☑ Ultrasonic scaling
☐ Subgingival curettage   ☐ Peridontal debridement
☑ Pumice-polishing   ☐ Air-polishing
☐ Periodontal surgery:

Oral surgery (Note sites on graph - X)
☐ Simple extraction(s):
☑ Surgical extraction(s): 204 RR, 409 RR, 309, 408, 107
☐ Incisional biopsy   ☐ Excisional biopsy
☑ Other/comments:
   Flaps replaced with 5/0 Monocryl®

Other dental procedures
1) Full-mouth radiographs (10 films)
2) Post-extraction radiographs (4 films)

Complications/comments
Institute homecare and book for concious
recheck in 3 weeks to evaluate

Right	109	108	107	406	104	103	102	101	201	202	203	204	205	207	208	209	Left
Buccal aspect																	Buccal aspect
Buccal aspect																	Buccal aspect
Right	409	408	407	404	403	402	401	301	302	303	304	307	308	309	Left		

Fig. 6.7, cont'd

Table 6.4 Modified Triadan system: a three-digit numbering system

Permanent dentition		Primary dentition	
Upper right = 1	Upper left = 2	Upper right = 5	Upper left = 6
Lower right = 4	Lower left = 3	Lower right = 8	Lower left = 7

Table 6.5 Common abbreviations

NAD	No abnormality detected
ORL	Odontoclastic resorptive lesion
GR	Gingival recession
GH	Gingival hyperplasia
UCF	Uncomplicated crown fracture
CCF	Complicated crown fracture
UCRF	Uncomplicated crown and root fracture
CCRF	Complicated crown and root fracture
W	Wear (abrasion or attrition) facet

rostral midline to the caudal end of each quadrant. In cats, where the complement of teeth is reduced (the 1st maxillary and the 1st and 2nd mandibular premolars are absent), some numbers are skipped in the premolar region.

On the dental record sheet, plaque and calculus can be noted, e.g. as low, moderate or heavy. We do not routinely score the degree of accumulation of plaque or calculus, as they will be removed during the periodontal therapy.

Abbreviations are used when filling in the record sheet. It is important that a list of abbreviation meanings is available. A list of commonly used abbreviations is found in Table 6.5.

The basic dental record sheet recommended by the European Veterinary Dental College (EVDC) can also be used in a general practice situation. The EVDC dental records can be downloaded from the EVDC website (www.EVDC.info) free of charge.

The dental record recommended by the EVDC is continuously updated. It also contains information that is not relevant to the general practitioner, e.g. case log entry numbers, plaque and calculus index for all teeth, staining scale for all teeth. I suggest using either my record sheet or the EVDC recommended record sheet as an example, and drawing up a dental record sheet suitable for the individual practice.

Digital recording systems are also available for dog and cat. The program is called Prodenta and is available from Accesia AB (www.accesia.se).

SUMMARY

◆ Full oral examination is only possible under general anesthesia.
◆ Oral examination should proceed in an orderly and structured fashion, using appropriate instrumentation.
◆ Adequate recording should take place at all stages, preferably on published or adapted dental charting systems.

◆ Several indices and measurements should be taken to complement visual assessments, e.g. gingival index, periodontal probing depth, periodontal/clinical attachment level.

REFERENCE

Löe, H., 1967. The gingival index, the plaque index and the retention index system. Journal of Periodontology 38, 610–616.

FURTHER READING

Gorrel, C., 1998. Radiographic evaluation. In: Holmstrom, S. (Ed.), Canine Dentistry. Veterinary Clinics of North America: Small Animal Practice. WB Saunders, Philadelphia, pp. 1089–1110.

Gorrel, C., 2008. Oral examination and recording. In: Saunders Solutions in Veterinary Practice – Small Animal Dentistry. Saunders/Elsevier, Philadelphia, pp. 13–21.

Robinson, J., Gorrel, C., 1995. Oral examination and radiography. In: Crossley, D.A., Penman, S. (Eds.), Manual of Small Animal Dentistry. BSAVA, Cheltenham, pp. 35–49.

Chapter | 7 |

Dental radiography

INTRODUCTION

Radiography is a vital diagnostic tool in veterinary dentistry. The bulk of the tooth, i.e. root and most of the periodontium, can only be visualized by means of radiographs. Consequently, a lot of pathology will remain undiscovered if clinical examination does not involve radiography. While lesions such as caries can be recognized without radiography, it is not possible to assess the full extent of the lesions or if there is pulpal and periapical involvement. In other words, a clinical examination is incomplete without radiography.

Periodontal disease, endodontic disease, caries, resorptive lesions, fractures, bone pathology and neoplastic conditions all require radiography for a more complete diagnosis, thus allowing optimal planning of treatment. It is also necessary to know the normal radiographic anatomy to be able to identify the abnormal. Many dental procedures can only be carried out under radiographic control. Checking adequacy of procedures and success of treatment also relies heavily on radiography. In short, radiographs are required to reach a diagnosis and thus plan treatment optimally, to be able to perform certain procedures, and to be able to assess the outcome of treatment performed. Practicing dentistry without radiography as a tool would be considered negligent in human dentistry. The same applies to veterinary dentistry.

Pathologic radiographic changes are usually discrete and therefore clarity and detail are essential. For a dental radiograph to be diagnostic, it should be an accurate representation of the size and shape of the tooth without superimposition of adjacent structures (Figs 7.1, 7.2). Intraoral radiographic techniques are therefore required – a parallel technique for the mandibular premolars and molars, and a bisecting angle technique for all other teeth. Contralateral (same teeth, opposite side) views should be taken as routine.

Intraoral radiographic techniques do require some time and patience to master, but once this has been achieved they provide invaluable information, with minimal loss of time, which allows optimal planning and performing of dental treatments. Attending a practical course is particularly valuable in learning these techniques.

EQUIPMENT AND MATERIALS (BOX 7.1)

Dental radiographs can be taken using conventional (film) or digital (digital sensors) methods. Digital radiography refers to computer-generated images of radiographs. In indirect digital systems the exposure is made on a photostimulatable phosphor plate (Fig. 7.3), rather than on a dental film. The latent image from the plate is then transferred to a computer. Direct-to-digital equipment uses a sensor (Fig. 7.4) as a data input device that sends the image directly to the computer. Most modern X-ray machines are compatible with most digital software and hardware packages. Older X-ray machines may not be capable of short enough exposure times (as low as 0.02 s for small patients).

Digital radiography has many advantages as compared to conventional. The main advantages of digital radiography are the following:

- Provides immediate/rapid image availability
- Eliminates the need for developing and fixing
- Eliminates errors associated with developing and fixing

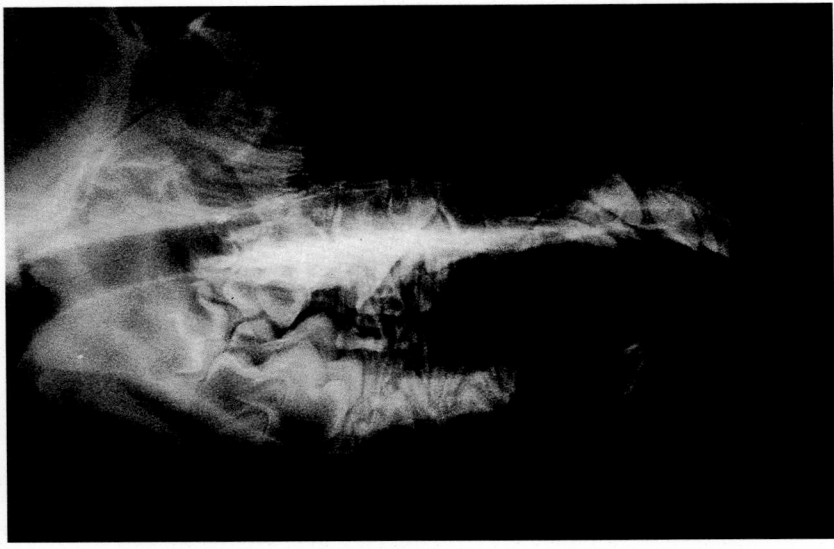

Fig. 7.1 A non-diagnostic view This lateral view (extraoral film positioning) is non-diagnostic for evaluation of teeth and associated tissues. There is superimposition of the right and left sides. In fact, it is not possible to say much more than that it is a radiograph of an immature dog and there are teeth present.

Box 7.1 Equipment and materials for intraoral radiography

Conventional

- X-ray machine
- X-ray film
- Processing facilities
- Mounts or envelopes for film storage

Digital

- X-ray machine
- Digital sensors
- Computer and software.

- Eliminates film mounting and storage issues
- Requires less radiation
- Allows digital enhancement to assist visualization:

  - Change contrast
  - Change brightness
  - Magnify
  - Invert image
  - Colorization.

I would strongly recommend that all veterinarians in small animal practice invest in a digital dental radiography system. The whole procedure of taking radiographs becomes so much simpler and quicker. In my experience, the resistance to using dental radiography as a diagnostic tool has been largely due to the 'hassle' factor (time consuming, messy, storage issues). With digital radiography, all these problems are removed and radiographs are thus more likely to be taken and disease processes identified and treated.

The X-ray unit

A dental X-ray machine is preferable to a veterinary X-ray machine. The dental unit has a freely maneuverable head that allows accurate positioning of the film with minimal adjustment in patient position. The cone of the dental unit will collimate the beam and provide the optimal film–focus distance.

Most veterinary X-ray machines can be used for dental radiography, but the film–focus distance will need to be adjusted to between 30 and 50 cm. The more maneuverable the head (in angulation and positioning) the better it is for intraoral techniques. With the less maneuverable units, it is necessary to position the animal differently for each area requiring investigation.

Ideally a dental X-ray machine should be installed in the designated dental theatre (Fig. 7.5). They are available as wall mounted or free-standing units. These machines are cost-effective and their outlay is rapidly recouped. They usually have a fixed potential of 50–70 kV and a fixed tube current of 8–10 mA. Electronic timers are used to set the desired exposure time. Modern dental X-ray machines are capable of exposures as low as 0.02 s, which is required for digital radiography. Do remember to ensure that the X-ray machine is compatible with the digital system you purchase.

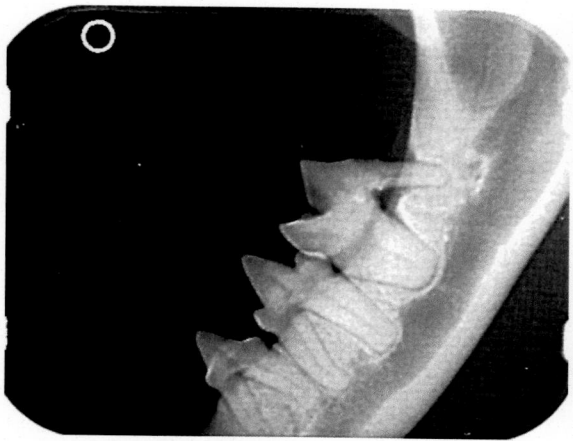

Fig. 7.2 **A diagnostic view** For a dental radiograph to be diagnostic, it should be an accurate representation of the size and shape of the tooth without superimposition of adjacent structures. Intraoral placement of dental film and parallel technique gives an accurate representation of the mandibular 3rd and 4th premolars and the 1st molar, as well as detail of the mandibular bone, in a cat. The mesial surface of the 3rd premolar is not on the film and a second view with the film placed further rostrally in the mouth is required to assess this tooth fully. In this view, the component structures of the tooth and its supporting tissues are well defined. The enamel is seen as an incompletely visualized radiodense band that covers the crown and tapers to a fine edge at the cervical margin of the tooth. The dentine is less radiodense than enamel and accounts for the bulk of the hard tissues of the tooth. The cementum is not visible. The pulp cavity is the continuous radiolucent space in the center of the tooth which extends from the coronal portion to the apex of the roots. The wall of the alveolar tooth socket (the lamina dura) is the radiodense line which runs parallel to the root of the tooth. The periodontal ligament space is the fine radiolucent line between the lamina dura and the root of the tooth. The cortical bone on the crest of the alveolar ridge is continuous with the lamina dura. The mandibular canal is clearly visible. The horizontal bone loss affecting the distal root of the molar is obvious.

X-ray film

Single emulsion, non-screen or screen film can be used to take dental radiographs. To allow intraoral film placement and achieve high definition, dental film should be used. Dental film is single emulsion, non-screen, and is available in three sizes (Fig. 7.6): occlusal, periapical and pediatric. The dental film is packed in either a paper or a plastic envelope and the film is flanked by black paper and backed by a thin lead sheet (foil) that reduces scattered radiation.

Dental film is available in a range of 'sensitivities' (film speeds) from A (least sensitive) to F (most sensitive). The sensitivity of the film determines the required exposure

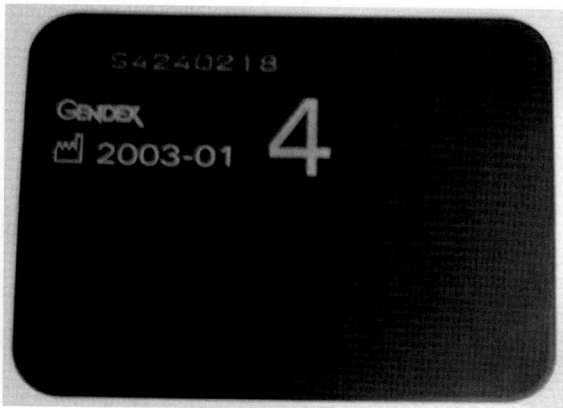

Fig. 7.3 **Indirect digital radiography** In indirect digital systems, the exposure is made on a photostimulatable phosphor plate rather than on a dental film. The latent image from the plate is then transferred to a computer.

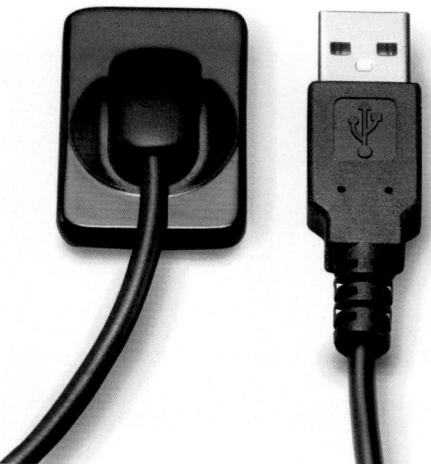

Fig. 7.4 **Direct digital radiography** In direct digital systems, a sensor is used instead of a dental film. The sensor sends the image directly to the computer.

time – faster speed (higher sensitivity) requires less radiation to expose (blacken) the film. The film sensitivity is increased by using larger silver halide crystals in the emulsion. Fast speed (higher sensitivity) produces images with a slightly lower image quality (*cf* larger and fewer pixels reduce the image quality of digital camera images). The decreased the image quality is only significant when the radiographs are viewed under magnification. In practice, depending on the type of processing used, D (ultra) and E (ekta) speeds are often used. D speed film requires slightly longer exposure and can be processed manually.

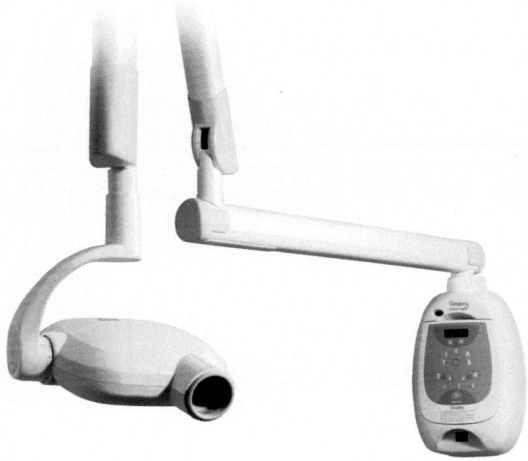

Fig. 7.5 A dental X-ray unit A dental X-ray unit installed in the designated dental theater is the ideal situation. They are available as free-standing or wall-mounted units. Wall mounting is usually preferable to save space.

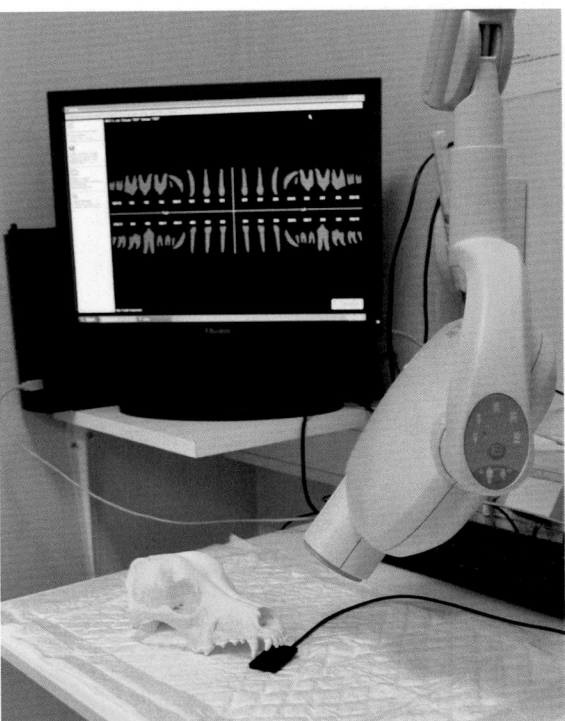

Fig. 7.7 Direct digital radiography In direct digital radiography a sensor replaces conventional film. The sensor sends the image directly to the computer.

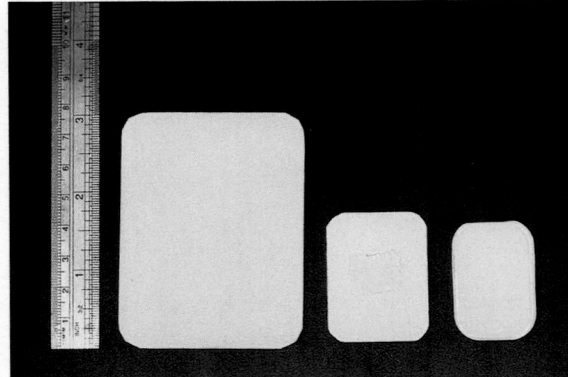

Fig. 7.6 Sizes of dental film Dental film is available in three sizes: occlusal (5×7 cm), periapical (3×4 cm) and pediatric (2×3 cm). The smallest film that depicts the area of interest should be used to facilitate film positioning in the mouth.

E speed film requires a lower exposure but can only be developed in an automatic processor.

Orientation

Ensure the correct side of the film envelope is facing the incident beam; the envelope is marked or labeled. If exposed through the back of the envelope, the lead sheet will absorb much of the X-ray beam, resulting in an under-exposed radiograph with the pattern of the lead sheet imposed on it.

Each film has a raised dot in one corner. The dot helps with orientation when viewing and mounting dental radiographs if the following procedure is adhered to. First, the dot should face the incident beam. Second, the film should be placed in the mouth so that the dot is always facing a specific direction. I position the dot so that it is always facing forward in the mouth. Another way is to ensure that the film is placed so that the dot is always in the same position, i.e. facing forward in the mouth on one side and backward in the mouth on the contralateral side.

Digital systems

In indirect digital systems the conventional film is replaced by a photostimulatable phosphor plate (Fig. 7.3). The plate is exposed and the latent image is transferred to a computer. The plates come in three sizes equivalent to dental film sizes. The plates are reusable in that the latent image can be cleared by placing them in light, e.g. against a viewing box.

In direct digital systems, the conventional film is replaced by a sensor that sends the X-ray image directly to the computer (Figs 7.4, 7.7). In my opinion, this is the easiest and most cost-efficient method of obtaining radiographs. The sensors are available in two sizes, equivalent to periapical and pediatric film. The occlusal size is not available. In my experience, the size 2 sensor is the only one needed for dogs and cats. The smaller, size 1 sensor may be useful in cats and small exotics.

There are several manufacturers of digital equipment. There are differences in quality images between sensors and the various software programs offer different capabilities with varying user-friendliness. Moreover, the field is constantly changing.

Exposure settings

Dental film requires higher exposure settings than screen film, but gives better definition. The actual settings required vary with different X-ray machines and with different film–focal distances. Digital systems require very low exposure settings, i.e. as low as 0.02 s for small animals.

Dental X-ray units provide guideline exposures for different size patients and different teeth. The X-ray unit is brought as close to the tooth that is being radiographed as possible, so setting the film–focus distance is not required. I strongly recommend the purchase of a modern dental X-ray unit. They are inexpensive and the cost is rapidly recouped.

For those of you who have not yet purchased a dental X-ray machine, it is possible to use a veterinary X-ray unit and D speed dental film to achieve dental radiographs. It is time-consuming and not cost-efficient, but it can be done. If you are using a veterinary X-ray unit and D speed dental film, set the film–focal distance to between 30 and 50 cm and try the exposures suggested in Table 7.1.

Irrespective of the type of X-ray unit available, it is advisable to take a series of trial exposures on animals of different size to make up exposure charts prior to undertaking dental radiography on patients.

Dental film processing

Automated processors are available for dental film processing, but excellent results can be obtained with the use of a chair-side processor (Fig. 7.8). These chair-side 'darkrooms' have four containers, one each for developing and fixing fluids and two for rinsing purposes. Care must be exercised during processing to prevent scratching of the film surface. Films must be adequately fixed so as not to lose quality during archiving. Thorough rinsing under running water (while gently rubbing the film surface with your fingers) after processing is essential to avoid fixation stains. Rinsing is complete when the film surface no longer feels 'soapy'. Remember that E speed film should not be processed using a chair-side processor.

Handling and mounting of dental radiographs

It is important to handle and mount processed dental films with care. Fingerprints can damage the emulsion on the film surface and the film is easily scratched. After rinsing thoroughly, adequate time should be allowed for the film to dry before being mounted, or else it will adhere to the mount. It is also important to archive the film in such a way that it can be easily retrieved and identified. Remember that these films make up part of the patient's clinical records.

Dental radiographs are viewed and mounted as if you were facing the animal and looking into its mouth. The raised dot should face you when viewing the film. Based on the anatomy of the jaws and teeth, it is then possible

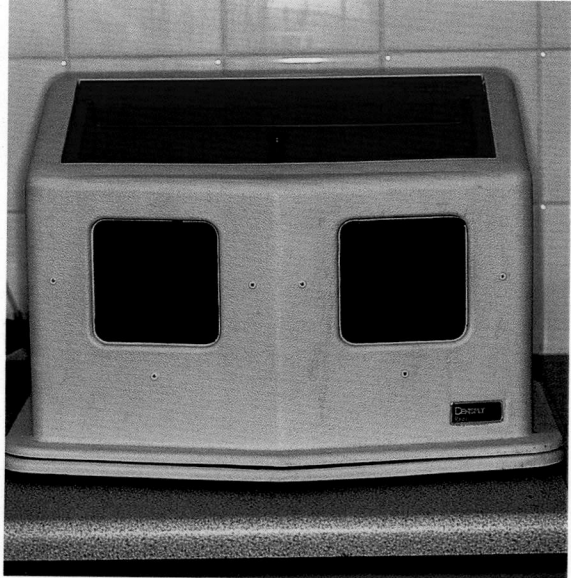

Fig. 7.8 The Rinn box A chair-side 'darkroom' (Rinn box) is a simple and inexpensive way of processing dental film. Thorough rinsing under running water (rubbing the film gently with your fingers until it no longer feels 'soapy') after developing and fixing is essential to avoid fixation stains.

Table 7.1 Suggested exposure settings using a veterinary X-ray machine (not recommended)		
Cat/small dog	60–70 kV	20–25 mA
Medium/large dog	70–80 kV	20–25 mA
Rabbit/guinea pig	50–60 kV	10–20 mA
Chinchilla	50–60 kV	5–15 mA

to identify upper and lower jaw views. If the films were always exposed with the dot facing forward in the mouth, then all views on the right side will have the dot in a different position from the left side views (Fig. 7.9). If the films were always exposed with the dot in the same position then all the views on one side will have the dot on the distal aspect of the teeth and the other side will have it on the mesial aspect of the teeth (Fig. 7.10).

Handling and mounting of digital images

Direct dental radiography offers a real advantage in that the images are immediately placed in the correct position in the mount as long as the sensor has been exposed correctly (Fig. 7.11).

In indirect systems, the image needs to be moved into its correct place in a dental mount.

Preparation of the patient

General anesthesia is required for dental radiography. Ideally, clinical examination and recording should precede the radiographic evaluation. It is also useful to clean the teeth before any radiographs are taken. Dental calculus, because it is radiodense, can obscure pathologic lesions on a radiograph.

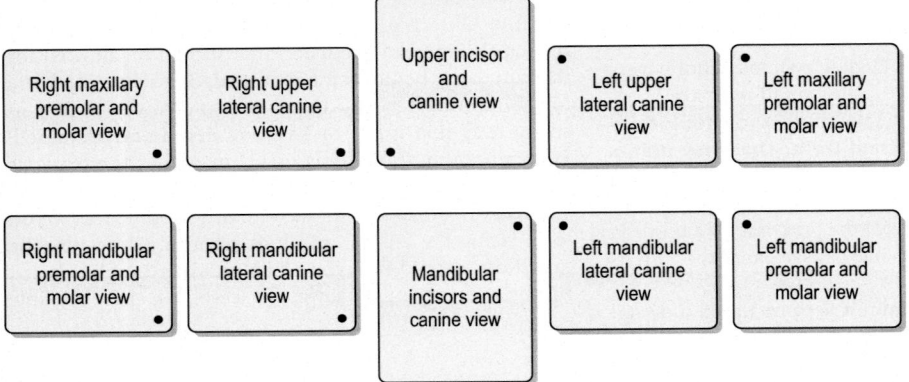

Fig. 7.9 Mounting if films are exposed with the dot facing forward in the mouth Dental radiographs are viewed and mounted as if you were facing the animal and looking into the mouth. The raised dot should face forward when viewing the film. Based on the anatomy of the jaws and teeth, it is then possible to identify upper and lower teeth views. If the films are always exposed with the dot facing forward in the mouth, then all views on the right side will have the dot in a different position from the left-side views. This diagram depicts how we would mount a full mouth series of cat radiographs when all the films have been exposed with the dot facing forward. This is my preferred method.

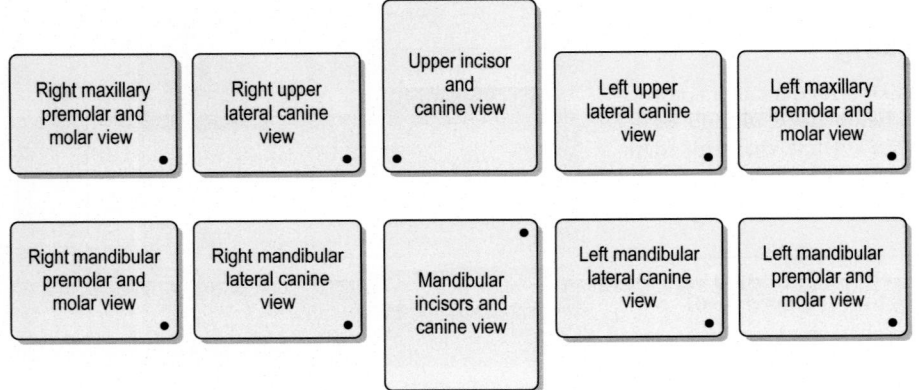

Fig. 7.10 Mounting if films are exposed with the dot in the same position If the films are exposed with the dot always in the same position, then all the views on one side will have the dot on the distal aspect of the teeth and the views on the other side will have them on the mesial aspect of the teeth. This diagram depicts how we would mount a full mouth series of cat radiographs if the films had been exposed with the dot always in the same position.

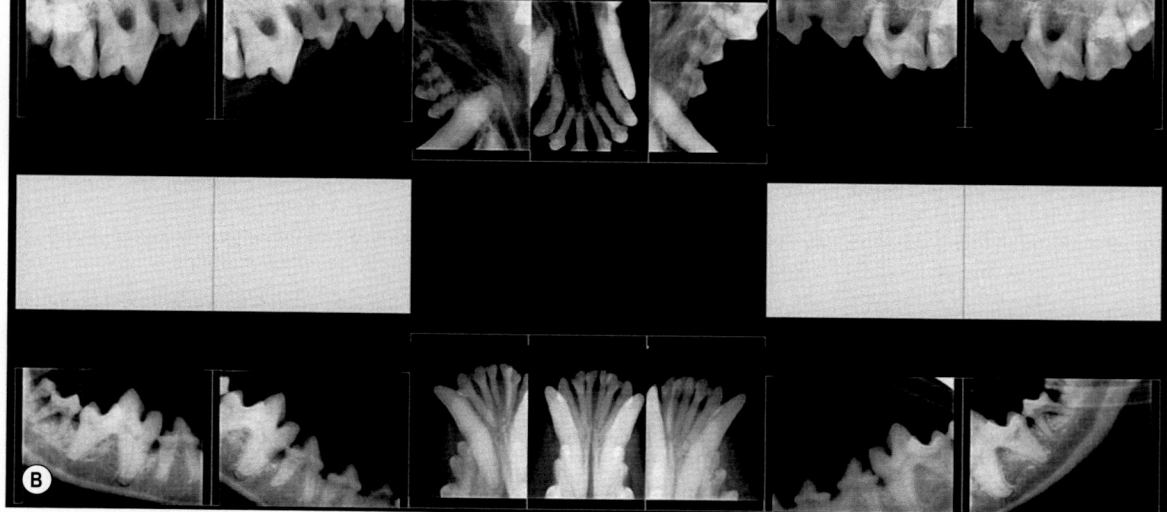

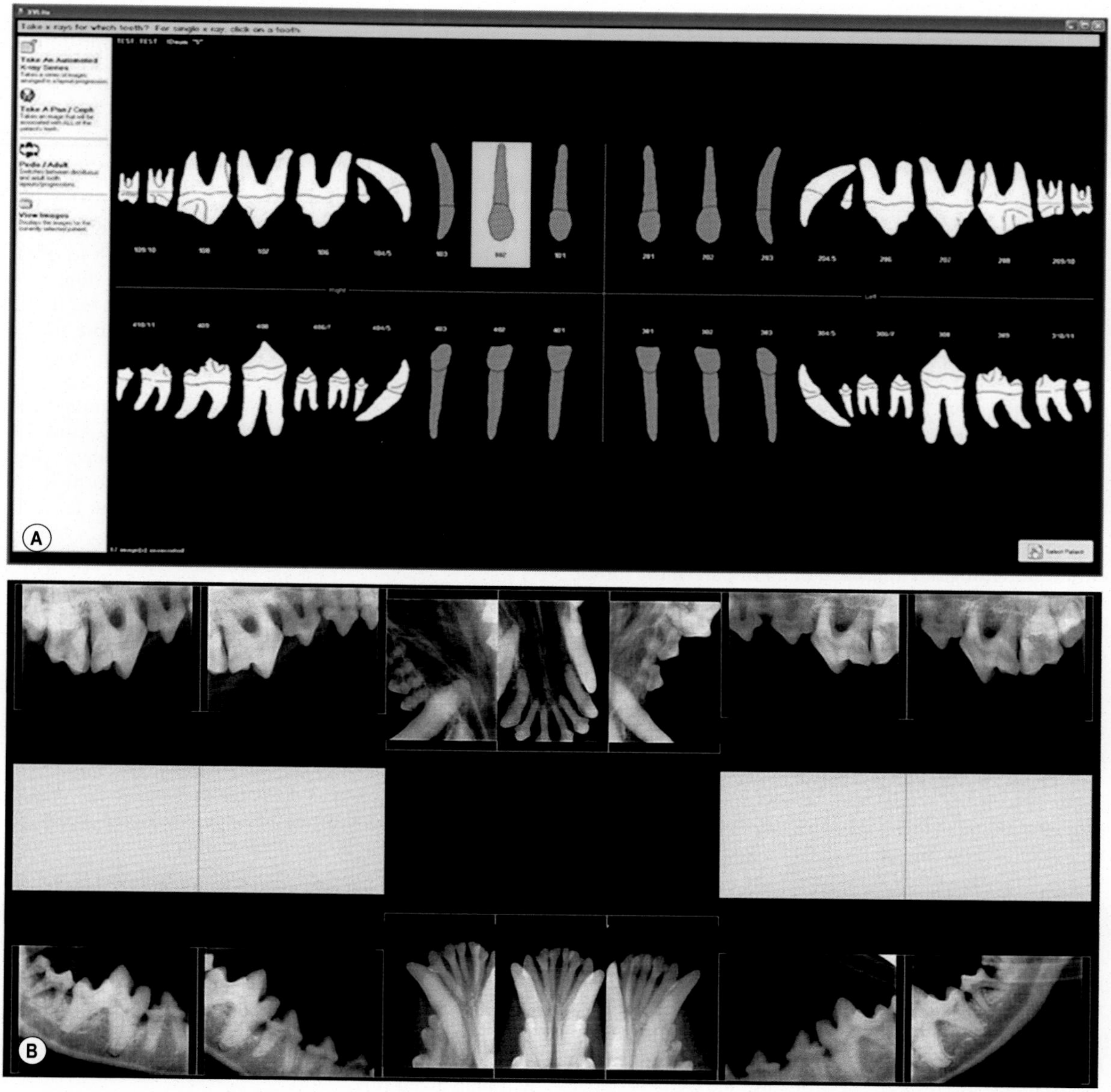

Fig. 7.11 Mounting using digital systems In indirect systems, the image needs to be moved into its correct place in a dental mount. In direct systems the images are immediately placed in the correct position in the mount as long as the sensor has been exposed correctly. The region that is being radiographed is highlighted on the computer (A), the sensor is activated and exposed and the resultant image is placed in that position in the mount (B).

INTRAORAL RADIOGRAPHIC TECHNIQUES

The film, phosphor plate or digital sensor is placed intraorally and the incident beam directed through the tooth onto it. For simplicity, in the following, the word 'film' will be used to mean dental film, phosphor plate or digital sensor. The easiest way to hold the 'film' in position is to place packing (foam wedge, swabs) behind it to sandwich the film against the tooth (Fig. 7.12). Various film holders are available but they can be difficult to use effectively.

Ensure that dental film or phosphor plate is not bent, as this will lead to distortion of the image, resulting in

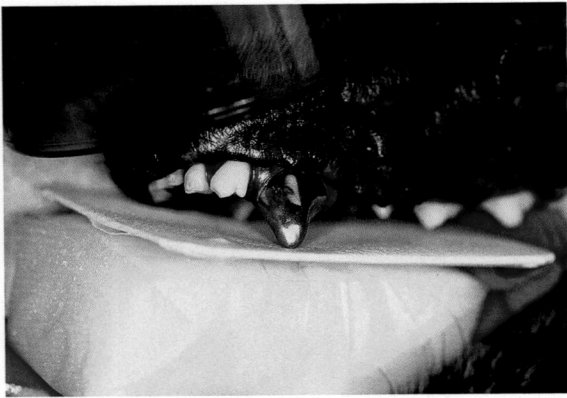

Fig. 7.12 Intraoral film placement The simplest way to hold a film in position in the oral cavity is to insert packing (in this case a pack of swabs) behind it to sandwich the film against the tooth. The pack should be replaced for each animal.

either shortening or elongation of all or part of the tooth. If it does bend, a tongue spatula inserted below it is usually sufficient to stabilize the 'film'. It should be borne in mind that superimposition of dental structures will also lead to the creation of artefacts and hence the meticulous positioning for each tooth is worth the time taken. The three-rooted teeth (4th premolars and molars in the upper jaw) have an added consideration, namely the palatal root. In these teeth, it is necessary to position the incident beam in such a way as to prevent superimposition of one root over another. Magnification is inevitable, but keeping the 'film' as close to the tooth as possible will minimize this. Changing the film–focal distance will also affect magnification.

The parallel technique is used to radiograph the mandibular premolars and molars. In this technique, the 'film' is placed parallel to the teeth and the incident beam strikes the film perpendicularly. All other teeth are radiographed using the bisecting angle technique. In this technique, the acute angle created by the tooth axis and the 'film' is bisected and the incident beam is directed perpendicular to this line.

The parallel technique

The parallel technique is used for the mandibular premolars and the molars. The patient is placed in lateral recumbency (with the side to be radiographed uppermost). The 'film' is placed between the tongue and the teeth and pushed as far down into the sublingual fossa as possible. The X-ray beam is then directed from lateral to medial at right angles to the long axis of the tooth, which is parallel to the 'film' (Fig. 7.13). The resulting image of the tooth has very little magnification or distortion.

Because of the anatomy of the oral cavity, this technique is only possible in the mandibular premolar and molar regions.

The bisecting angle technique

The bisecting angle technique is required to minimize distortion when taking radiographs of the teeth in the upper jaw and the mandibular incisors and canines. The 'film' is positioned at an angle behind the tooth in question. If the X-ray beam is directed at 90° to the 'film', the image would then be foreshortened (Fig. 7.14). If the beam is directed at 90° to the long axis of the tooth, the image would then be elongated (Fig. 7.15). To avoid these problems, an imaginary plane is drawn half way between the plane of the 'film' and a plane through the long axis of the tooth, i.e. at the *bisecting angle*, and the X-ray beam is directed perpendicular to this plane (Fig. 7.16). In this way, both sides of the triangles formed are the same length and the resulting image of the tooth is similar to the real tooth.

To achieve correct positioning requires a mental image of the normal orientation, length and morphology of the tooth roots. Two tongue spatulas, fingers or instrument handles can be used to visualize these planes outside the mouth and so aid the positioning of the beam. A common problem is to 'miss the apex' of a tooth (especially on canine teeth) owing to poor estimation of root length or position.

It may be helpful to position the patient as follows:

- Sternal recumbency for the incisors in the upper jaw
- Lateral or sternal recumbency for the canines, premolars and molars in the upper jaw
- Dorsal recumbency for the mandibular incisors
- Dorsal or lateral recumbency for the mandibular canines.

The premolar and molar views of the upper jaw of the cat are difficult. Often the zygomatic arch is superimposed over the roots and apices of the teeth. Placing a foam wedge or small sandbag under the nose, thus tilting the head up so that the dental arch is parallel with the table, will help avoid this.

Another common problem is superimposition of the mesiobuccal and mesiopalatal roots of the upper 4th premolar in both dogs and cats. It is often necessary to take more than one view, changing the angle of the incident beam slightly (either rostrally or caudally), to be able to visualize both roots separately.

Extraoral film placement

When intraoral dental radiography is not available, extraoral views of the teeth may have to be used. Extraoral views are not ideal for dental examination, mainly because of superimposition of the contralateral side, which

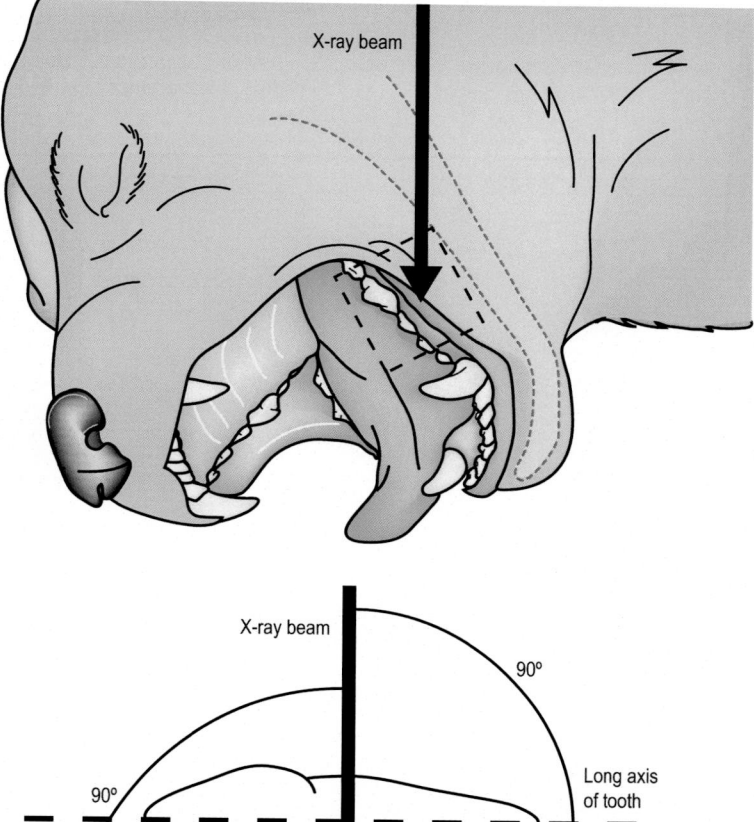

Fig. 7.13 The parallel technique
With the patient in lateral recumbency
(with the side to be radiographed
uppermost), the film is placed between
the tongue and the teeth and pushed
as far down into the sublingual fossa as
possible. The X-ray beam is then directed
from lateral to medial at right angles
to the long axis of the tooth, which is
parallel to the film.

obscures, and causes distortion of, the image. However, it may be possible to obtain diagnostic radiographs of the maxillary and mandibular premolars and molars using extraoral film placement, especially in dogs with wide skulls. Some examiners routinely use extraoral film placement to radiograph the maxillary premolars and molars in the cat.

The technique is depicted in Figure 7.17. The film is placed on the table and the animal is placed in dorsolateral recumbency with the side to be radiographed closest to the film, i.e. the lower side of the animal's head. The mouth is held wide open using a radiolucent device, e.g. plastic needle cap. Tilting the head rotates the contralateral side away and an open mouth should mean the beam passes only through the soft tissue of the contralateral side. The tilting will place maxillary teeth almost parallel to the film but in reality the beam still requires adjustment according to the bisecting angle technique to reduce image distortion.

The parallax effect

As a radiograph is two dimensional, it is not possible to tell which of two objects in the image is nearer to the viewer. It is, however, often necessary to know at what depth an object is, e.g. in locating an ectopic unerupted tooth. When a second image is taken, after rotating the beam position around the object's axis, the image of the object will move relative to other structures. When the object appears to move in the same direction as the shift in the X-ray head, it is placed lingually (nearer to the film); if it moves in the opposite direction it is more buccally positioned (further from the film). This technique is also useful to separate and identify two overlying roots, e.g. the mesiobuccal and palatal roots of an upper carnassial tooth in carnivores.

The SLOB rule (Same direction Lingual, Opposite direction Buccal) may help you remember the parallax effect. To use the SLOB rule you need to know the original and

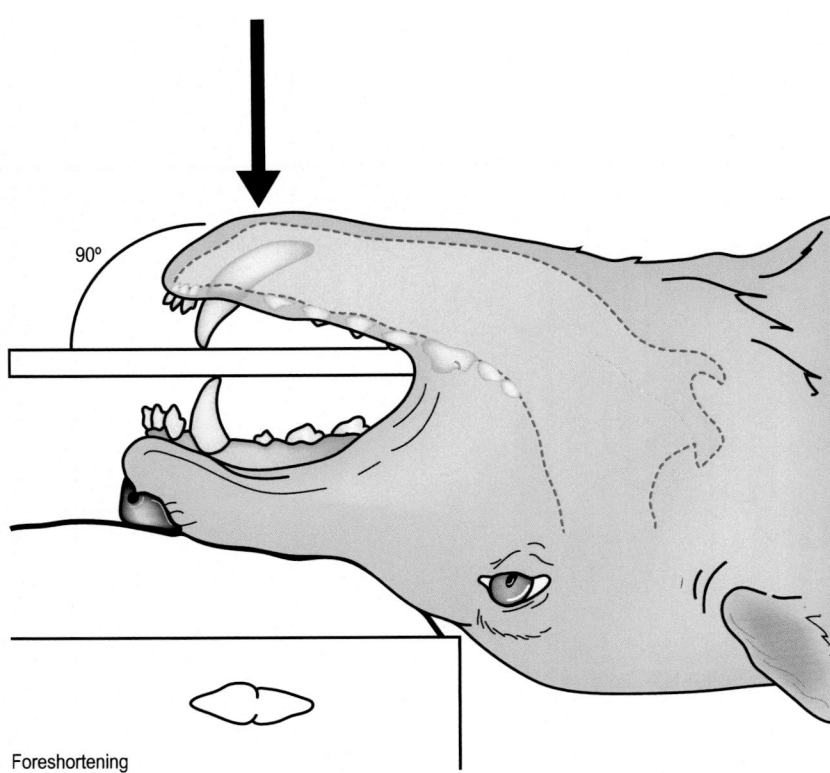

Fig. 7.14 Foreshortening of the image If the X-ray beam is directed at 90° to the film the image is foreshortened.

90°

Foreshortening

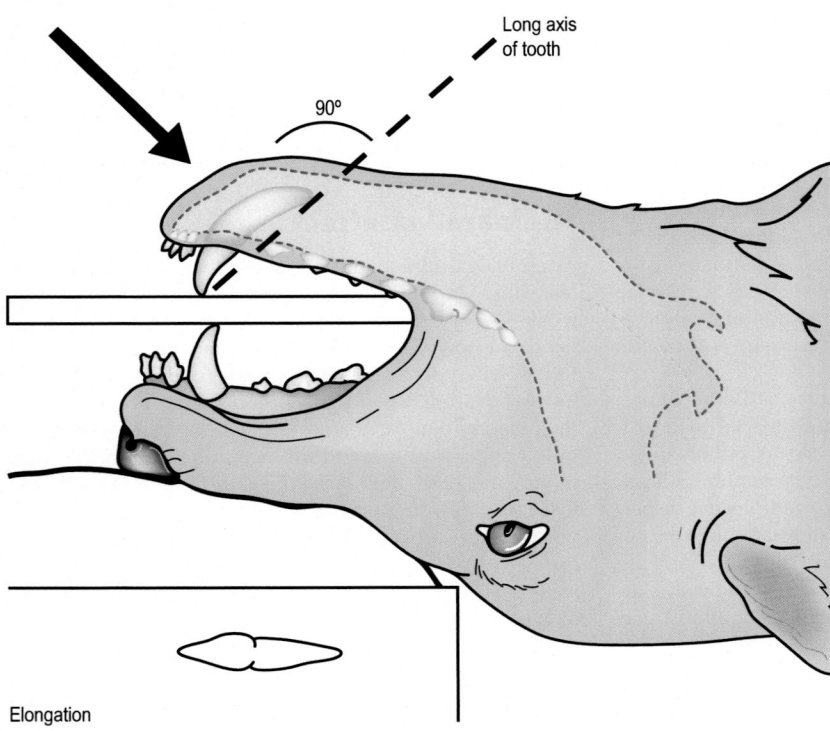

Fig. 7.15 Elongation of the image If the beam is directed at 90° to the long axis of the tooth the image is elongated.

Long axis of tooth

90°

Elongation

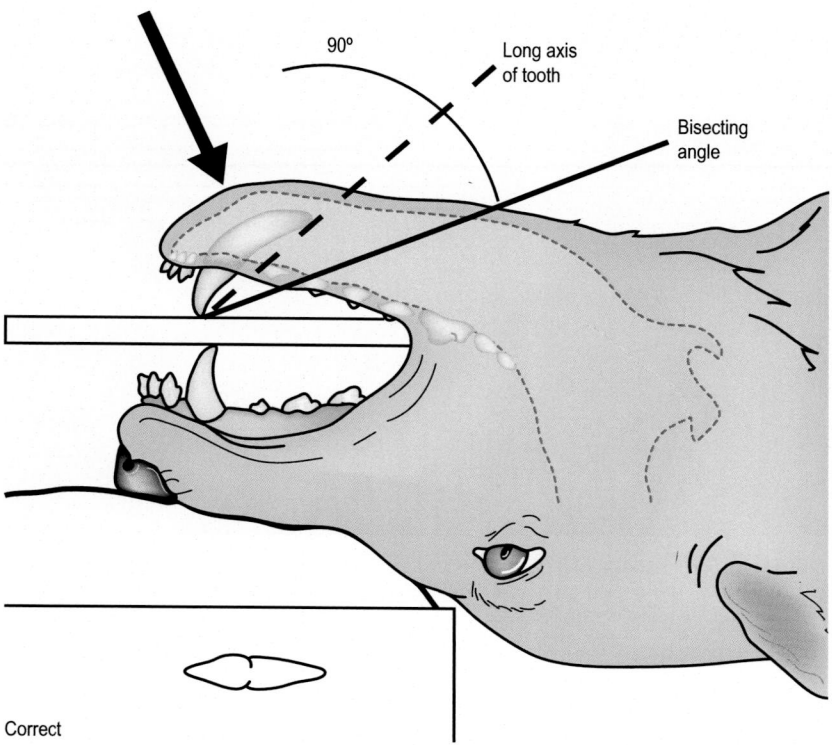

Correct

Fig. 7.16 Bisecting angle technique To avoid foreshortening or elongating the image, an imaginary plane is drawn half way between the plane of the film and a plane through the long axis of the tooth, i.e. at the bisecting angle, and the X-ray beam is directed perpendicular to this plane. In this way, both sides of the triangle formed are the same length and the resulting image of the tooth is similar to the real tooth.

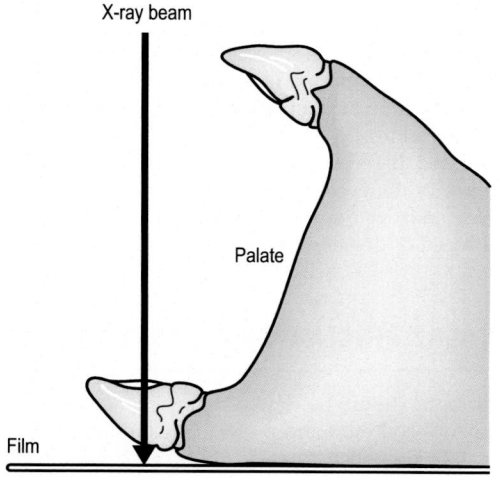

Fig. 7.17 Extraoral film placement The film is placed on the table and the animal is placed in dorsolateral recumbency with the side to be radiographed closest to the film, i.e. the lower side of the animal's head. The mouth is held wide open using a radiolucent device, e.g. plastic needle cap. Tilting the head rotates the contralateral side away and an open mouth should mean the beam passes only through the soft tissue of the contralateral side. The tilting will place maxillary teeth almost parallel to the film, but the beam still requires adjustment according to the bisecting angle technique to reduce image distortion.

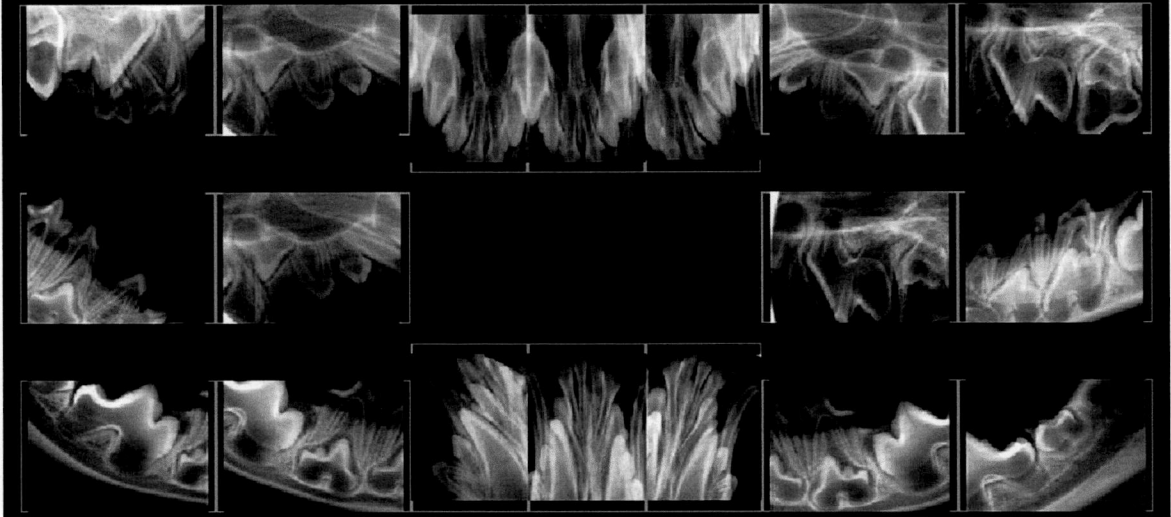

Fig. 7.18 A series of full mouth radiographs Full mouth radiographs describes a series of 'films', where each tooth of the dentition is accurately depicted in at least one view. The depicted series is from a puppy with a mixed dentition. The reason for taking the series was to evaluate if all permanent teeth were present.

second beam position. An object that has moved in the same direction as you have moved the incident beam is lingually located. Conversely, an object that has moved in the opposite direction to that which the incident beam has been moved is buccally located.

Full mouth radiographs

Full mouth radiographs describes a series of films where each tooth of the dentition is accurately depicted in at least one view (Fig. 7.18). A full mouth radiographic series of all animals undergoing dental examination provides valuable information, but is not always practically or financially viable. However, it is strongly recommended that all adult cats have full mouth radiographs taken as part of the oral and dental examination. Resorptive lesions are common in cats and clinical examination without radiography will only detect end-stage lesions.

In cats, it is necessary to take a minimum of eight views, but 10 views are recommended, to ensure that all teeth are properly visualized. These are as follows:

Essential views in cats

- Incisor view in the upper jaw.
- Lateral view for each of the canines of the upper jaw.
- Left and right maxillary premolar and molar views.
- Mandibular incisor and canine view.

- Left and right mandibular premolar and molar views.

Recommended views in cats

- Lateral view for each of the canines of the mandible (in addition to the eight essential views).

The choice of film size for each view is subjective. The smallest film that will depict the area of interest should be used to facilitate film positioning. We use periapical size film for all cat views.

In the case of dogs, full mouth radiographs are encouraged, especially at first examination. If this is not possible (time or financial restrictions), then radiographs are taken where indicated, based on the findings during the clinical examination. In the event of full mouth radiographs, the size of film and the number of films used will depend upon the breed of dog and the shape of its face.

RADIOGRAPHIC INTERPRETATION

The radiographs should be viewed on a viewing box with minimal peripheral light and preferably using magnification. It is recommended to radiograph the contralateral structures for comparative purposes. A good knowledge of the radiographic appearance of normal structures of the upper jaw and mandible is imperative to avoid misdiagnosis. The radiographic features of normal structures are outlined below. Pathologic radiographic features are covered in Chapters 8, 9, 11, and 12.

Normal radiographic anatomy

All normal anatomic landmarks are by no means demonstrable in any given radiograph. In fact, there are those that are visualized in a small percentage of cases only. It is, however, important to be familiar with them so that they can be identified and correctly interpreted when they are visualized. There are also wide structural variations which are within normal limits. This is well exemplified by the trabecular structure of bone, which presents a variable picture depending on the size of the bone, size of its medullary space and thickness of its cortex. The pattern will also vary with use, disuse and age of the patient. With disuse and advancing age, the trabeculations tend to become fewer and finer in structure.

The tooth and its supporting tissues

The component structures of the tooth and its supporting tissues are usually well defined radiographically (Fig. 7.2). The enamel of the tooth is seen as a very radiodense band that covers the crown and tapers to a fine edge at the cervical margin of the tooth. The enamel of dogs and cats is very much thinner than in humans and is often incompletely visualized on radiographs. The dentine is less radiodense than enamel and accounts for the bulk of the hard tissues of the mature tooth. The cementum, which covers the surface of the root of the tooth, is even less radiodense than dentine and is usually only visible when it has undergone hyperplasia. The pulp cavity, i.e. pulp chamber and the root canal(s), is visualized as a continuous radiolucent space in the center of the tooth which extends from the coronal portion to the apex of the root(s).

The size and width of the pulp chamber and root canal(s) will vary with the age of the animal. An immature tooth can be present in a mature animal where early trauma has caused pulp necrosis and thus stopped further development of the tooth. The lamina dura represents the wall of the alveolar tooth socket. It is seen as a radiodense line which runs parallel to the root of the tooth. The lamina dura is not always visible on radiographs but a break in the path of a visible lamina dura usually implies periodontal pathology. Contralateral radiographs, however, should always be taken for comparison. The periodontal ligament space is depicted by a fine radiolucent line that is situated between the lamina dura and the root of the tooth. The cortical bone on the crest of the alveolar ridge is continuous with the lamina dura.

The largest number and variety of anatomic structures appear in radiographs of the upper jaw. Superimposition of nasal structures over the apices of the premolar and molar roots will make it impossible to assess the periapical status of these teeth. Consequently, an intraoral bisecting angle technique to avoid superimposition and give an accurate reproduction of the teeth is required.

Nutrient canals

The nutrient canals referred to here are those that contain blood vessels and nerves that supply the teeth, interdental spaces and gingiva. In radiographs, these are seen as radiolucent lines of uniform width, which sometimes have radiodense borders. The most easily identified nutrient canal is the mandibular canal (Fig. 7.2). Nutrient canals that arise from the mandibular canal are those that extend upward into the interdental space, and those that extend directly to the periapical foramina at the root of the tooth. Other nutrient canals, which may be seen, are the canal or groove that occupies the posterior superior alveolar artery and the anterior palatine (incisive) canal.

Foramina

Foramina may sometimes be mistaken for periapical lesions. Important foramina to remember are: the anterior palatine (incisive) foramen, the infraorbital foramina and the mental foramina.

SUMMARY

- ◆ Radiography is mandatory for good dental practice.
- ◆ Intraoral technique employing parallel and bisecting angle views is essential for meaningful results to be obtained.
- ◆ Dental X-ray machine and digital software and hardware are ideal and such equipment proves convenient and cost-effective.
- ◆ Full mouth radiographs (8–10 views) are strongly advocated in cats in order to detect odontoclastic resorptive lesions. The technique is recommended in dogs also.

FURTHER READING

Aller, M.S. (Ed.), 1998. Atlas of Canine and Feline Dental Radiography. Veterinary Learning Systems, Trenton.

DeForge, D.H., Colmery III, B.H. (Eds), 2000. An Atlas of Veterinary Dental Radiology. Iowa State University Press, Ames.

DuPont, G.A., DeBowes L.J., 2009. Atlas of Dental Radiography in Dogs and Cats. Elsevier, London.

Gorrel, C., 1998. Radiographic evaluation. In: Holmstrom, S. (Ed.), Canine Dentistry. Veterinary Clinics of North America: Small Animal Practice. WB Saunders, Philadelphia, pp. 1089–1110.

Gorrel, C., 2008. Saunders Solutions in Veterinary Practice – Small Animal Dentistry. Saunders/Elsevier, Philadelphia.

Gracis, M., Harvey, C.E., 1998. Radiographic study of the maxillary canine tooth in mesaticephalic dogs. Journal of Veterinary Dentistry 15 (2), 73–78.

Robinson, J., Gorrel, C., 1995. Oral examination and radiography. In: Crossley, D.A., Penman, S. (Eds.), Manual of Small Animal Dentistry. BSAVA, Cheltenham, pp. 35–49.

Chapter | **8** |

Common oral conditions

INTRODUCTION

This chapter deals with common oral conditions. Some of these conditions may require no professional intervention; others can be managed successfully in general practice (often by extraction) and some need referral to a specialist for treatment. The general practitioner needs to recognize the conditions, be able to perform the diagnostic work-up, realize the clinical significance and institute treatment (in-house or referral) as required.

Periodontal disease is covered in Chapter 9. All dog and cat teeth require a combination of homecare (daily toothbrushing and dental diet/dental hygiene chew) and professional cleaning. Preventive dentistry is indicated for every dog and cat and is detailed in Chapter 10. Odontoclastic resorptive lesions are covered in Chapter 11. Conditions that require prompt management, e.g. traumatic tooth injuries, jaw fracture, and can thus be viewed as 'emergencies', are covered in Chapter 12. Extraction is detailed in Chapter 13.

DEVELOPMENTAL DENTAL DISORDERS

Developmental dental disorders may be due to abnormalities in the differentiation of the dental lamina and the tooth germs (anomalies in number, size and shape) or to abnormalities in the formation of the dental hard tissues (anomalies in structure).

Anomalies in number, size and shape

Congenitally missing teeth

Congenital absence of teeth is common in the dog. Radiographs are required to determine whether teeth missing on clinical examination are actually absent or unerupted (Fig. 8.1). This is often of interest for the owner of a dog meant for the show ring.

Absence of teeth can be an inherited abnormality or can result from disturbances during the initial stages of tooth formation. The primary teeth give rise to the permanent tooth buds, so if there is no primary tooth the permanent counterpart will also be missing. It is possible, however, for the primary tooth to be present and the permanent counterpart absent.

In humans, anodontia (total absence of teeth) and oligodontia (congenital absence of many but not all teeth) are associated with ectodermal dysplasia (Shafer et al. 1974a). In dogs, anodontia and oligodontia are rare and can be associated with ectodermal dysplasia or occur in dogs with no apparent systemic problem or congenital syndrome (Skrentary 1964; Andrews 1972; Harvey and Emily 1993). Hypodontia (absence of only a few teeth) is, however, a relatively common finding in dogs. It is especially common in purebred and linebred dogs, as the genetic fault will have been perpetuated. It is also more common in small breed dogs. The premolar teeth are the most commonly missing (Harvey and Emily 1993).

In general, missing teeth are of no clinical significance other than that plaque accumulation may be more extensive as the cleaning of teeth associated with chewing is likely to be reduced.

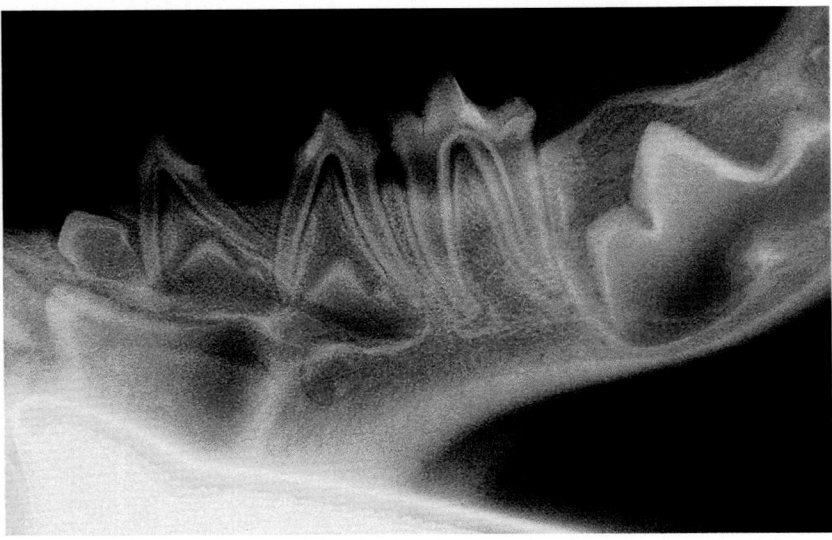

Fig. 8.1 Congenitally missing teeth Radiographs are required to determine whether teeth missing on clinical examination are actually absent or unerupted. This puppy has a missing permanent 4th premolar.

Supernumerary teeth

Supernumerary teeth (Fig. 8.2) are common in certain dog breeds (Harvey and Emily 1993). They are the result of either a genetic defect or a disturbance during tooth development. The duplication of teeth may affect the primary as well as the permanent dentition. Many supernumerary teeth resemble normal teeth, others have a conical shape, and some bear no resemblance to any normal tooth form. The most common complications caused by supernumerary teeth are malpositioning and non-eruption of other teeth (Aitchison 1963; Harvey and Emily 1993). As with other teeth that remain embedded, there is the possibility of cyst formation (Shafer et al. 1974b; Stafne and Gibilisco 1975a; Harvey and Emily 1993). Eruption and shedding disorders are covered later in this chapter. In addition, tooth crowding may contribute to severe plaque accumulation and predispose to periodontal disease.

Supernumerary teeth that contribute to malocclusion or crowding should be extracted (Harvey and Emily 1993; Gorrel and Robinson 1995a). Radiographic evaluation allows differentiation between primary and permanent teeth. Primary teeth are smaller than their permanent counterparts, with long, slender roots. Compared with permanent teeth, the roots of primary teeth are relatively long in relation to the crown. The radiographs will also allow you to plan and perform the extractions in a tissue-friendly fashion.

Fusion and gemination

Fusion is the developmental union of two or more teeth in which the dentine and one other dental tissue are

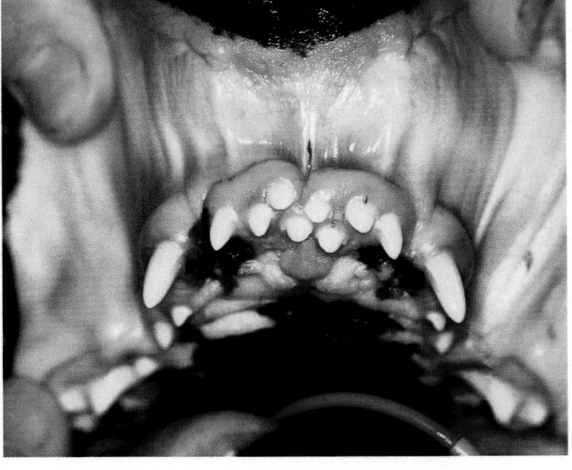

Fig. 8.2 Supernumerary teeth Supernumerary teeth commonly cause crowding and malocclusion. In this dog, the supernumerary permanent teeth were involved in an incisor malocclusion, resulting in excessive wear of the mandibular incisor teeth and gingival trauma in the upper incisor arch (radiographs were taken to elucidate whether the supernumerary teeth were primary or permanent). Treatment consisted of extraction of the upper incisor teeth that were grossly out of alignment and had abnormal occlusion with the mandibular incisor teeth.

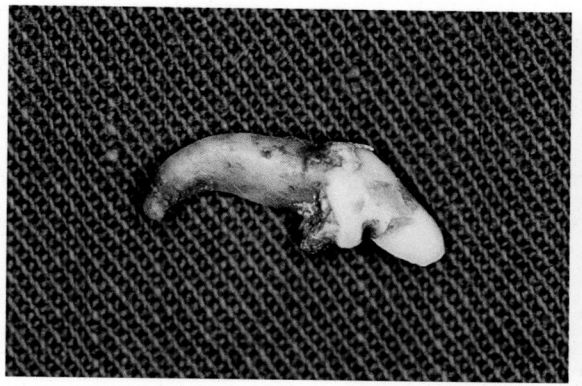

Fig. 8.3 Abnormalities in root shape The upper 3rd incisor depicted has a marked curvature at its apex. Preoperative radiographs should be taken of all teeth where extraction is planned. Identification of an abnormality in root morphology allows selection of the optimal extraction technique. In this case an open (surgical) extraction technique was chosen.

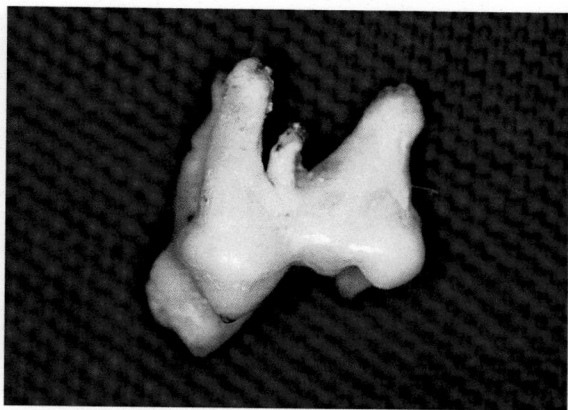

Fig. 8.4 Abnormalities in the number of roots The upper 1st molar depicted has a small extra root. It was identified on preoperative radiographs. The tooth was extracted owing to severe periodontitis and could thus be removed without sectioning.

united. There may be a complete union resulting in one abnormally large tooth, or union of the crowns, or union of the roots only. A supernumerary tooth is frequently one of the teeth involved. Gemination is an attempt to make two teeth from one enamel organ, without complete division. Fusion and gemination affect primary teeth as well as permanent ones.

If these teeth do not cause any functional problem, they may not need to be extracted. When they do require extraction, radiography will give information as to the extent of fusion or gemination and allow planning of the best extraction technique.

Root abnormalities

Common root abnormalities include aberrations in shape (Fig. 8.3) and in the number of roots present (Figs 8.4, 8.5). They are not detected without radiographs. The identification of an abnormally shaped root or an extra root is not an indication for treatment *per se*. However, if the tooth is affected by pathology that requires extraction, it is essential to have prior knowledge of an existing anatomic abnormality, so that the extraction can be planned accordingly. Radiographs should always be taken prior to extraction of a tooth.

Anomalies in structure

Enamel hypoplasia (dysplasia)

Enamel hypoplasia (dysplasia) may be defined as an incomplete or defective formation of the organic enamel matrix of teeth. The result is defective (soft, porous)

enamel. It can be caused by local, systemic or hereditary factors. Depending on the cause, the condition can affect one or only a few teeth (localized form), or all teeth in the dentition (generalized form). It is essential to remember that enamel hypoplasia results only if the injury occurs during the formative stage of enamel development, i.e. during amelogenesis. Thus, the defect occurs before the tooth erupts into the oral cavity. Crown formation lasts from the 42nd day of gestation through to the 15th day postpartum for the primary teeth and from the 2nd week through to the 3rd month postpartum for the permanent teeth of dogs and cats (Arnall 1960). Depending on the time of the insult, enamel dysplasia will affect primary and/or permanent teeth.

Teeth with enamel dysplasia may appear normal at the time of eruption, but they soon become discolored as the defective (porous) enamel soaks up pigments (from food, soil, etc.). In more severely affected teeth, the defective enamel may flake off with use. In very severe cases, the enamel is visibly deficient, discolored in patches or partly missing already at the time of eruption.

As already mentioned, enamel dysplasia may be caused by local, systemic or hereditary factors (Shafer et al. 1974a). Local factors include trauma to the developing crown, e.g. a blow to the face or an infection. Infection is often a consequence of a bite injury. Periapical disease of a primary tooth may cause enamel dysplasia in adjacent developing permanent teeth. Usually only one or a few teeth are affected. Systemic factors include nutritional deficiencies, febrile disorders, hypocalcemia and excessive intake of fluoride during the period of enamel formation. Usually most teeth are affected. Historically, enamel dysplasia in dogs occurred as a result of distemper infection.

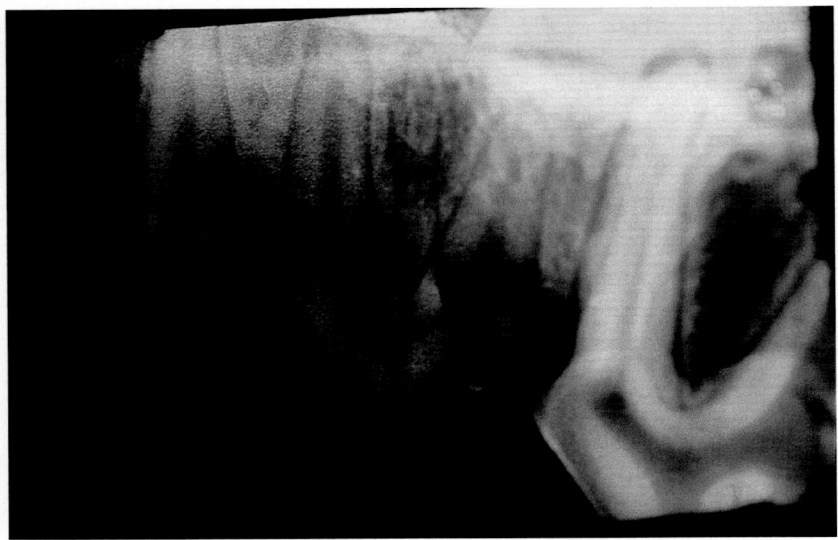

Fig. 8.5 Abnormalities in the number of roots The maxillary 3rd premolar depicted on the radiograph has a palatal root as well as the expected mesial and distal roots. This was an incidental finding on full mouth radiographs. It was bilateral, i.e. both left and right maxillary 3rd premolars had an extra palatal root. If this tooth were to require extraction, it would need to be sectioned into three single-rooted segments rather than the usual two single-rooted segments.

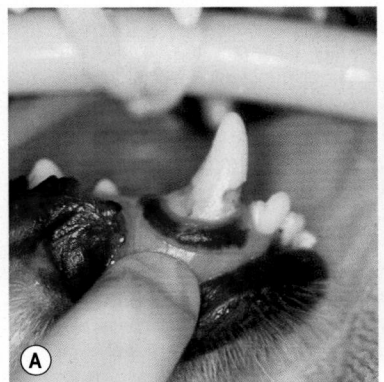
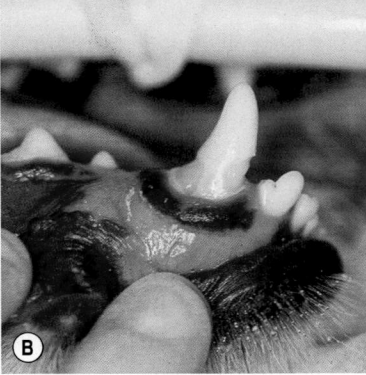
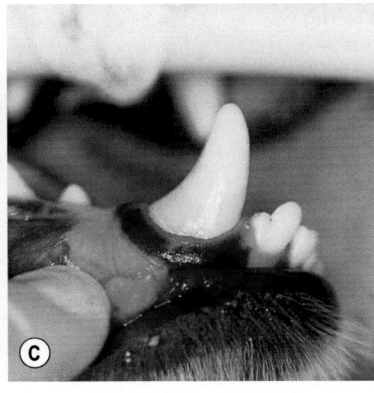

Fig. 8.6 Localized enamel dysplasia (A) Localized region of defective enamel of the right mandibular canine tooth. This was the only affected tooth in the dentition. This type of enamel dysplasia is likely to be the result of local trauma, e.g. blow to the face. Only the region of enamel undergoing active formation at the time of the trauma is defective, appearing as a band at the gingival third of the crown. The rest of the crown is covered by normal enamel. (B) The defect has been debrided (discolored dysplastic enamel was removed with a round bur in a slow-speed hand piece with water cooling) and prepared to accept a restorative material. (C) Completed restoration using a white filling material (compomer).

This is rare today as most dogs are vaccinated against distemper. Hereditary types of enamel dysplasia have been described in humans. The incidence in cats and dogs is unknown.

If the enamel dysplasia is the result of a local trauma (Fig. 8.6A) or systemic pyrexia (Fig. 8.7A) that resolves within a period of time, only those areas undergoing active formation during the period of the insult will be affected. This is seen clinically as bands of dysplastic enamel encircling the crown, with areas of normal enamel elsewhere on the tooth. Banding is evident in both Figures 8.6A and 8.7A.

Poorly protected or exposed dentine is painful. These teeth do become less sensitive with increasing age of the animal since secondary dentine is laid down continuously

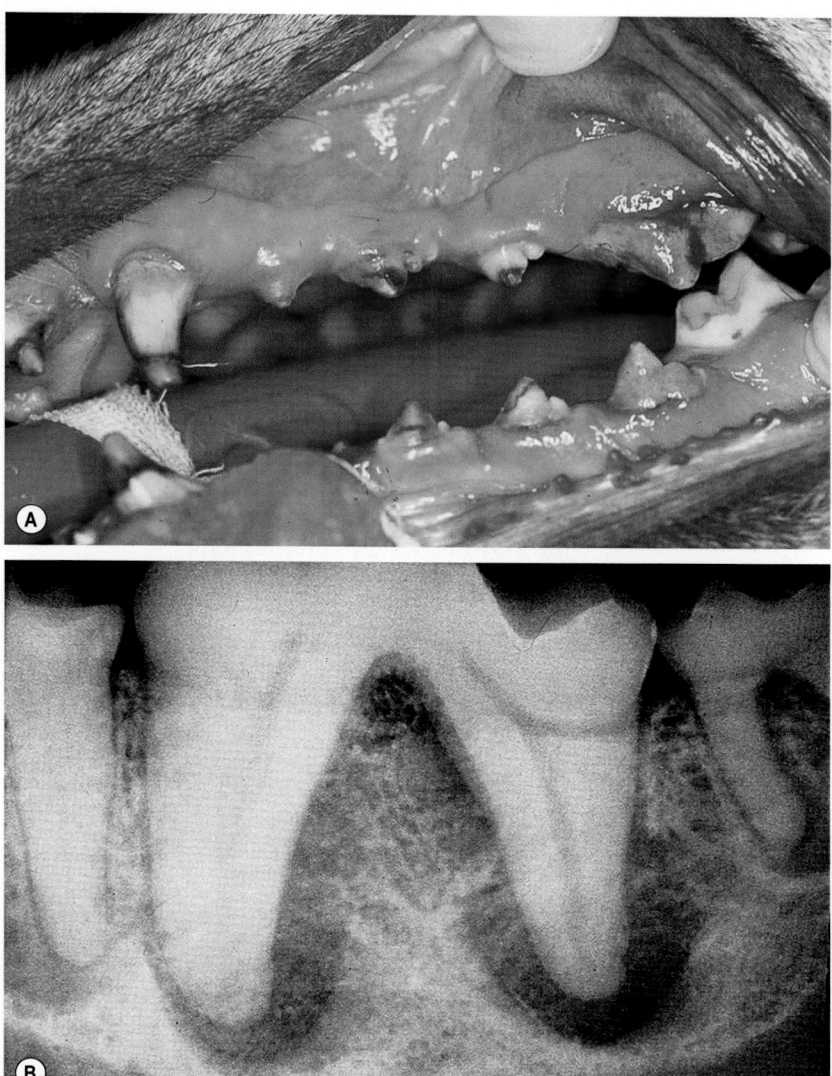

Fig. 8.7 Generalized enamel dysplasia (A) Enamel dysplasia affecting all teeth of the dentition. This type of enamel dysplasia is likely to be caused by systemic factors, e.g. pyrexia, at the time of active enamel development. Only the areas actively forming at the time of the insult will be affected as is seen by the obvious banding with areas of normal enamel elsewhere on the tooth. (B) A radiograph of the caudal left mandible of the same dog reveals pulp and periapical disease affecting the mandibular 4th premolar and the 1st and 2nd molars. The full mouth radiographic series showed that almost all teeth of the dentition had evidence of pulp and periapical pathology. The dog was referred to me because her teeth were discolored and the enamel had seemed to 'crumble' on ultrasonic scaling. She was 5 years old at the time of referral. Treatment consisted of extraction of all teeth except the incisors and canines as these were unaffected by pulp and periapical disease. Homecare was recommended and annual radiographic examination was instituted. The dog was not amenable to toothbrushing, and further extractions due to pulp and periapical pathology have been performed.

by the pulp. Another consideration is that dysplastic enamel harbors dental plaque. In severe cases of generalized enamel hypoplasia, where the dentine is effectively exposed to the oral environment, chronic pulp disease and potentially periapical disease may occur as a result of pulpal irritation via the poorly protected or exposed dentine tubules (Fig. 8.7B). Teeth affected by such pathology require treatment, i.e. either extraction or referral to a specialist for endodontic therapy (outlined in the Appendix), if they are to be maintained.

In the management of patients affected by enamel dysplasia, oral hygiene is of paramount importance. Daily plaque removal will promote periodontal health and possibly reduce pulpal irritation. Affected animals require radiographic assessment and monitoring to detect complications such as pulp and periapical disease. In fact, a series of full mouth radiographs at regular intervals is indicated. In young animals exhibiting signs of discomfort, topical fluoride application may be beneficial. Topical fluoride application will enhance enamel remineralization and 'harden' the enamel. The main effect of fluoride incorporation into the enamel is that it makes the enamel more resistant to acid dissolution that occurs with caries. It must be remembered that fluoride is potentially toxic and the risk of systemic administration of fluoride products meant for topical application is greater in the dog and cat as they will swallow these products.

The use of professionally applied varnishes and gels associated with a moderate rise in plasma fluoride concentrations may well be safer than daily use of fluoride-containing toothpastes. In other words, it is useful to apply fluoride varnishes or gel at regular intervals. The best time to do this is following a dental cleaning. The product is applied while the animal is under general anesthesia and excess is removed before the animal is allowed to recover. In severely affected cases, the enamel is so soft that it is removed on scaling. In these patients, gross calculus accumulation is carefully removed with hand instruments (a scaler or curette) rather than powered scalers (sonic or ultrasonic). The crowns are polished with a fine grain (to reduce abrasion) prophy paste. Restoration of lost enamel, i.e. debriding the defect and replacing lost tissue with a suitable filling material, is useful for smaller lesions (Fig. 8.6B,C), as it protects against dentine sensitivity. It is not practical for extensive, generalized lesions. Restoration requires referral to a specialist.

DISORDERS OF ERUPTION AND SHEDDING

Unerupted teeth can be detected and evaluated by radiographic examination only (Fig. 8.8). Embedded teeth are those that have failed to erupt and remain completely or partially covered by bone or soft tissue or both. Those that have been obstructed by contact against another erupted or non-erupted tooth in the course of their eruption are

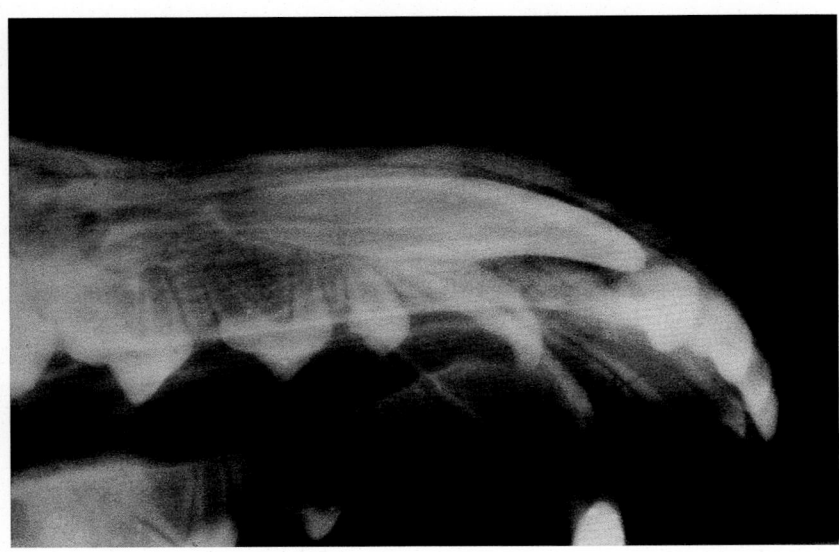

Fig. 8.8 Unerupted teeth Unerupted teeth can only be detected and evaluated by radiographic examination. In this patient, the right permanent maxillary canine tooth has not erupted. The right primary maxillary canine tooth is persistent. The owner was not amenable to the regular radiographic evaluation indicated if the unerupted permanent tooth were to be maintained. The chosen treatment in this case therefore consisted of extracting (open/surgical technique) both the persistent primary canine and the unerupted permanent canine.

referred to as impacted teeth (Shafer et al. 1974a; Stafne and Gibilisco 1975b).

The causes for non-eruption of teeth are numerous (Andrews 1972; Stafne and Gibilisco 1975b). In humans, the most common cause is lack of space. Another common cause is obstruction, either by persistent (retained beyond their normal time for exfoliation) primary teeth or by supernumerary teeth. In dogs, persistent primary teeth more commonly result in abnormal positioning of the permanent tooth rather than non-eruption (Harvey and Emily 1993). Cysts and tumors may also obstruct eruption of the teeth. Other possible causes for non-eruption of teeth include infection, trauma, anomalous conditions affecting the jaws and teeth (e.g. abnormal primary displacement of the tooth bud) and systemic conditions, which cause underdevelopment of the jaws, structural defects of the teeth or poor quality of bone.

Unerupted teeth may cause no pathology, in which case they do not require any treatment. If an obstruction to eruption can be clearly identified, e.g. supernumerary tooth, it should be removed. An increased risk of cyst formation has been reported with unerupted teeth (Stafne and Gibilisco 1975a). The follicle of the unerupted tooth undergoes cystic transformation. The resultant follicular (dentigerous) cyst may cause extensive alveolar bone resorption as it increases in size. These cysts expand as an osmotic gradient develops between the cyst lumen and the surrounding tissues. The pressure of the expanding cyst stimulates resorption of the bone. Follicular cysts can become large and cause extensive resorption of the surrounding alveolar bone. Consequently, unerupted teeth that are maintained require regular radiographic monitoring to identify development of a follicular cyst at an early stage. Treatment then consists of removing the unerupted tooth and its associated cyst. Some clinicians choose to extract unerupted teeth as a prophylactic measure.

WEAR OF DENTAL HARD TISSUE

Attrition is the loss of tooth substance that results from wear that is produced by opposing teeth coming into contact with one another, i.e. teeth that have occlusal contact. Attrition is therefore also called occlusal wear. Incisal wear is the term used when describing attrition of the incisor region. There is progressive attrition with increasing age, resulting in the wearing away of the cusps and exposure of the dentine (Fig. 8.9). The deposition of secondary dentine keeps pace with the loss of tooth substance and there is rarely pulpal exposure. In fact, the crown pulp may come close to obliteration. In other words, attrition is a physiologic event that occurs, to varying degrees, in all animals. Factors such as loss of teeth, malocclusion and habits such as stone chewing may produce excessive attrition, i.e. attrition that is so rapid

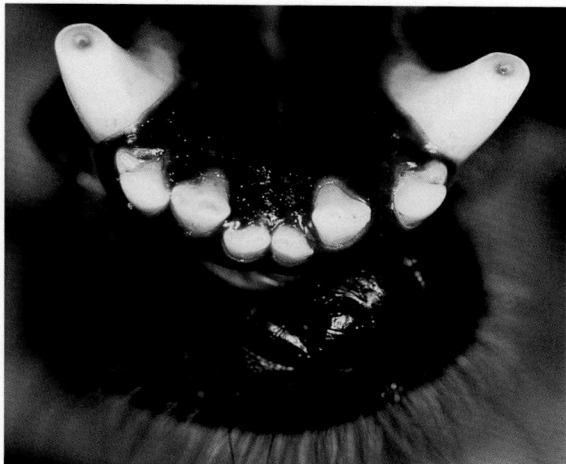

Fig. 8.9 Attrition Attrition is the normal wear on tooth surfaces that are in occlusion. As the enamel is worn away, the dentine is exposed to the oral environment. The deposition of secondary dentine keeps pace with the loss of tooth substance and there is rarely pulpal exposure. The exposed dentine is yellow to brown and has a hard surface on exploration with a dental probe/explorer.

that the formation of secondary dentine cannot keep pace with it, and pulp exposure results (Stafne and Gibilisco 1975c).

Abrasion is the wearing away of tooth structure, which is not caused by incisal or occlusal wear. In other words, wear of tooth surfaces that are not in contact. In humans, the most common cause of abrasion is incorrect use of a toothbrush, resulting in abrasion of the buccal tooth surfaces, usually just above the gingival margin. In dogs, the most common cause of abrasion is cage biting. The hard tissues on the distal aspect of the maxillary canine teeth are progressively lost, weakening the tooth, until the crown fractures (generally with pulpal exposure).

The consequences of pulpal exposure, whether caused by excessive attrition or abrasion, are detailed on pages 91–94. An exposed pulp always requires treatment, either by extraction of the affected tooth or by endodontic therapy, which allows the tooth to be maintained. Measures to prevent excessive attrition and abrasion should be instituted – these are detailed in Chapter 10.

CARIES

Caries (dental decay) occurs in dogs. In our experience, medium and large breed dogs are more commonly affected and the lesions usually affect the teeth that have true occlusal tables, namely the molar teeth. Caries has not been described in cats.

While both periodontal disease and caries are caused by the accumulation of dental plaque on the tooth surfaces, the pathogenesis of the two diseases is completely different. Periodontal disease is a plaque-induced inflammation of the periodontium and caries is a plaque-induced destruction of the hard tissues of the tooth. Caries starts as an inorganic demineralization of the enamel. The demineralization occurs when plaque bacteria use fermentable carbohydrate (notably sugar) from the diet as a source of energy. The fermentation products are acidic and demineralize the enamel. Once the enamel has been destroyed, the process extends into the dentine. In the dentine, the process accelerates as an organic decay and will eventually involve the pulp causing pulpitis and possibly pulp necrosis and/or periapical pathology. Dental caries stimulates the formation of secondary dentine on the surface of the pulpal wall, which is directly beneath it (Shafer et al. 1974c,d; Stafne and Gibilisco 1975c,d). If the carious lesion is progressing slowly, the deposition of secondary dentine may keep pace with its advance and prevent exposure of the dental pulp.

The initial inorganic demineralization can be halted as long as the process has not reached the enamel–dentine junction. Meticulous dental hygiene in combination with topical fluoride treatment and dietary restrictions (reducing the frequency of intake of easily fermentable carbohydrate) can lead to remineralization of the initial defect. An enamel 'scar' will, however, always be present (Shafer et al. 1974c; Stafne and Gibilisco 1975c). If the process has entered the dentine it becomes irreversible and progressive. Treatment (restoration or extraction) becomes mandatory.

In dogs caries is very rarely diagnosed at the early enamel demineralization stage. It is usually diagnosed only when the process already involves the dentine (Fig. 8.10) or the pulp is exposed (Figs 8.11, 8.12). The reason why caries is rarely diagnosed at the enamel demineralization stage in dogs is two-fold. First, the occlusal surfaces are not generally explored with a sharp explorer during clinical examination. Moreover, dog enamel is comparatively thinner than human enamel and the process is thus likely to extend into the dentine more rapidly than in human patients.

Caries can occur on any tooth surface. However, the occlusal (grinding) surfaces of the molar teeth seem predisposed in dogs. Clinically, caries manifests as softened, often discolored (dark brown or black) areas in the enamel (Fig. 8.10). A dental explorer will 'catch' in the softened carious tooth surface. A small enamel defect covers a large cavern of decayed dentine. Note that not all lesions are grossly discolored and all occlusal surfaces, whether discolored or not, should be meticulously examined with a dental explorer. If the explorer sticks in the tooth surface, then caries should be suspected and radiographs are indicated. Radiographically, radiolucent defects are seen in the affected area of the crown. Radiographs will also give an

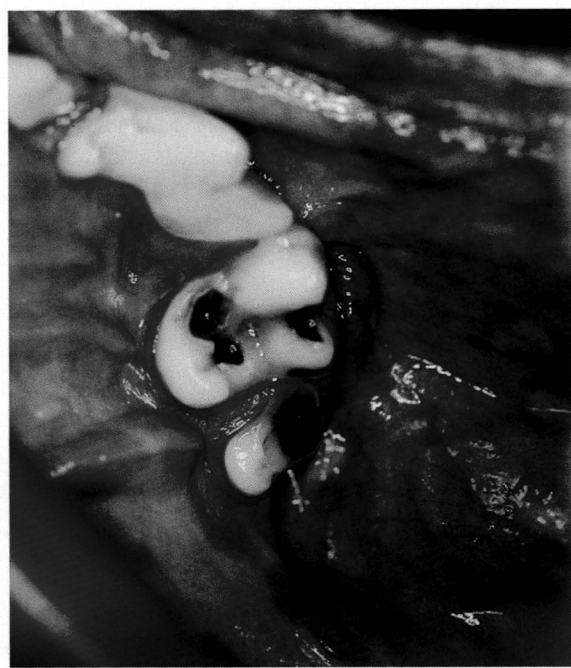

Fig. 8.10 Caries The clinical appearance of dental caries affecting the left 1st and 2nd molars is depicted. The black areas were soft on exploration, with the explorer readily 'catching' in the tooth surface. Radiographs are indicated to assess the full extent of the lesions and select appropriate treatment, i.e. extraction or referral.

indication of how close to the pulp chamber a carious lesion extends (the extent of secondary dentine formation and the amount and thickness of dentine that separates the pulp from the carious lesion), which allows selection of the most appropriate treatment. Discolored areas that are hard and in which the explorer does not 'catch' are not caries – they could be exposed dentine due to attrition or stain.

Diagnosed caries requires treatment. The options are extraction or referral to a specialist for restoration (if the process involves the pulp tissue, as in Figure 8.12, endodontic therapy prior to restoration is required). If the process has resulted in gross loss of tooth substance at the time of diagnosis, then extraction is the only option (Fig. 8.11). Measures to prevent new lesions must be instituted in animals with diagnosed caries. In addition to homecare and dietary modifications as detailed in Chapter 10, these dogs may benefit from regular professional fluoride applications. Fluoride enhances remineralization and makes the enamel more resistant to the acid dissolution that occurs with caries.

PULP AND PERIAPICAL DISEASES

The pathophysiology of pulp and periapical diseases caused by traumatic tooth injuries is also covered in Chapter 12. A tooth affected by pulp and periapical diseases should always be treated, i.e. it cannot just be ignored. In general terms, treatment is either extraction or endodontic therapy. The principles of endodontic therapy, which allows a tooth to be maintained, are outlined in the Appendix.

Pulpal reactions

The immature tooth has a wide pulp cavity. As the tooth matures, secondary dentine is laid down and the pulp cavity becomes narrower. Note that the contours of the pulp chamber mimic the shape of the crown so that the pulpal horns are always relatively close to the surface. Consequently, crown fracture very often involves exposure of the pulp in the older animal as well as in the young.

Apart from the reduction in size of the pulp cavity, which is associated with continued deposition of secondary dentine as the animal gets older, there are also conditions that accelerate the rate of deposition of secondary dentine, thus prematurely reducing the size of the pulp

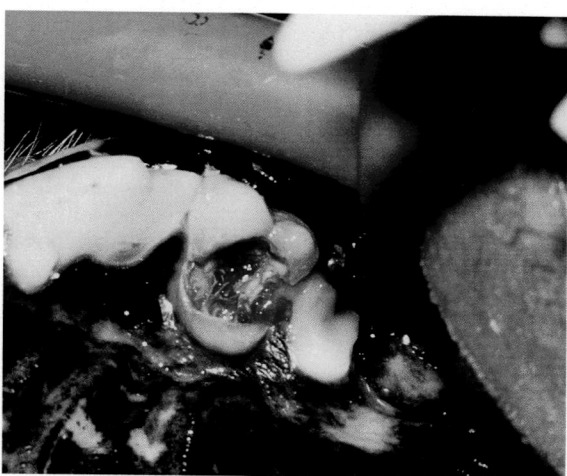

Fig. 8.11 Caries The carious lesion of the maxillary 1st molar depicted here has resulted in extensive loss of enamel and dentine and has exposed the pulp chamber to the oral cavity. The pink tissue seen in the centre of the occlusal table is inflamed and hyperplastic pulp tissue (pulp granuloma). Radiographs reveal that the dentine destruction has been so extensive that the furcation of the roots has been broached, i.e. the three roots are unconnected to the crown. Extraction is the only treatment possible for this tooth!

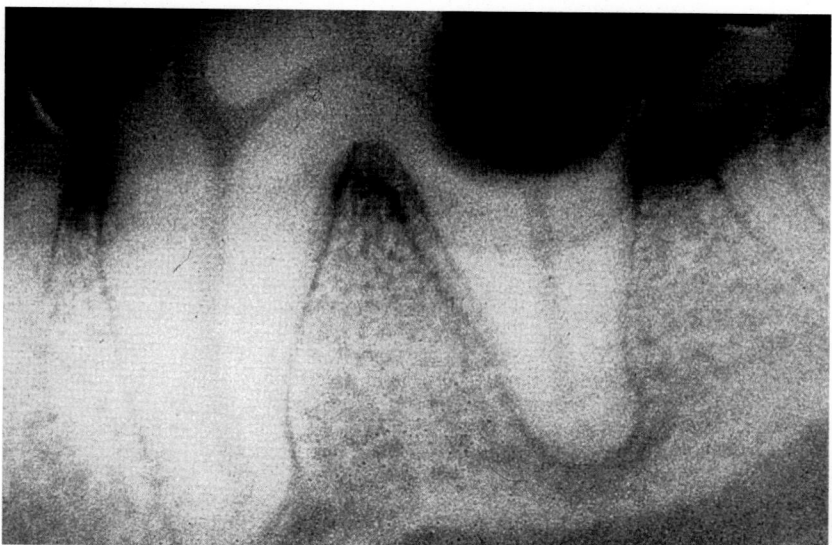

Fig. 8.12 Caries The radiograph of the left mandibular 1st molar shows an extensive carious lesion on the distal occlusal surface. The process extends into the root pulp. Periapical lesions of both roots are obvious. Treatment consists of extraction or referral. From the specialist's point of view, there are two options available if the tooth is to be maintained. One option is to perform endodontic therapy and restoration. The restoration of the distal occlusal surface will be large and likely to have subgingival margins, which complicates plaque control. A second option involves sectioning the tooth and extracting the distal portion (crown and root). The mesial section of the tooth is maintained following endodontic therapy of the mesial root and restorations of the crown (endodontic access point and at the point of sectioning). For either option, homecare is mandatory. The owner needs to brush the teeth on a daily basis.

cavity. Attrition and abrasion are two common conditions resulting in a narrow pulp cavity. Alterations and decrease of the pulp chamber and canals can occur with injury or disease. In some instances, injury to a tooth will result in complete obliteration of the pulp chamber and root canals. More unusually, the obliteration is partial with the pulp chamber retaining the size and shape it had at the time of the injury, and the root canals becoming completely obliterated. Orthodontic force can result in partial or complete obliteration of the pulp cavity (Shafer et al. 1974b; Stafne and Gibilisco 1975b). Injuries that cause inflammation and degeneration/necrosis of the pulp account for many abnormally large pulp cavities (Stafne and Gibilisco 1975c) as dentine production ceases when the pulp is chronically inflamed or necrotic.

Calcifications in the pulp tissue are sometimes seen (Fig. 8.13). In humans, their presence has been attributed to local irritants of long standing, such as abrasion, erosion and gingival recession, but they also occur in normal teeth where such factors are absent. The present consensus is that calcification of the pulp is of no great significance if one excludes the few instances where pathologic calcification occurs as a result of inflammation or necrosis of the pulp (Stafne and Gibilisco 1975c). Calcifications associated with pulpal inflammation require extraction of the tooth or referral for endodontic therapy.

Periapical lesions

Pathology in the area surrounding the apex of a root, i.e. periapical pathology, is most commonly a sequel to chronic pulpitis or pulp necrosis. The source of the infection may be blood-borne, but such cases are rare (Shafer et al. 1974d; Stafne and Gibilisco 1975e; Gorrel and Robinson 1995b). The earliest radiographic evidence of periapical pathology is widening of the periodontal ligament space in the apical region. This widening is due to inflammation of the apical periodontal ligament. If untreated, the apical periodontitis progresses to involve the surrounding bone resulting in destruction of the bone, which is replaced by soft tissue. This is evident as an apical rarefaction on a radiograph (Figs 8.7B, 8.12, 8.14). The soft tissue may be granulation tissue (periapical granuloma), cyst (periapical or radicular cyst) or abscess (periapical abscess) (Shafer et al. 1974d; Gorrel and Robinson 1995b). Definitive differentiation between these three possibilities requires histopathology of the tissue. In veterinary dentistry, histopathology of periapical lesions is rarely performed.

Treatment for all three entities is the same, i.e. endodontic therapy or if there are complicating factors, e.g. advanced periodontitis, then extraction. Remember that not all apical rarefaction is pathologic in the dog and cat. The periapical bone of normal canines often appears radiolucent in the dog. Comparison should always be made with other teeth of the same type in the same animal. A distinctly round radiolucent area, however, is usually pathologic. Periapical sclerosis, instead of radiolucency, as a result of a chronically inflamed/necrotic pulp can sometimes be seen (Shafer et al. 1974d).

The periapical cyst usually occurs as a sequel to the periapical granuloma (Shafer et al. 1974d; Gorrel and

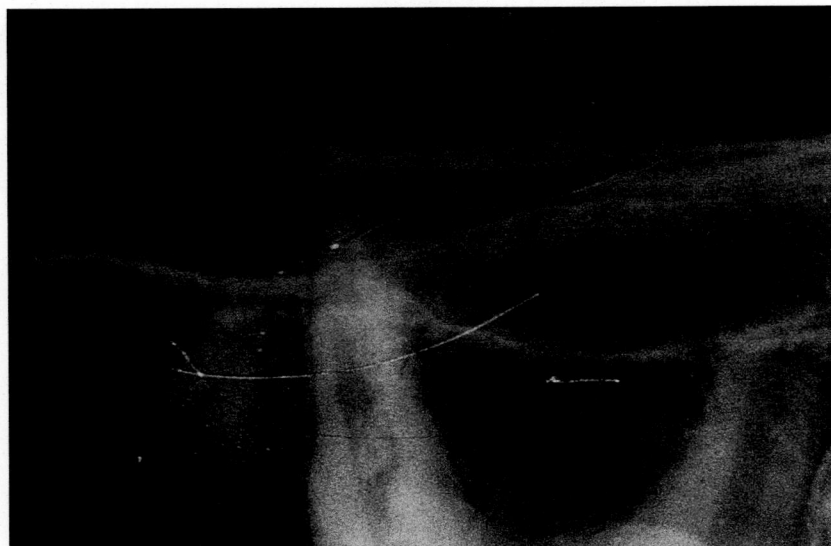

Fig. 8.13 Calcifications in the pulp Calcifications in the pulp tissue have been attributed to local irritants of long standing, e.g. abrasion. They also occur in normal teeth as incidental findings on radiography. These require no treatment. Calcifications associated with pulpal inflammation require extraction of the tooth or referral for endodontic therapy.

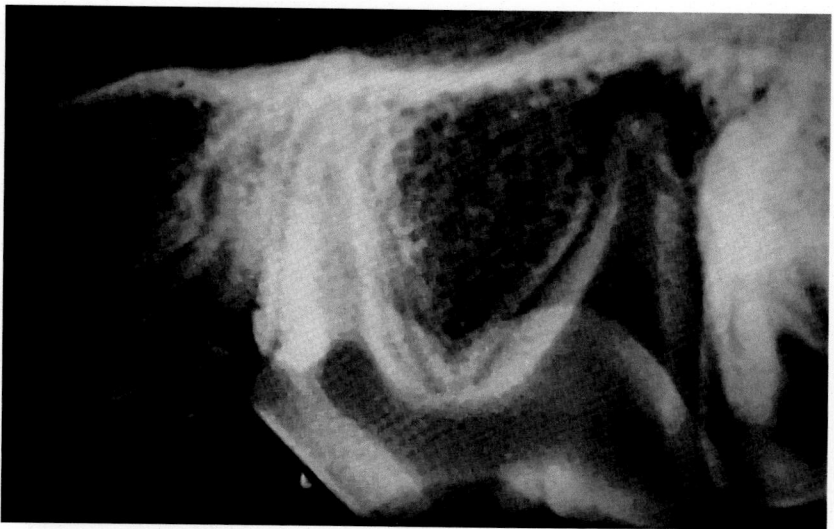

Fig. 8.14 Periapical lesions Destruction of the bone surrounding the apex of the tooth is evident as rarefaction on a radiograph. In the radiograph depicted, there is an obvious periapical lesion of the distal root of the left maxillary 4th premolar. This tooth requires referral for endodontic therapy if it is to be maintained. Extraction is the other option.

Robinson 1995b). It is a true cyst, since the lesion consists of a pathologic, often fluid-filled, cavity that is lined by epithelium. Periapical cysts enlarge as a result of the osmotic gradient set up between the lumen of the cyst and tissue fluids in the surrounding connective tissue. These lesions can become very large at the expense of the adjacent bone tissue, which is resorbed (owing to pressure from the cyst).

An untreated periapical abscess can lead to complications such as osteomyelitis and cellulitis through spread of the infection. A fistulous tract opening on the skin or oral mucosa may develop (Shafer et al. 1974d; Stafne and Gibilisco 1975e; Gorrel and Robinson 1995b).

Periapical lesions may be entirely asymptomatic or excruciatingly painful. The periapical granuloma and periapical cyst rarely cause severe discomfort but they may undergo exacerbation and develop into a periodontal abscess, which usually is an extremely painful condition. The clinical signs indicative of periapical pathology are often insidious and not noticed by the owner. It is often only after completion of treatment that the owner reports a dramatic improvement in the animal's general demeanor. Consequently, periapical lesions confirmed by radiography should be treated even if the animal is not showing obvious signs of pain or discomfort. Similarly, discolored teeth with a necrotic pulp need to be treated before periapical pathology develops. Once diagnosed, patients with necrotic pulps and periapical pathology should receive endodontic treatment (referral) or extraction of the affected tooth as soon as possible (Gorrel and Robinson 1995b).

Combined periodontic and endodontic lesions

There are possible pathways of communication between the pulp and the periodontium. These are denuded dentine tubules, lateral and/or accessory pulp canals and at the apical foramen. Consequently, a periapical lesion may have a periodontal origin and a periodontal-type lesion may originate from the pulp. Another possibility is that a lesion is the result of a combination of endodontic and periodontal pathology (Shafer et al. 1974d; Bergenholtz 1992). The lesions are classified according to etiology as follows:

- A Class I lesion, or endodontic–periodontic lesion, is endodontic in origin, i.e. pathology begins in the pulp and progresses to involve the periodontium.
- Class II lesion, or periodontic–endodontic lesion is periodontic in origin, i.e. pathology begins in the periodontium and progresses to involve the pulp.
- A Class III lesion, or true combined lesion, is a fusion of independent periodontic and endodontic lesions.

Diagnosis depends on clinical examination and radiography. The prognosis for long-term retention of the tooth is based on the above classification. Class I lesions have a better prognosis as endodontic treatment may lead to resolution of the periodontal extension of the inflammation. In contrast, Class II and Class III lesions require endodontic treatment as well as extensive periodontal

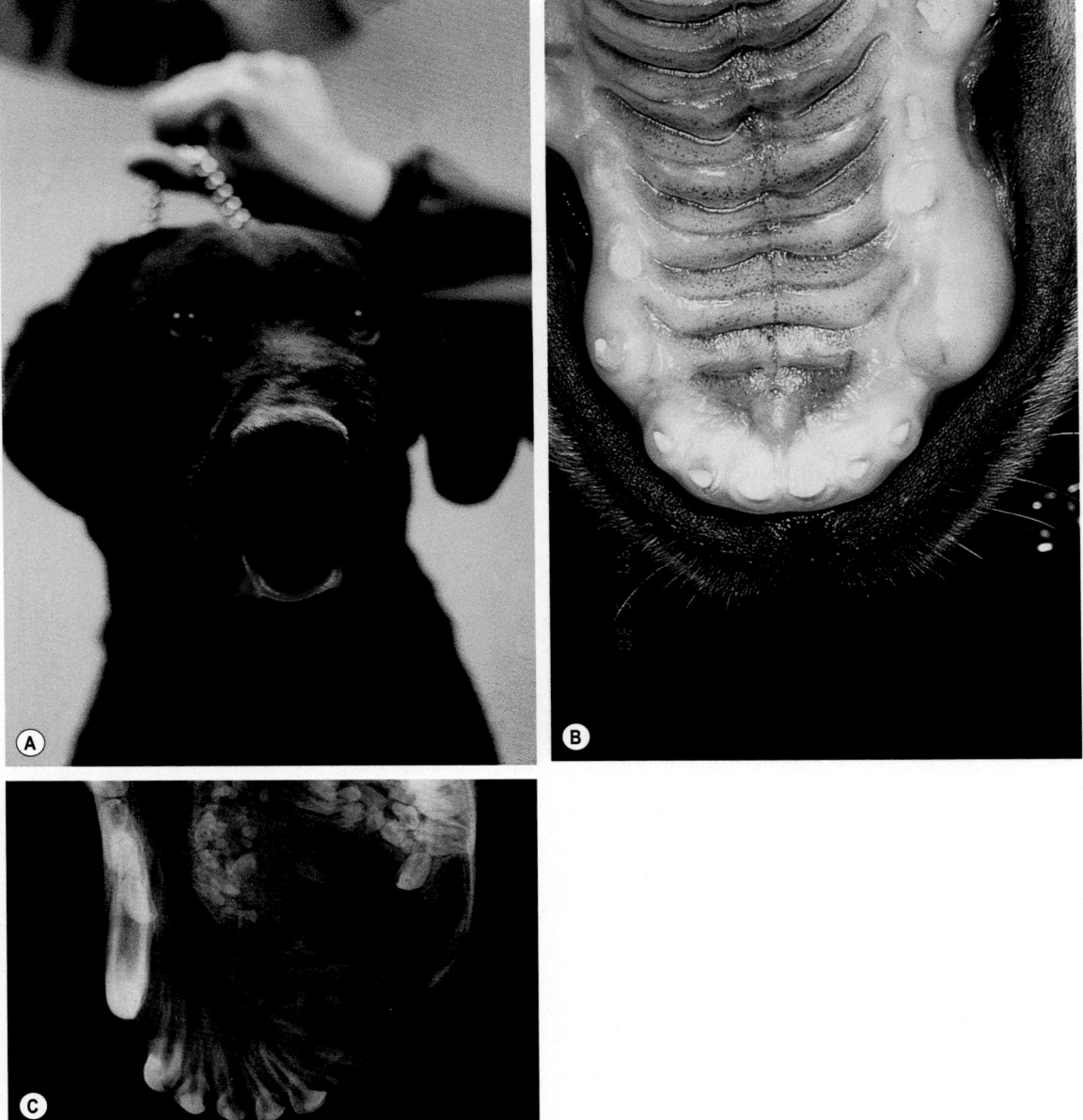

Fig. 8.15 Odontoma (A) A swelling on the left side of the nose in this young dog is obvious. The mass is slightly fluctuant on palpation. (B) The intraoral examination reveals that there is also an intraoral swelling extending from the left canine in a caudal direction. (C) The radiograph reveals that the swelling comprises a cyst-like lesion that contains tooth-like material. This radiograph is pathognomonic for odontoma, i.e. histopathology is not required for diagnosis. Treatment consists of shelling out the cyst-like lesion and its contents.

therapy and the periodontal destruction is often too extensive to be amenable to treatment.

Teeth with severe destruction of the periodontium should be extracted whatever the original cause (Gorrel and Robinson 1995a,b). Other treatment options are endodontic therapy and/or periodontal therapy depending on the classification. Referral to a specialist is recommended.

OSTEOMYELITIS

Osteomyelitis of the jawbones is not a particularly common disease in dogs and cats. Infection of dental origin is not the only cause of osteomyelitis in the upper jaw or mandible, but it is probably the most frequent one. Osteomyelitis then occurs as an extension of pulp and periapical pathology. The disease may be acute, subacute or chronic and presents a different clinical course depending on its nature (Stafne and Gibilisco 1975e).

Osteomyelitis can be very difficult to differentiate from neoplastic bone lesions on radiography. Biopsy and histopathologic examination of the bone is really the only way to reach a definitive diagnosis. Once diagnosed, osteomyelitis is treated by removing the cause (extraction or possibly endodontic therapy of teeth with pulp and periapical disease) in combination with antibiotic therapy. The choice of antibiotic should be based on the results of culture and antibiogram. The duration of antibiotic treatment required is usually longer than for other oral infections.

ORAL TUMORS

A variety of neoplastic lesions (benign and malignant) occurs in the oral cavity. These can be odontogenic or non-odontogenic in origin. In addition, non-neoplastic lesions and swellings, e.g. gingival hyperplasia and infective conditions, can be confused with neoplasia. Conversely, oral neoplasms may present as non-healing ulcerative lesions rather than as masses. Also, the so-called epulides constitute a variety of pathologic entities.

Malignant neoplasms of the mouth and pharynx constitute 5–7% of all canine tumors (Verstraete 1995). The most common malignant neoplasms are malignant melanoma (30–35%), squamous cell carcinoma (20–30%) and fibrosarcoma (1–20%) (Verstraete 1995). Osteosarcoma is also relatively common.

The term 'epulid' (epulis) is a clinically descriptive term referring to a localized swelling on the gingiva. A number of distinct histopathologic entities can thus present as an epulis, including malignant tumors. However, most epulides are non-neoplastic lesions or odontogenic

tumors. In one study (Verstraete et al. 1992), it was found that 44% of epulides were focal fibrous hyperplasia. Peripheral odontogenic fibromas were also common (17%) and peripheral ameloblastoma accounted for 18% of epulides examined histologically.

Odontogenic tumors are benign neoplasms that arise from odontogenic tissue. They are classified based on the type of neoplastic tissue (epithelial or mesodermal) and whether they are inductive or non-inductive (i.e. whether an interaction similar to that seen during odontogenesis takes place between epithelial and mesenchymal tissues or not). The odontoma (Fig. 8.15) is an example of an inductive tumor and the peripheral ameloblastoma and the peripheral odontogenic fibroma are examples of non-inductive tumors.

Radiography, while not diagnostic of the tumor type, will provide information about the extent of bony involvement of oral neoplasms (Fig. 8.16). Such information, in

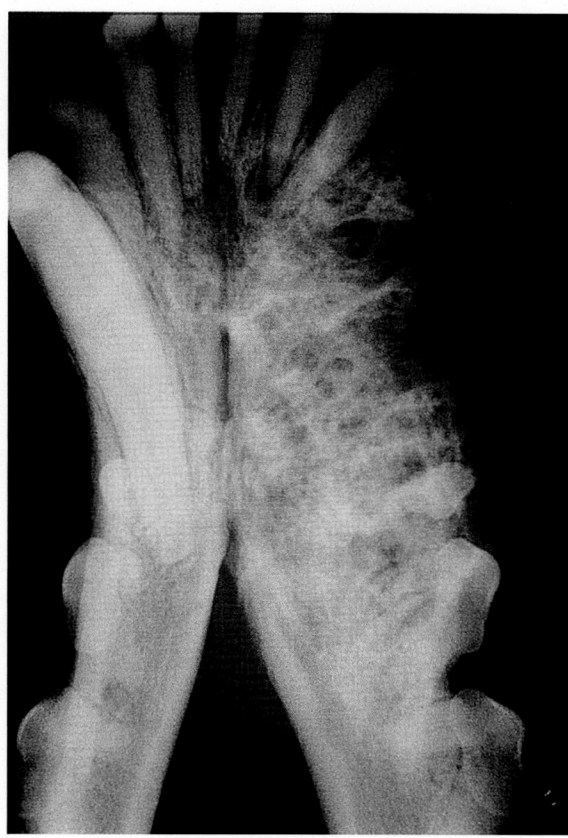

Fig. 8.16 Bony extension of neoplasia Radiography will provide information about the extent of bony involvement of oral neoplasms. This information, in combination with the histopathologic diagnosis, is important in planning management.

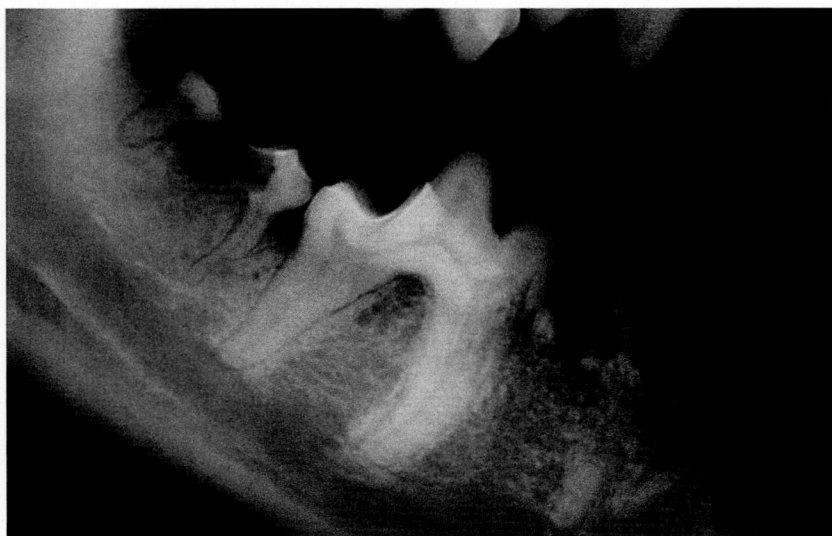

Fig. 8.17 External root resorption The right mandibular 3rd and 4th premolars and the 1st and 2nd molars depicted in this radiograph are affected by external root resorption. The periodontal ligament space of the affected roots cannot be identified. In fact, it is impossible to differentiate between root and bone in some locations. At these locations, the crown appears to be separated from its roots by a layer of bone. The distal roots of the 4th premolar and the 2nd molar cannot be identified. The root resorption has extended into the crown dentine resulting in loss of hard tissue and communication with the oral environment. Histologically, this was diagnosed as external root resorption with bony replacement of destroyed dental hard tissues. The resorption was mediated by odontoclasts.

conjunction with the histopathologic diagnosis, is important in planning tumor management.

ROOT RESORPTION

Hard tissues are protected from resorption by their surface layer of cells (Lindskog and Hammarström 1980; Gunnraj 1999). Internal root resorption (when the root is resorbing from the pulp side towards the external tooth surface) is triggered by pulpal inflammation. External root resorption (when the root is resorbing from the cementum towards the pulp) may follow any damage to the protective periodontal ligament and cementoblast layer. Inflammatory external root resorption is seen as a complication to orthodontic treatment, in periodontitis and in conjunction with periapical pathology.

External root resorption (odontoclastic resorptive lesions) of unknown etiology is common in cats and is detailed in Chapter 11. Similar lesions (Arnbjerg 1996) have been reported in dogs (Fig. 8.17).

SUMMARY

◆ Common oral conditions should be readily appreciated so that appropriate treatment (conservative, in-house or referral) can be instituted.
◆ A variety of developmental disorders occur commonly, including missing teeth, supernumerary teeth, fused teeth, aberrant root shapes and numbers, and enamel hypoplasia.
◆ Caries (dental decay) is a recognized entity in dogs but not in cats.
◆ Pulp and periapical conditions always require treatment by extraction or endodontic therapy.
◆ Osteomyelitis requires differentiation from neoplasia.
◆ The commonest malignant oral tumors are malignant melanoma and squamous cell carcinoma.
◆ Most epulides are non-neoplastic.
◆ Odontogenic tumors are benign neoplasms arising from odontogenic tissues.

REFERENCES

Aitchison, J., 1963. Changing incisor dentition of bull dogs. Veterinary Record 75, 153.

Andrews, A.H., 1972. A case of partial anodontia in a dog. Veterinary Record 90, 144–145.

Arnall, L., 1960. Some aspects of dental development in the dog. II. Eruption and extrusion. Journal of Small Animal Practice 1, 259.

Arnbjerg, J., 1996. Idiopathic dental root replacement resorption in old dogs. Journal of Veterinary Dentistry 13 (3), 97–99.

Bergenholtz, G., 1992. Periodontics and endodontics. In: Lindhe, J. (Ed.), Textbook of Clinical Periodontology, second ed. Munksgaard, Copenhagen, pp. 258–281.

Gorrel, C., Robinson, J., 1995a. Periodontal therapy and extraction technique. In: Crossley, D.A., Penman, S. (Eds.), Manual of Small Animal Dentistry. BSAVA, Cheltenham, pp. 139–149.

Gorrel, C., Robinson, J., 1995b. Endodontics in small carnivores. In: Crossley, D.A., Penman, S. (Eds.), Manual of Small Animal Dentistry. BSAVA, Cheltenham, pp. 168–181.

Gunnraj, M.N., 1999. Dental root resorption. Oral Surgery 88, 47–53.

Harvey, C.E., Emily, P., 1993. Occlusion, occlusive abnormalities and orthodontic treatment. In: Small Animal Dentistry. Mosby, Missouri, pp. 266–296.

Lindskog, S., Hammarström, L., 1980. Evidence in favour of an anti-invasion factor in cementum or periodontal membrane. Scandinavian Journal of Dental Research 88, 161–163.

Shafer, W.G., Hine, M.K., Levy, B.M., 1974a. Developmental disturbances of oral and paraoral structures. In: A Textbook of Oral Pathology, third ed. WB Saunders, Philadelphia, pp. 2–80.

Shafer, W.G., Hine, M.K., Levy, B.M., 1974b. Cysts and tumors of odontogenic origin. In: A Textbook of Oral Pathology, third ed. WB Saunders, Philadelphia, pp. 236–284.

Shafer, W.G., Hine, M.K., Levy, B.M., 1974c. Dental caries. In: A Textbook of Oral Pathology, third ed. WB Saunders, Philadelphia, pp. 366–432.

Shafer, W.G., Hine, M.K., Levy, B.M., 1974d. Diseases of the pulp and periapical tissues. In: A Textbook of Oral Pathology, third ed. WB Saunders, Philadelphia, pp. 433–462.

Skrentary, T.T., 1964. Preliminary study of the inheritance of missing teeth in the dog. Wiener Tierarztliche Monatsschrift 51, 231.

Stafne, E.C., Gibilisco, J.A., 1975a. Cysts of the jaws. In: Oral Roentgenographic Diagnosis, fourth ed. WB Saunders, Philadelphia, pp. 147–168.

Stafne, E.C., Gibilisco, J.A., 1975b. Malposition of teeth. In: Oral Roentgenographic Diagnosis, fourth ed. WB Saunders, Philadelphia, pp. 44–56.

Stafne, E.C., Gibilisco, J.A., 1975c. The pulp cavity. In: Oral Roentgenographic Diagnosis, fourth ed. WB Saunders, Philadelphia, pp. 61–70.

Stafne, E.C., Gibilisco, J.A., 1975d. Dental caries. In: Oral Roentgenographic Diagnosis, fourth ed. WB Saunders, Philadelphia, pp. 71–73.

Stafne, E.C., Gibilisco, J.A., 1975e. Infections of the jaws. In: Oral Roentgenographic Diagnosis, fourth ed. WB Saunders, Philadelphia, pp. 74–85.

Verstraete, F.J.M., 1995. Advanced oral surgery in small carnivores. In: Crossley, D.A., Penman, S. (Eds.), Manual of Small Animal Dentistry. BSAVA, Cheltenham, pp. 193–207.

Verstraete, F.J.M., Ligthelm, A.J., Weber, A., 1992. The histological nature of epulides in dogs. Journal of Comparative Pathology 106, 169–182.

Chapter | 9 |

Periodontal disease

INTRODUCTION

Periodontal disease is the result of the inflammatory response to dental plaque, i.e. oral bacteria, and is limited to the periodontium. It is the most common oral disease seen in dogs (Hamp et al. 1984). It is also common in cats (Reichart et al. 1984). In fact, periodontal disease is probably the most common disease seen in small animal practice with the great majority of dogs and cats over the age of 3 years having a degree of disease that warrants intervention.

In addition to periodontal disease, a spectrum of inflammatory responses to agents other than plaque (e.g. toxic, viral and unknown) also occurs in the oral cavity. These generally affect the oral mucous membrane, but may also involve the periodontium. Inflammation of the oral mucosa is called stomatitis. Table 9.1 lists the most important oral inflammatory conditions, other than periodontal disease. This chapter will deal with periodontal disease and feline gingivostomatitis.

Periodontal disease is a collective term for a number of plaque-induced inflammatory lesions that affect the periodontium. The term infection refers to the presence and multiplication of a microorganism in body tissues. Periodontal disease is a unique infection in that it is not associated with a massive bacterial invasion of the tissues. Gingivitis is inflammation of the gingiva and is the earliest sign of disease. Individuals with untreated gingivitis *may* develop periodontitis. The inflammatory reactions in periodontitis result in destruction of the periodontal ligament and alveolar bone. The result of untreated periodontitis is ultimately exfoliation of the affected tooth. Thus, gingivitis is inflammation that is not associated with destruction (loss) of supporting tissue. It is reversible. In contrast,

periodontitis is inflammation where the tooth has lost a variable degree of its support (attachment). It is irreversible. The salient features of gingivitis and periodontitis are depicted in diagrammatic form in Figure 9.1.

Periodontal disease can cause discomfort to affected individuals. Moreover, there is strong circumstantial evidence that a focus of infection in the oral cavity may cause disease of distant organs (DeBowes et al. 1996). Consequently, prevention and treatment of periodontal disease is important for the general health of companion animals. It is not a cosmetic issue. Prevention of periodontal disease is detailed in Chapter 10. This chapter details etiology, pathogenesis, diagnosis and treatment. Successful management of periodontal disease relies on a comprehensive understanding of the etiology and pathogenesis of the disease.

ETIOLOGY

The *primary cause* of gingivitis and periodontitis is accumulation of dental plaque on the tooth surfaces. Contrary to common belief, calculus (tartar) is only a secondary etiologic factor.

Dental plaque

Dental plaque is a biofilm composed of aggregates of bacteria and their by-products, salivary components, oral debris and occasional epithelial and inflammatory cells (Fig. 9.2). Plaque accumulation starts within minutes on a clean tooth surface. The initial accumulation of plaque occurs supragingivally but will extend into the sulcus and populate the subgingival region if left undisturbed. As

Table 9.1 Non-periodontal oral inflammatory diseases

Conditions associated with immune system depression or dysfunction	Necrotizing ulcerative gingivostomatitis Mycotic infections, commonly candidiasis Neutrophil dysfunction, gray collie syndrome, drug therapy, viral infection, e.g. feline immunodeficiency virus
Autoimmune disorders	Vesiculobullous skin diseases, e.g. pemphigus and pemphigoid Systemic or discoid lupus erythematosus Sjögren-like syndrome
Hypersensitivity	Drug eruptions Insect stings
Viral infections	Feline leukemia virus Calicivirus
Miscellaneous conditions	Eosinophilic granuloma complex Chronic gingivostomatitis

demonstrated in a study where dogs were fed by intubation, the formation of dental plaque occurs whether food passes through the oral cavity or not, i.e. food debris does not attach to the teeth to form plaque (Egelberg 1965). Supragingival plaque bacteria derive their main nutrients from dietary particles dissolved in saliva. Within the sulcus or pathologic periodontal pocket, the major nutritional source for bacterial metabolism comes from the periodontal tissues and blood.

Classic experiments have demonstrated that accumulation of plaque on the tooth surfaces reproducibly induces an inflammatory response in associated gingival tissues, and that removal of the plaque leads to disappearance of the clinical signs of this inflammation (Löe et al. 1965; Theilade et al. 1966). At first, a direct relationship was assumed to exist between the total number of bacteria that accumulated on a tooth surface and the amplitude of the pathogenic effect. Such a view of dental plaque as a biomass is referred to as the *non-specific plaque hypothesis* (Theilade 1986). As it became evident that not all gingivitis lesions invariably developed to periodontitis lesions, the *specific plaque hypothesis* was developed. In this hypothesis, the view is that periodontitis is caused by specific pathogens (Loesche 1979). Differences in the composition of the subgingival plaque have been attributed in part to the local availability of blood products, pocket depth, redox potential and PO_2. Therefore, the question of whether the presence of specific microorganisms in patients or distinct sites may be the cause or consequence of disease is still a matter of dispute (Socransky et al. 1987). Many periodontopathogens are strict anaerobes and, as such, may contribute little to the initiation of periodontitis in shallow periodontal pockets. Instead, these organisms are linked to progression of disease in sites with pre-existing periodontitis.

The formation of plaque involves two processes, namely the initial adherence of bacteria and then the continued accumulation of bacteria due to a combination of multiplication and further aggregation of bacteria to those cells that are already attached. As soon as a tooth becomes exposed to the oral cavity, its surfaces are covered by the pellicle (an amorphous coating of salivary proteins and glycoproteins). The pellicle alters the charge and free energy of the tooth surfaces, which increases the efficiency of bacterial adhesion. Specific bacteria such as *Streptococcus sanguis* and *Actinomyces viscosus* can adhere to the pellicle. These bacteria produce extracellular polysaccharides, which aggregate other bacteria that are not otherwise able to adhere.

The plaque associated with healthy gingiva mainly comprises aerobic and facultative anaerobic bacteria. As gingivitis develops, plaque extends subgingivally. Aerobes consume oxygen and a low redox potential is created, which makes the environment more suitable for growth of anaerobic species. The aerobic population does not decrease, but with increasing number of anaerobes, the aerobic/anaerobic ratio decreases. The subgingival flora associated with periodontitis is predominantly anaerobic and consists of *Porphyromonas* spp, *Prevotella* spp, *Peptostreptococcus* spp, *Fusobacterium* spp and spirochetes (Hennet and Harvey 1991). High levels of *Porphyromonas* spp and spirochetes are consistently associated with progressive periodontitis in the dog. The bacterial flora of the normal feline gingival margin, as well as the bacteria found in subgingival plaque of cats with gingivitis and periodontitis, are similar to those found in humans and dogs under similar conditions (Mallonee et al. 1988; Love et al. 1990).

SUMMARY FOR TREATMENT OF DENTAL PLAQUE

- ◆ The first bacteria to adhere to the pellicle are aerobic Gram-positive organisms.
- ◆ In dogs and cats, the main bacteria in supragingival plaque are *Actinomyces* and *streptococci*.
- ◆ As the plaque thickens, matures and extends further down the gingival sulcus, the environment becomes suitable for growth of anaerobic organisms, motile rods and spirochetes.

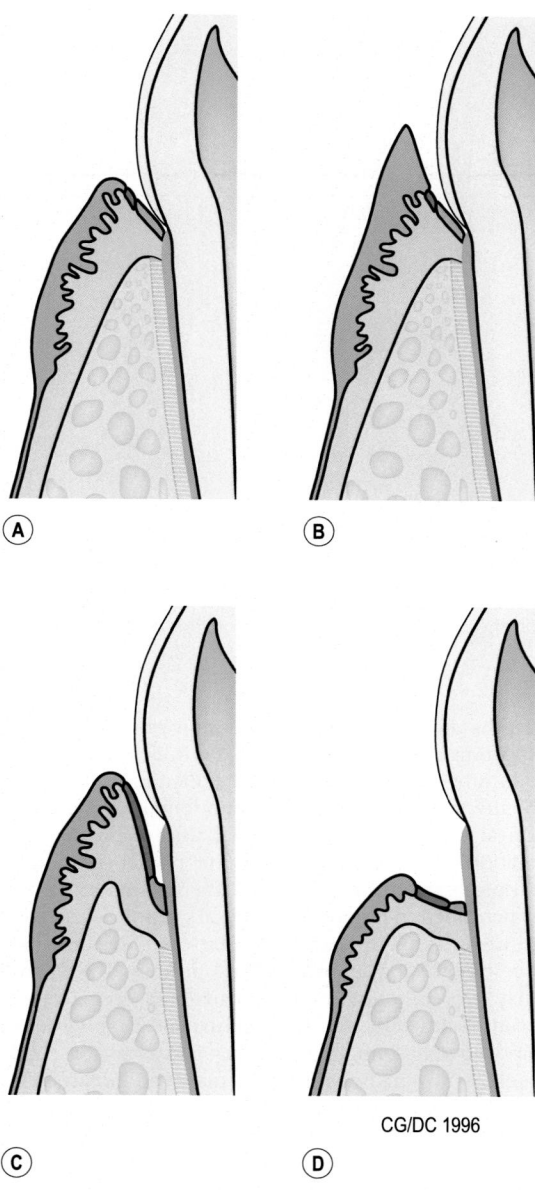

CG/DC 1996

Fig. 9.1 Periodontal disease Periodontal disease is a collective term for plaque-induced inflammation of the gingiva. (A) *Gingivitis*. The inflammation is limited to the gingiva with no associated destruction of the periodontium. Gingivitis is reversible. (B) *Gingival hyperplasia*. Gingival hyperplasia may be the result of plaque-induced inflammation (hyperplastic gingivitis), but may also be of idiopathic or familial origin. It can also be induced by certain drugs. Gingival hyperplasia results in increased periodontal probing depths, initially with no loss of periodontal support, i.e. there is no attachment loss. (C) *Periodontitis with vertical bone loss*. The plaque-induced inflammation results in irreversible destruction of the periodontal ligament and alveolar bone. The junctional epithelium (epithelial attachment) migrates apically and attaches on the root surfaces. If the gingival margin does not recede, the apical migration of the epithelial attachment results in increased periodontal probing depth, i.e. a pathologic pocket is formed. Destruction of the alveolar bone can be horizontal or vertical. Shown here is vertical bone loss, resulting in the formation of a periodontal pocket where the apical extension of the pocket is below the margin of the alveolar bone, i.e. infrabony pocket. (D) *Periodontitis with horizontal bone loss*. The periodontal destruction is evidenced by loss of periodontal ligament and horizontal bone loss. The junctional epithelium has migrated apically and attached to the root surfaces. However, the gingival margin has receded, so periodontal probing depths do not increase.

Dental calculus

Dental calculus is mineralized plaque. However, a layer of plaque always covers calculus. Both supragingival and subgingival plaque becomes mineralized. Supragingival calculus *per se* does not exert an irritant effect on the gingival tissues. In fact, it has been shown in monkeys that a normal attachment may be seen between the junctional epithelium and calculus if the calculus surface had been disinfected using chlorhexidine (Listgarten and Ellegaard 1973). It has also been shown that sterilized calculus may be encapsulated in connective tissue without causing marked inflammation or abscess formation (Allen and Kerr 1965). It has been speculated that calculus may exert a detrimental effect on the soft tissue owing to its rough surface. However, it has clearly been established that surface roughness alone does not initiate gingivitis (Waerhaug 1956). The main importance of calculus in periodontal disease thus seems to be its role as a plaque-retentive surface. This is supported by well-controlled

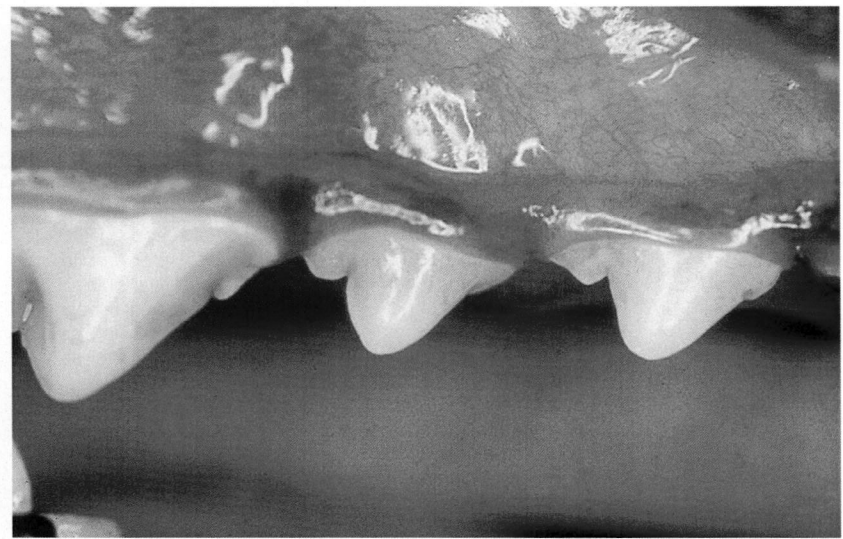

Fig. 9.2 Dental plaque Dental plaque is a biofilm composed of aggregates of bacteria and their by-products, salivary components, oral debris and occasional epithelial and inflammatory cells. It starts accumulating within minutes on a clean tooth surface Plaque may be difficult to see with the naked eye and the use of plaque-disclosing solutions (dyes that stain plaque) is recommended for visualization.

animal (Nyman et al. 1986) and human (Nyman et al. 1988; Mombelli et al. 1995) studies that have shown that the removal of subgingival plaque on top of subgingival calculus will result in healing of periodontal lesions and the maintenance of healthy periodontal tissues.

PATHOGENESIS

The pathogenic mechanisms involved in periodontal disease include:

* Direct injury by plaque microorganisms
* Indirect injury by plaque microorganisms via inflammation.

The microbiota in periodontal pockets is in a continual state of flux; periodontitis is a dynamic infection caused by a combination of bacterial vectors that change over time. As a result, the molecular events that trigger and sustain the inflammatory reactions constantly change. Many microbial products have little or no direct toxic effect on the host. However, they possess the potential to activate non-immune and immune inflammatory reactions that cause the tissue damage. It is now well accepted that *it is the host's response to the plaque bacteria, rather than microbial virulence* per se *that directly causes the tissue damage* (Kinane and Lindhe 1997).

In gingivitis, the plaque-induced inflammation is limited to the soft tissue of the gingiva (Fig. 9.1A). Sulcus

depths are normal (i.e. periodontal probing depths are 1–3 mm in the dog and 0.5–1.0 mm in the cat). As periodontitis occurs (Fig. 9.1C), the inflammatory destruction of the coronal part of the periodontal ligament allows apical migration of the epithelial attachment and the formation of a pathologic periodontal pocket (i.e. periodontal probing depths increase). If the inflammatory disease is permitted to progress, the crestal portion of the alveolar process begins to resorb. Alveolar bone destruction type and extent are diagnosed radiographically. The resorption may proceed apically on a horizontal level. Horizontal bone destruction is often accompanied by gingival recession, so periodontal pockets may not form (Fig. 9.1D). If there is no gingival recession, the periodontal pocket is supra-alveolar, i.e. above the level of the alveolar margin. The pattern of bone destruction may also proceed in a vertical direction along the root to form angular bony defects. The periodontal pocket is now intra- or subalveolar, i.e. below the level of the crestal bone.

Disease progression is generally an episodic occurrence rather than a continuous process. Tissue destruction occurs as acute bursts of disease activity followed by relatively quiescent periods. The acute burst is clinically characterized by rapid deepening of the periodontal pocket as periodontal ligament fibers and alveolar bone are destroyed by the inflammatory reactions. The quiescent phase is not associated with clinical or radiographic evidence of disease progression. However, complete healing does not occur during this quiescent phase, because subgingival plaque remains on the root surfaces and inflammation persists in the connective tissue. The inactive phase can last for extended periods.

Other conditions, such as physical or psychologic stress and malnutrition, may impair protective responses such as the production of antioxidants and acute phase proteins, and can aggravate periodontitis but do not actually cause destructive tissue inflammation. A genetic predisposition to destructive inflammation of the periodontium may be important in some individuals. In humans, a strong association has been observed between the severity of periodontitis and a specific genotype of the interleukin-1 (IL-1) gene cluster (Kornman et al. 1997). Patients carrying this periodontitis-associated genotype may demonstrate phenotypic differences, as indicated by elevated levels of IL-1β in gingival sulcular (crevicular) fluid (Engebretson et al. 1999). No similar data are available for the dog or cat.

Significance

Undisturbed plaque accumulation results in gingivitis. While some individuals with untreated gingivitis will develop periodontitis, not all untreated animals will do so. It cannot be predicted which individuals with gingivitis will develop periodontitis. However, animals in which clinically healthy gingivae are maintained will not develop periodontitis. Consequently, *the aim in periodontal disease prevention and treatment is to establish and maintain clinically healthy gingivae to prevent periodontitis.*

DIAGNOSIS

General considerations

Diagnosis of periodontal disease relies on clinical examination of the periodontium in the anesthetized animal. In addition, radiography is mandatory if there is evidence of periodontitis on clinical examination. It is essential to differentiate between gingivitis and periodontitis in order to institute appropriate treatment. In individuals with gingivitis, the aim is to restore the tissues to clinical health; in individuals with established periodontitis, the aim of therapy is to prevent progression of disease.

Oral examination and recording of findings are detailed in Chapter 6.

The following parameters need to be assessed and recorded for *each tooth* in *all patients*:

1. Gingivitis and gingival index
2. Periodontal probing depth (PPD)
3. Gingival recession (GR)
4. Furcation involvement
5. Mobility.

Periodontal probing depth, gingival recession, furcation involvement and mobility measure the extent of destruction of the periodontium, i.e. assess the presence and severity of periodontitis.

I do not assess and record the extent of plaque and calculus accumulation in patients that are seen for the first time. These deposits will be removed during periodontal therapy. Instead, I assess and record plaque at follow-up visits to assess the efficacy of the homecare regimen that has been instituted. Plaque accumulation is visualized using a plaque-disclosing solution and the teeth that have plaque at the gingival margin are noted and recorded. The amount of plaque is graded subjectively as mild, moderate or severe depending on the depth of staining achieved by the plaque-disclosing solution.

Gingivitis

Gingivitis is defined as a *reversible* plaque-induced inflammation limited to the gingiva (i.e. no loss of periodontal attachment).

Clinical signs and diagnostic methods

Gingivitis manifests clinically as swelling, reddening and often bleeding of the gingival margin (Fig. 9.3). It may be accompanied by halitosis. It is diagnosed clinically by means of a combination of visual inspection and tactile examination. The presence and degree of gingival inflammation is assessed based on a combination of redness and swelling, as well as presence or absence of bleeding on gentle probing of the gingival sulcus. Various indices can be used to give a numerical value to the degree of gingival inflammation present. In the clinical situation, a simple bleeding index may be the most useful. Using this method the gingival sulcus of each tooth is gently probed at several points and given a score of 0 if there is no bleeding and a score of 1 if the probing elicits bleeding. The patient with uncomplicated gingivitis will have normal periodontal probing depths (1–3 mm in the dog and 0.5–1.0 mm in the cat) and show no evidence of gingival recession, furcation involvement or tooth mobility. Radiography is not mandatory if the clinical examination reveals no evidence of periodontal destruction, i.e. periodontitis.

Gingival hyperplasia (Figs 9.1B, 9.4) may be the result of plaque-induced inflammation, i.e. hyperplastic gingivitis. It may also be of idiopathic or familial origin, and it can be induced by certain drugs, e.g. hydantoin, ciclosporins. Gingival hyperplasia is common in some breeds, e.g. Boxer, Springer Spaniel. There is an increase in periodontal probing depths owing to the gingival overgrowth.

Consequences to affected animal

Uncomplicated gingivitis is generally not associated with discomfort or pain in humans. In fact, it is an insidious process and the patient may be unaware of its existence.

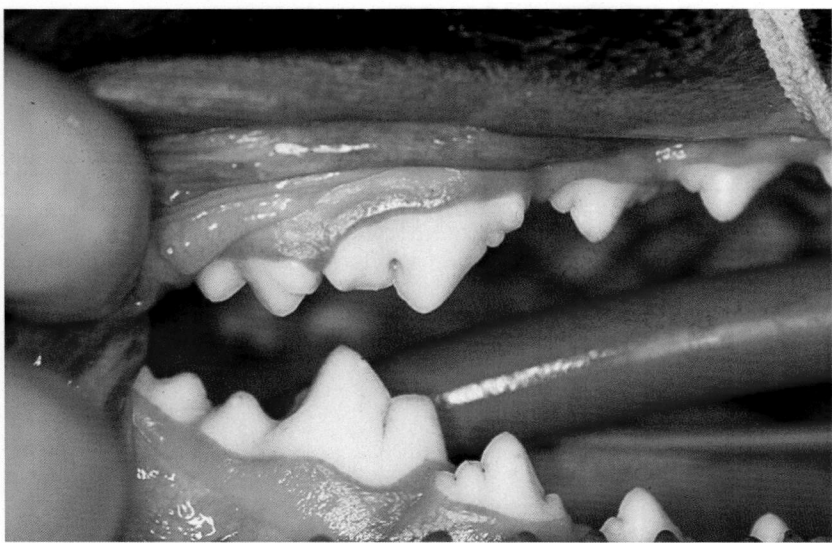

Fig. 9.3 Gingivitis Gingivitis manifests clinically as swelling and reddening of the gingival margin.

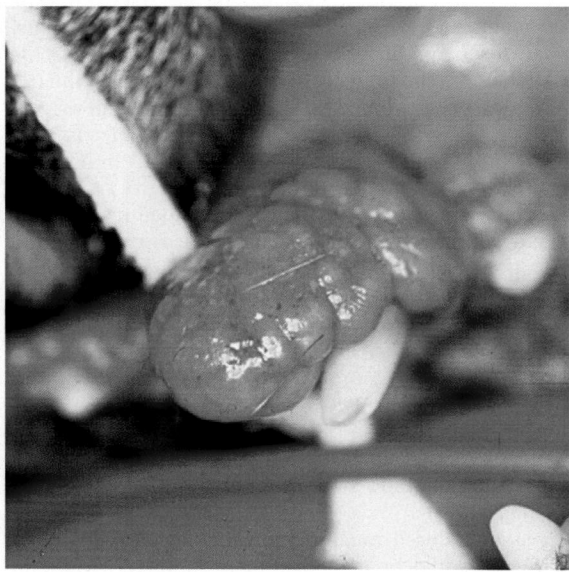

Fig. 9.4 Gingival hyperplasia The hyperplastic gingival tissue almost covers the crowns, resulting in the formation of pseudopockets.

The significance of gingivitis is that, if untreated, periodontitis may develop, as described earlier.

Gingival hyperplasia does pose an additional concern. The hyperplastic gingiva alters the position of the gingival margin and results in a false or pseudopocket. It is called a pseudopocket because the increased periodontal probing depth is not due to destruction of periodontal ligament and alveolar bone with apical migration of the junctional epithelium, as in periodontitis. Instead, the increased periodontal probing depth is due to the overgrowth of the gingiva. The presence of hyperplastic gingiva compromises tooth cleaning and may predispose to periodontitis. Radiography, to identify and thus treat concurrent periodontitis, is mandatory for patients with gingival hyperplasia.

Periodontitis

Individuals with untreated gingivitis *may* develop periodontitis. The inflammatory reactions in periodontitis result in destruction of the periodontal ligament and alveolar bone. The result of untreated periodontitis is eventually exfoliation of the affected tooth. It is important to remember that periodontitis is a *site-specific disease*, i.e. it may affect one or more sites of one or several teeth. Periodontitis can generally be considered irreversible. *The aim of treatment is thus to prevent development of new lesions at other sites and to prevent further tissue destruction at sites which are already affected.*

Clinical signs

Halitosis is common and is often the first sign noted by the pet owner. Large amounts of dental deposits are usually present. These deposits need to be removed to allow a detailed examination of the periodontium. Ulcers affecting mucous membranes of lips and cheeks may be present in areas where these tissues are exposed to plaque-covered tooth surfaces (Fig. 9.5).

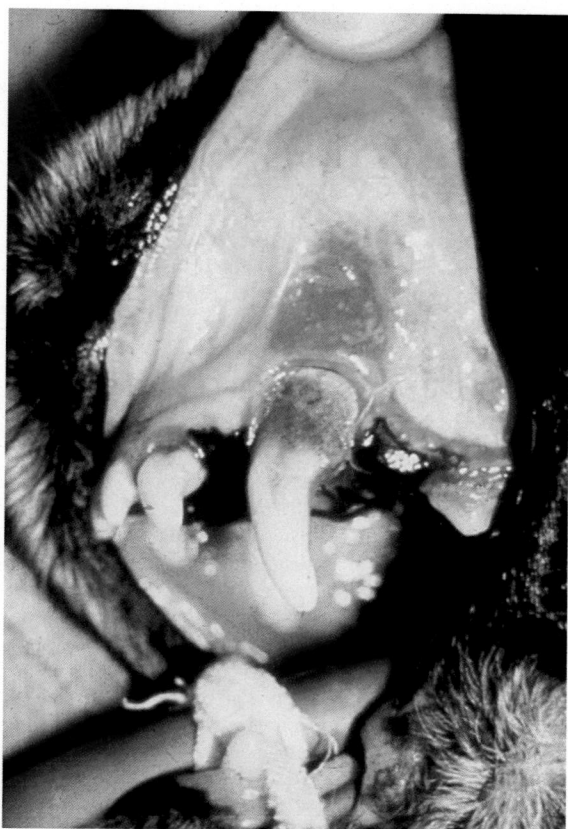

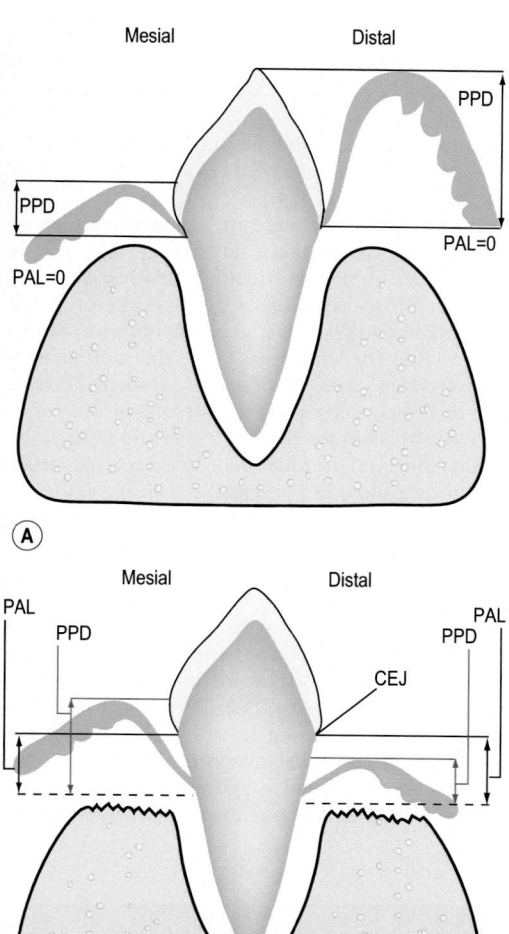

Fig. 9.5 Gingival recession and mucous membrane ulceration The periodontal ligament and alveolar bone on the labial aspect of the left upper canine has been destroyed. The gingival margin has receded. Periodontal probing depth is 1 mm, i.e. there is no pathologic pocket. A mucous membrane ulcer has developed on the lip surface that is in contact with the plaque-covered tooth surface. *Note*: While uncomplicated periodontitis is not associated with severe discomfort, these mucous membrane ulcers are known to be painful.

Diagnostic methods

Tissue destruction in periodontitis is assessed by measuring periodontal probing depth, gingival recession, furcation involvement and degree of tooth mobility. In many cases, measuring or calculating the periodontal attachment level (PAL) is also useful. The PPD is not necessarily correlated with severity of attachment loss (Fig. 9.6). Gingival hyperplasia may contribute to a deep pocket (or pseudopocket if there is no attachment loss), while gingival recession may result in the absence of a pocket but also minimal remaining attachment. PAL records the distance from the cemento-enamel junction (or from a fixed point on the tooth) to the base or apical extension of the

Fig. 9.6 Attachment loss (A) The epithelial attachment on both sides of the tooth is at the cemento-enamel junction (CEJ), so there is no loss of periodontal attachment (PAL = 0). The surface labeled mesial depicts normal gingival attachment; periodontal probing depth (PPD) is 1–2 mm. The surface labeled distal has an increased PPD, e.g. 8 mm. However, this is not periodontitis as there has been no loss of periodontal support. (B) PPD on the surface labeled mesial is increased, e.g. 6 mm. PPD on the side labeled distal is normal, i.e. 1–2 mm, due to the gingival recession. PAL, i.e. the extent of periodontal ligament and alveolar bone destruction, is the same.

pathologic pocket. It is thus a more accurate assessment of tissue loss in periodontitis. PAL can either be measured with a periodontal probe or it can be calculated (e.g. PPD + gingival recession).

Radiography to assess the type and extent of alveolar bone destruction is mandatory for periodontitis patients. Consequently, full mouth radiographs should be performed prior to the institution of any therapy. In addition, radiographs need to be taken at regular intervals to monitor outcome of any treatment. A detailed examination of the periodontal ligament space and interproximal alveolar margin requires the use of an intraoral radiographic technique (detailed in Ch. 7). The radiographic changes associated with periodontal disease include resorption of the alveolar margin, widening of the periodontal space, a break in the path or loss of the radiopacity of the lamina dura and destruction of alveolar bone resulting in supra- or infrabony pockets.

Radiographs using a parallel technique (see Ch. 7) will demonstrate more accurately the features of periodontitis because this technique provides a better view of the alveolar margin and reveals more accurately the actual extent or depth of the periodontal lesion in relation to the root of the tooth. Radiographs produced with a bisecting angle technique may show greater destruction of the alveolar bone than is actually present, because the central ray is directed obliquely to the long axis of the teeth and jaw, which produces dimensional distortion. Moreover, with the bisecting angle technique, subgingival calculus may be superimposed on alveolar bone and would thus not be detected. Views taken using a parallel technique will demonstrate deposits of subgingival calculus and defects of the cementum but may not cover a sufficient area to demonstrate extensive periodontitis lesions adequately. In the maxilla and anterior mandible, bisecting angle and parallel views of the same region may be required to visualize the extent of the tissue destruction more accurately.

As periodontitis develops, the crestal portion of the alveolar process begins to resorb. Radiographically, the destruction is evident as a cup-shaped notch or as scalloping of the alveolar margin. The resorption may proceed apically on a horizontal level (Fig. 9.7). Beyond this, the lamina dura appears to be normal and there is no widening of the periodontal space. Horizontal bone destruction (Fig. 9.1D) is often accompanied by gingival recession (Fig. 9.5), so periodontal pockets may not form. If there is no gingival recession, the periodontal pocket is supra-alveolar, i.e. above the level of the alveolar margin. The pattern of bone destruction may also proceed in a vertical direction along the root to form angular bony defects. Radiographically these are usually evidenced by a vertical or V-shaped flaw, with the root of the tooth forming one side of the defect (Fig. 9.8). The periodontal pocket is now infra- or subalveolar, i.e. below the level of the crestal bone (Fig. 9.1C).

Infrabony defects are diagnosed by a combination of exploration with a periodontal probe (the probe meets the firm resistance of bone when angled away from the tooth) and radiography. They are described by depth and by the extent of the bony circumference involved. The

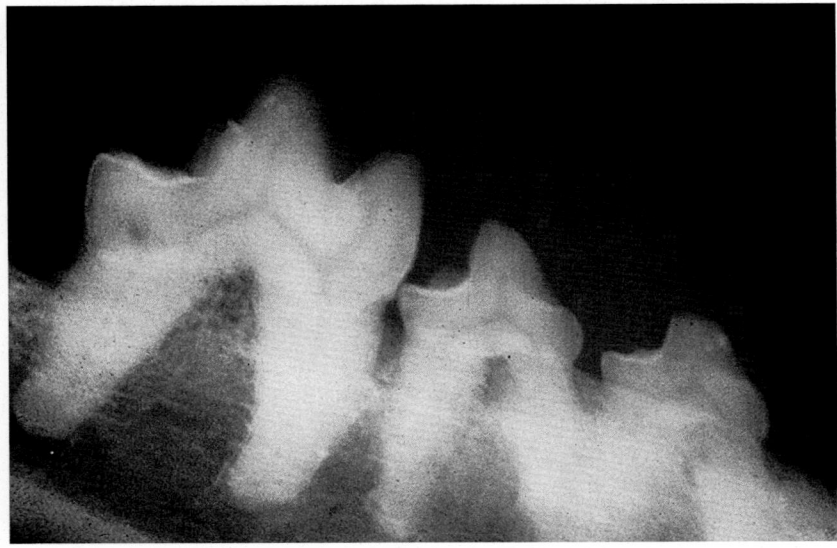

Fig. 9.7 Horizontal bone loss In this dog, resorption of the alveolar bone has proceeded apically in a horizontal fashion. The right mandibular 3rd premolar is unaffected, i.e. the height of the alveolar margin is normal. The right mandibular 4th premolar and 1st molar have lost around 2 mm of alveolar bone.

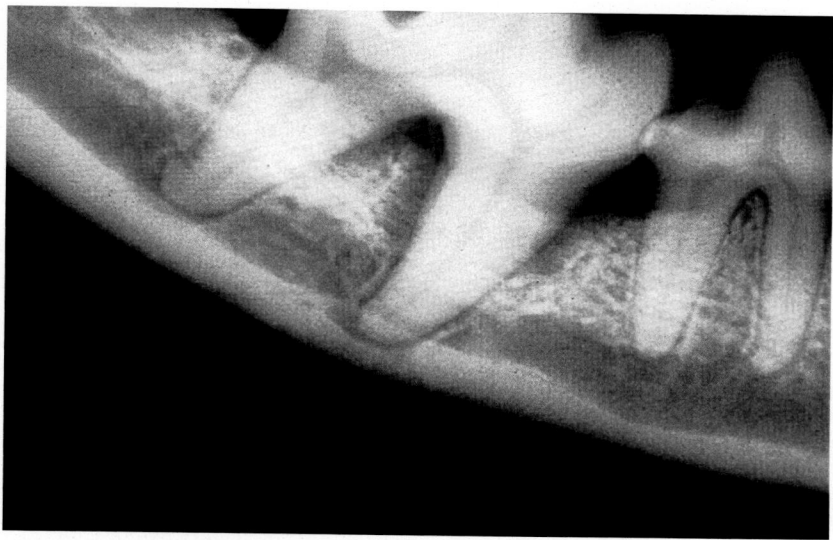

Fig. 9.8 Vertical bone loss The pattern of bone destruction has proceeded in a vertical direction along the root to form angular bony defects at the mesial and distal aspects of the mesial root of the right mandibular 1st molar tooth and at the mesial aspect of the distal root of the same tooth.

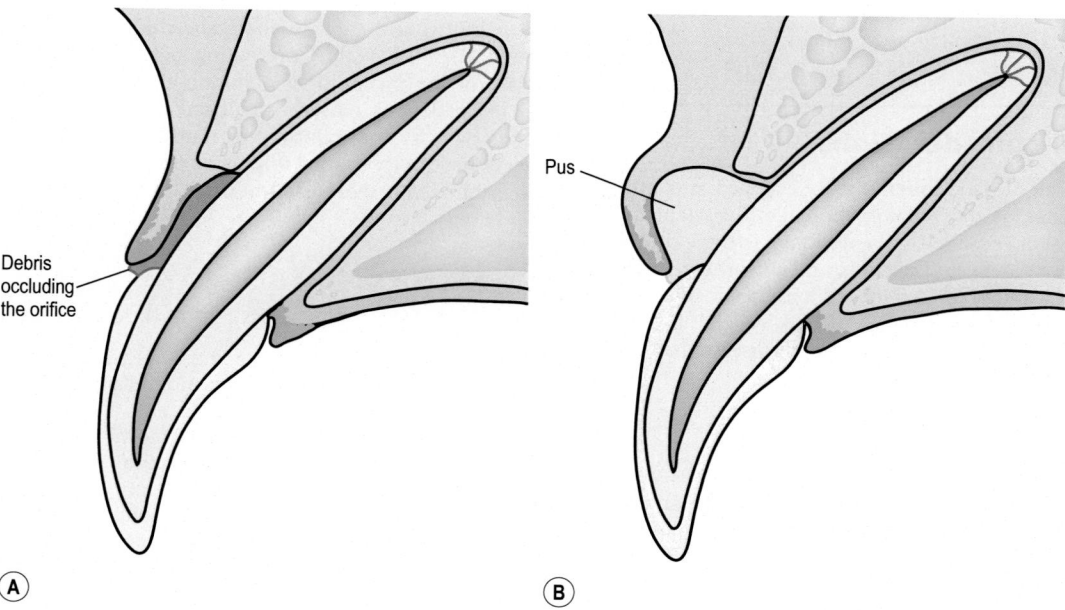

Debris
occluding
the orifice

Pus

(A)   (B)

Fig. 9.9 The formation of a lateral periodontal abscess (A) Occlusion of the orifice of an existing periodontal pocket. (B) An abscess has formed.

surrounding alveolar bone is thought of as forming four walls (mesial, buccal, distal, palatal/lingual). When bone is present around the entire circumference of the pocket, a four-wall defect is present. When bone is missing on one face, a three-wall defect is present. Two- and one-wall defects have two and three surfaces of the tooth root without bony support, respectively.

A periodontal abscess is an acute exacerbation of the process occurring in a chronic periodontal pocket (Fig. 9.9). It usually occurs from partial or complete obstruction of the orifice of the pocket. Multiple acute periodontal abscesses may occur in some cases of advanced generalized periodontitis. An abscess may also develop in the healthy periodontium if a foreign body is forced beyond the epithelial attachment. Grass seeds embedded in the gingival sulcus have been identified as causing acute periodontal abscessation in the dog. The acute periodontal abscess may produce rapid and extensive bone loss. In some instances, the bone loss will extend beyond the apices of the roots of the teeth.

Consequences to affected animal

Based on feedback from human patients, uncomplicated periodontitis is not associated with severe pain or discomfort. In contrast, complications such as the development of a lateral periodontal abscess or ulcers in the mucous membranes are very painful.

It has been shown that a severe infection in the oral cavity, as with extensive periodontitis, will lead to a transient bacteremia on chewing (Thoden van Velzen et al. 1984). In fact, an association has been demonstrated between periodontal disease and histopathologic changes in kidney, myocardium, and liver in the dog (DeBowes et al. 1996).

TREATMENT

General considerations

The treatment of periodontal disease is aimed at controlling the cause of the inflammation, i.e. dental plaque. Conservative or cause-related periodontal therapy consists of removal of plaque and calculus, and any other remedial procedures required, under general anesthesia, in combination with daily maintenance of oral hygiene. In other words, the treatment of periodontal disease has two components:

1. Maintenance of oral hygiene
2. Professional periodontal therapy.

Maintenance of oral hygiene is performed by the owner and is often called homecare. Its effectiveness depends on the motivation and technical ability of the owner and the cooperation of the animal. Homecare is detailed in Chapter 10.

Professional periodontal therapy is performed under general anesthesia and includes:

- Supra- and subgingival scaling
- Root planing
- Tooth crown polishing
- Subgingival lavage
- Sometimes periodontal surgery.

The term 'dental prophylaxis' or 'prophy' has been used to encompass clinical examination and professional periodontal therapy. This is misleading since the real prophylaxis, i.e. steps taken to prevent disease development and progression, is not the professional periodontal therapy carried out under general anesthesia but the daily homecare regime to remove plaque. If no homecare is instituted, then plaque will rapidly reform after a professional periodontal therapy procedure and the disease will progress. Before any treatment is instituted, the owner must be made aware that homecare is the most essential component in both preventing and treating periodontal disease. Whenever possible it is useful to institute a homecare programme before any professional periodontal therapy is performed.

The aim of treatment differs whether the patient has gingivitis only or whether the patient also has periodontitis.

Gingivitis

Gingivitis is, by definition, reversible. Removal or adequate reduction of plaque will restore inflamed gingivae to health. Once clinically healthy gingivae have been achieved, these can be maintained by daily removal or reduction in the accumulation of plaque. In short, the treatment of gingivitis is to restore the inflamed tissues to clinical health and then to maintain clinically healthy gingivae (Fig. 9.10), thus preventing periodontitis. The purpose of the professional periodontal therapy in the gingivitis patient is removal of dental deposits, mainly calculus (which is not removed by toothbrushing). Once the teeth have been cleaned it remains up to the owner to remove the plaque that re-accumulates on a daily basis.

SUMMARY FOR TREATMENT OF GINGIVITIS

- ◆ Educate the owner to understand the disease process.
- ◆ Train and motivate the owner to perform daily homecare.
- ◆ Institute daily homecare regimen by the owner – ideally, toothbrushing with a pet toothpaste in conjunction with a dental hygiene product.
- ◆ Professional periodontal therapy (supra- and subgingival scaling and polishing) under general anesthesia to remove dental deposits (plaque and calculus).
- ◆ Regular check-ups to ensure that the owner is following recommendations and to boost the owner's motivation.

Periodontitis

Untreated gingivitis may progress to periodontitis. In most instances in a practice situation, periodontitis is

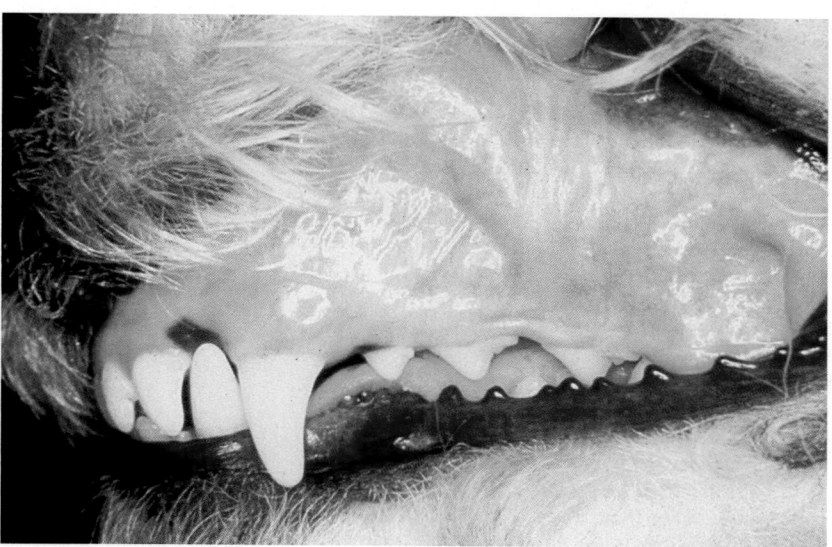

Fig. 9.10 Clinically healthy gingivae With good homecare, clinically healthy gingivae can be maintained for the life span of the animal. An animal with clinically healthy gingivae will not develop periodontitis.

irreversible. It is important to remember that periodontitis is a site-specific disease, i.e. it may affect one or more sites of one or several teeth. The aim of treatment is thus to prevent development of new lesions at other sites and to prevent further tissue destruction at sites which are already affected.

Professional periodontal therapy removes dental deposits above and below the gingival margin. It then rests with the owner to ensure that plaque does not re-accumulate. Meticulous supragingival plaque control, by means of daily toothbrushing and adjunctive antiseptics when indicated, will prevent migration of the plaque below the gingival margin. If the subgingival tooth surfaces are kept clean, the sulcular epithelium will reattach.

In patients with suspected periodontitis, I recommend instituting daily toothbrushing 3–4 weeks prior to the planned professional periodontal therapy if the animal will allow it. This will result in less inflamed tissue at the time of professional therapy and will allow assessment of the ability of the owner to perform homecare. If homecare is not possible, the professional treatment will need to be more radical, e.g. extraction of teeth that could potentially have been retained with good homecare.

The term 'periodontal surgery' is used to encompass specific surgical techniques aimed at achieving normal anatomic relationships to allow optimal homecare. The techniques allow reattachment or regeneration of periodontal attachment. Periodontal surgery includes various flap procedures, gingivoplasty, guided tissue regeneration and implants. Periodontal surgery is never first-line treatment for periodontal disease. Conservative management of periodontal disease, i.e. a thorough supra- and subgingival scale, root planing, polishing and irrigation in combination with daily meticulous homecare, is the first step. Periodontal surgery should only be performed where the owner has shown the ability to keep the mouth clean. If a client cannot maintain good oral hygiene measures in their pet then in the interest of the wellbeing of the animal there is no indication for surgery.

SUMMARY FOR TREATMENT OF PERIODONTITIS

◆ Educate the owner to understand the disease process.
◆ Train and motivate the owner to perform daily homecare.
◆ Institute daily toothbrushing regimen by the owner.
◆ Professional periodontal therapy: this includes supra and subgingival scaling and polishing, root planing and extraction of unsalvageable teeth under general anesthesia.
◆ Regular check-ups to ensure that the owner is following recommendations and to boost the owner's motivation.
◆ Periodontal surgery may be indicated, but only if optimal homecare is in place.

PROFESSIONAL PERIODONTAL THERAPY

General considerations

Professional periodontal therapy must be performed under general anesthesia. Anesthesia and special care of the patient undergoing dentistry and/or oral surgery is covered in Chapter 2. The basic instrument requirements for periodontal therapy are covered in Chapter 1. Antibiotics should not be used to treat periodontal disease in the absence of mechanical debridement. The prudent use of antibiotics and antiseptics is detailed in Chapter 3.

The degree of discomfort or pain caused by dental and/or oral surgery procedures is usually not considered. Domestic pets have a dental anatomy and nerve paths similar to our own. Their perception of pain may well be different but a reasonable assumption is to assume that procedures that cause discomfort in humans are likely to do the same in dogs and cats. The recommended use of analgesics is covered in Chapter 2.

To master the technical skills required for dentistry and oral surgery, attending practical courses is recommended. In general, dental instruments are held in a modified pen grip (Fig. 9.11A) and the 4th and 5th fingers are placed on adjacent structures (neighboring teeth, opposite jaw) for stability and support. A periosteal elevator may be worked using a modified pen grip, or it can be held as depicted in Figure 9.11B.

The procedures

Supragingival scaling

Supragingival scaling is the removal of plaque and calculus above the gingival margin. It can be performed using hand instruments alone or a combination of hand instruments and powered scalers.

The recommended procedure is as follows:

1. Remove gross dental deposits (plaque-covered calculus) using rongeurs, extraction forceps or calculus-removing forceps (Fig. 9.12).
2. Remove residual supragingival dental deposits with sharp hand instruments (either a sickle-shaped scaler or a curette), as demonstrated in Figure 9.13.
3. A powered scaler (either an ultrasonic or a sonic scaler) is then used to remove residual dental deposits (Fig. 9.14).

Powered scalers generate heat and have the potential to cause iatrogenic damage if not used properly. Overheating a tooth will cause desiccation of the dentine and consequent damage to the underlying pulp tissue. Pulp damage may be a reversible pulpitis but it can become severe enough to cause pulp necrosis, which would necessitate endodontic treatment of the affected tooth. The etiology

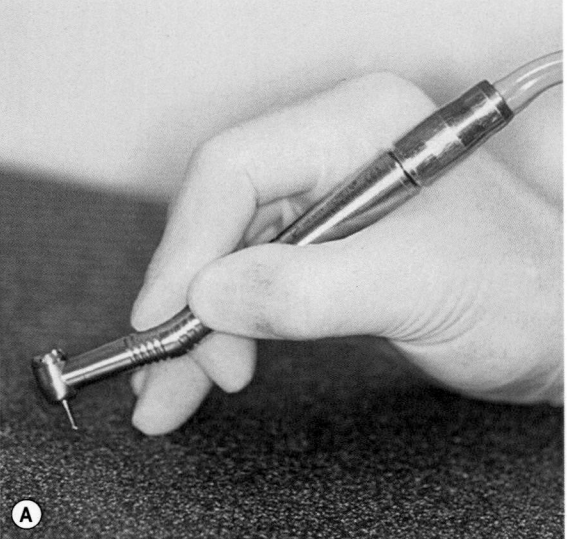

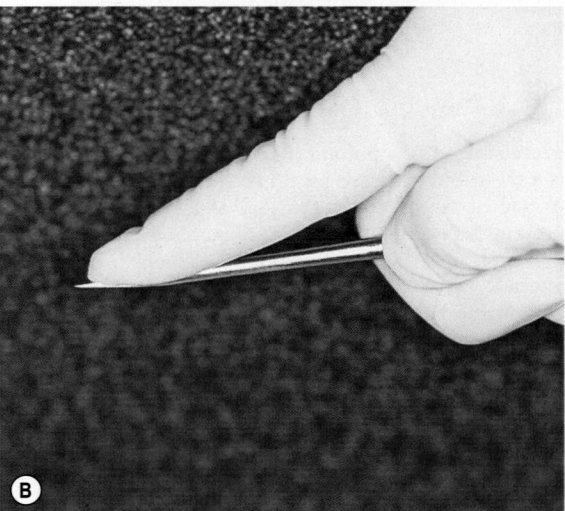

Fig. 9.11 How to hold dental instruments (A) Dental instruments are generally held using a modified pen grip, as depicted here. Resting the 4th and 5th fingers on adjacent structures gives stability and support, reducing the risk of slippage and iatrogenic injuries. (B) Periosteal elevators can be held using either the modified pen grip or as depicted. The advantage of grasping the instrument handle inside the palm of the hand and placing your index finger close to the working end is that should you slip your index finger will stop the slippage and minimize iatrogenic damage.

and pathogenesis of pulp and periapical disease are covered in Chapter 8.

An ultrasonic or sonic scaler should be used by gently stroking the tooth with the side of the tip and with continuous movement over the tooth surface. A plentiful

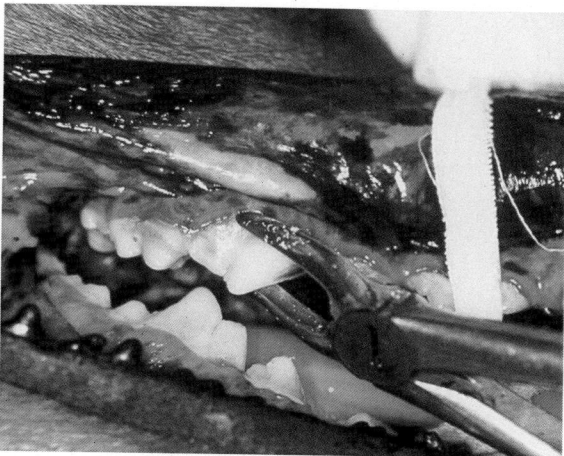

Fig. 9.12 Removing gross supragingival dental deposits with extraction forceps Do not traumatize the gingival margin with the forceps.

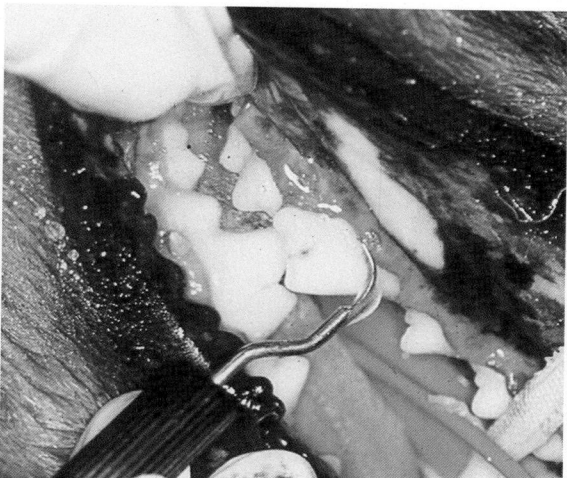

Fig. 9.14 Removing supragingival dental deposits with an ultrasonic scaler The use of a fine perio (sickle, universal) insert is recommended for both ultrasonic and sonic scalers.

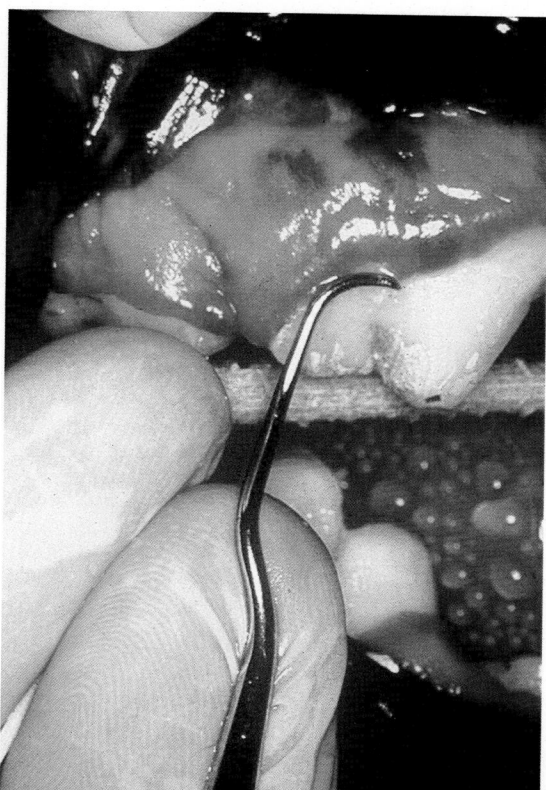

Fig. 9.13 Removing supragingival dental deposits with hand instruments Here, a universal scaler is being used to remove calculus.

supply of water is essential to cool the oscillating tip and flush away debris. Using the tip of the instrument or applying excessive pressure will cause gouging of the tooth surface as well as generating excessive heat. As an arbitrary rule, it is suggested that no more than 15 s of continuous scaling should be performed on any one tooth. If the tooth is not clean in that period of time, then return to it after scaling a few other teeth. This will allow the original tooth time to cool down.

Both sonic and ultrasonic scalers should be used with a thin pointed tip, sometimes called a perio, sickle or universal insert. The large (wide) tip is not recommended. A fine tip will remove dental deposits more accurately, with less likelihood of damage to the tooth enamel.

Subgingival scaling and root planing

Subgingival scaling is the removal of plaque, calculus and other debris from the tooth surface below the gingival margin, i.e. within the gingival sulcus or periodontal pocket. There is no need to perform extensive subgingival scaling if there is no calculus below the gingival margin. However, the presence of subgingival deposits should always be investigated with a dental explorer and removed if any are identified. Root planing is the removal of the superficial layer of toxin-laden cementum from the root surfaces. Root planing produces a smooth root surface which is less likely to accumulate plaque and more likely to permit epithelial reattachment. The healing process after subgingival scaling and root planing is depicted diagrammatically in Figure 9.15. Scaling and planing are achieved simultaneously using a curette. The procedure can be performed using either a closed (without raising an

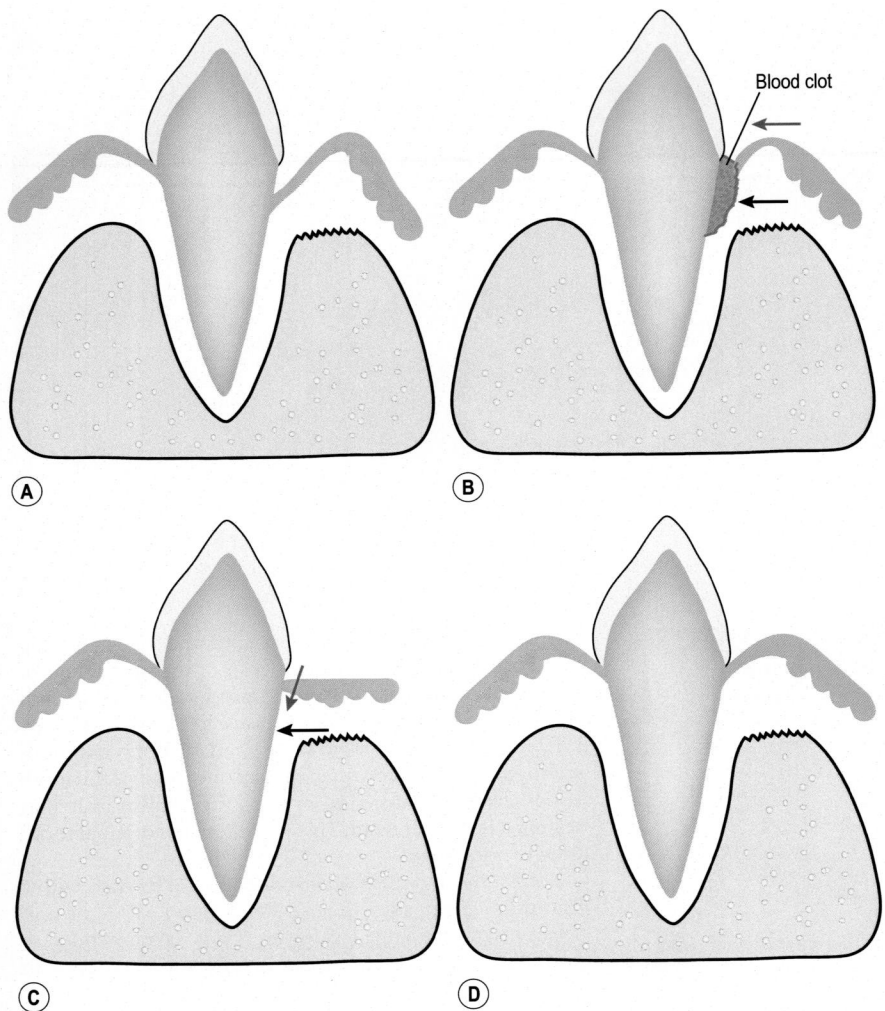

Fig. 9.15 Healing after subgingival debridement (A) Before subgingival debridement. (B) Irrespective of whether a closed or open technique has been used for subgingival debridement, the epithelial attachment and pocket epithelium will have been removed during the procedure and a blood clot will have formed between the tooth and the connective tissue of the gingiva. As healing starts both the epithelium and connective tissue are activated. The oral gingival epithelium will start to grow across to cover the exposed connective tissue (red arrow) and the connective tissue starts to form a new attachment with the clean root surface (black arrow). (C) Once the oral epithelium has reached the tooth surface it will start to grow apically (red arrow) and the situation becomes a race between the epithelium growing apically and the connective tissue attaching to the root surface (black arrow). The result of the race will determine at which level the epithelium's apical attachment will be. (D) The final stage of the healing process is the reformation of the normal epithelial attachment and gingival sulcus.

access flap) or open (raising an access flap) technique. An open technique is recommended for pockets deeper than 4 mm, as it is difficult even for a skilled operator to ensure that all subgingival deposits have been removed without raising a gingival flap for direct access and visualization. However, an open technique is only indicated in patients with proven sufficient homecare, i.e. it is not first-line treatment.

Ultrasonic and sonic scalers are designed for supragingival work. Once inserted into the gingival sulcus or periodontal pocket the water will no longer reach to cool the tip. This then results in thermal damage of both hard and soft tissues. Quick subgingival excursions are permissible only if the gingiva is edematous, or held mechanically out of the way to allow the water to reach the tip. Scalers with specially designed working tips where the water exits at the very end are safer to use under the gingival margin, but the removal of established subgingival deposits can only be adequately performed with meticulous use of sharp curettes. The curette has a sharp working or cutting edge on the curved blade and has a rounded tip. Most curettes are double ended. They are used as a pair to enable instrumentation of the whole root circumference. Many different sizes and shapes are available. My preferred curettes are the Gracey 7/8 and the Columbia 13/14.

Closed subgingival debridement. The procedure for closed subgingival debridement is as follows:

1. The curette is inserted to the bottom of the gingival sulcus or periodontal pocket without engaging the cutting edges of the instrument (Fig. 9.16A).
2. The cutting edges of the instrument are then engaged against the tooth root and sulcular epithelium and the curette is pulled out of the sulcus or periodontal pocket in this position (Fig. 9.16B).
3. The instrument is moved circumferentially around the tooth using overlapping vertical strokes. Oblique or horizontal strokes are also used, particularly in the furcation area of multirooted teeth.

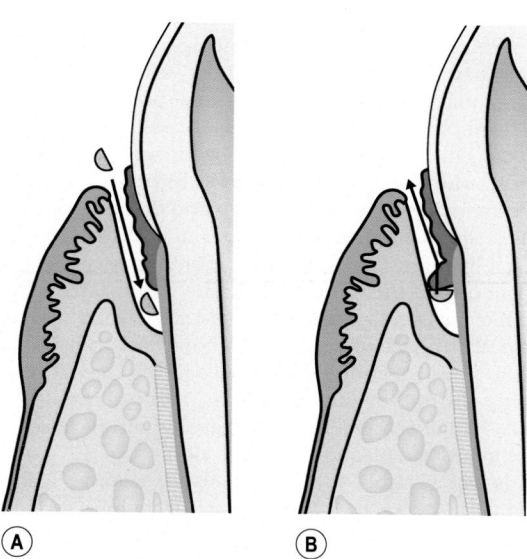

Fig. 9.16 Procedure for closed subgingival debridement (A) The curette is inserted to the bottom of the periodontal pocket without engaging the cutting edges of the instrument. (B) The cutting edges of the curette are then engaged (by turning the handle of the instrument) against the root surface and pocket epithelium and the curette is pulled out of the pocket in this position. The instrument is worked in this way around the whole circumference of the tooth using overlapping strokes (mainly vertical, but oblique and horizontal strokes are also used, particularly in the furcation area of multirooted teeth).

4. The process is repeated around all the teeth.
5. A dental explorer is run over the root surface (Fig. 9.17) to ensure that all deposits have been removed. The instrument will catch against or skip over any areas of remaining calculus, which must be removed.

A curette with two cutting edges will also remove the sulcular lining. Removing the inflamed sulcular epithelium is called subgingival curettage. It has been shown that subgingival curettage is not essential in controlling periodontal disease. The vital step is the removal of all subgingival deposits, i.e. subgingival scaling, and restoring the root surface to smoothness, i.e. root planing.

Subgingival debridement (scaling and root planing) takes time. A thorough procedure in an animal with extensive pocketing and subgingival deposits may well take an hour and often more. It must be emphasized that removing subgingival plaque, calculus and debris as well as the superficial layer of toxin-laden cementum and restoring the root surfaces to smoothness is a most important step. Removing only the supragingival debris at a periodontitis site does not have any therapeutic benefit. It will not prevent disease progression as the cause of the disease, namely subgingival plaque, is still present.

Open subgingival debridement. The procedure for open subgingival debridement (Fig. 9.18) is as follows:

1. The epithelial attachment is cut by inserting a scalpel blade (No. 11 or 15) into the gingival sulcus, pointing apically, and cutting down to the level of the crestal bone. Using the scalpel blade in a handle gives better control.
2. Vertical releasing incisions are made at either end of the primary incision.
3. The attached gingiva is freed from the underlying periosteum using a periosteal elevator. The flap

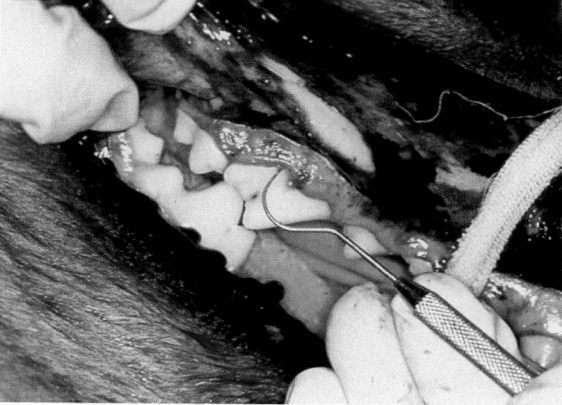

Fig. 9.17 Checking adequacy of subgingival debridement A dental explorer is inserted below the gingival margin and run over the root surface to identify the presence of residual subgingival calculus, which needs to be removed.

111

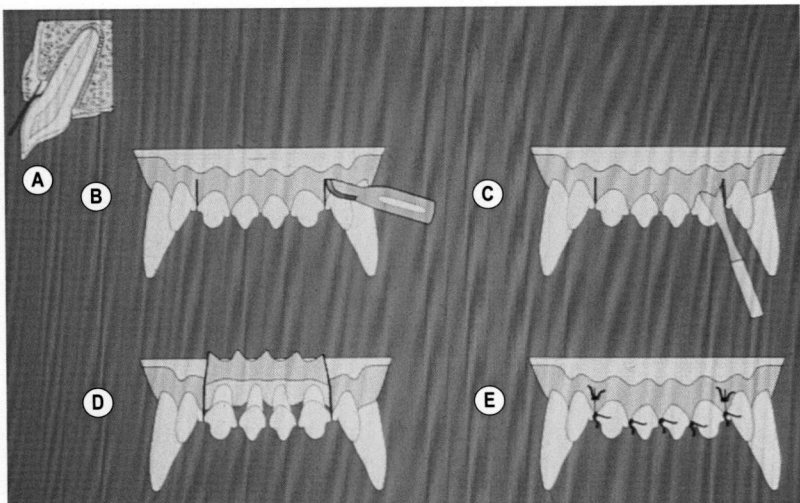

Fig. 9.18 Procedure for open subgingival debridement (A) Cutting the epithelial attachment. (B) Releasing incisions are made on either side of the primary incision. (C) A periosteal elevator is used to free the attached gingiva from the underlying periosteum. (D) The flap is gently retracted to expose the root surfaces and alveolar bone. The exposed root surfaces can now be scaled and polished. Minor osteoplasty can also be performed. (E) The flap is replaced and sutured in its original position.

should generally not be raised beyond the mucogingival line.

4. The flap is gently retracted to expose the root surfaces and the alveolar bone. The gingival flap should be handled gently throughout the procedure.

5. The exposed root surfaces can now be scaled, using either hand instruments or a combination of hand instruments and powered scalers, and then polished. Minor osteoplasty, e.g. removing sharp bony spicules, can be carried out using either bone-cutting forceps or a bur in a slow- or high-speed hand piece with copious water cooling.

6. The area is flushed clean using either saline or dilute chlorhexidine solution, and the flap replaced and sutured in its original position. The buccal flap is joined to the palatal or lingual gingiva by means of simple interrupted sutures placed in the interproximal spaces. The releasing incisions are sutured. The suture material should be resorbable. The use of a swaged on needle is recommended to avoid tearing the gingiva.

Polishing

Scaling, even when done correctly, will cause minor scratches of the tooth. A rough surface will facilitate plaque retention. Polishing smoothes this roughness and helps remove any remaining plaque and stained pellicle.

Polishing is performed by applying a mildly abrasive prophylaxis paste to the tooth surface with a prophylaxis cup mounted in a slowly rotating low-speed hand piece. The hand piece should be running at less than 1000 rpm to avoid generating excessive heat by friction. The amount of heat, which can easily result from incorrect polishing, can certainly cause severe pulpal pathology. A surplus of paste is applied to the tooth surface in a soft rubber cup using a light force, i.e. just enough force to cause the cup to flare out on the tooth surface. The prophylaxis cup is kept moving over the entire tooth surface for a few seconds per tooth. The flared edge of the prophylaxis cup can be used to polish slightly subgingivally, taking care to avoid causing any further gingival damage. This is illustrated in Figure 9.19. It is useful to check that all tooth surfaces are clean by using a plaque-disclosing solution.

It is not possible to polish the root surfaces within subgingival pockets (unless an open technique for sub-gingival debridement is used), so their smoothness must be assured by thorough (but not overzealous) root planing.

Sulcular lavage

Sulcular lavage involves gently flushing the gingival sulcus and pathologic pockets with saline or dilute chlorhexidine to remove any free-floating debris. This step is particularly important in a deep periodontal pocket as free-floating debris may occlude the orifice of the pocket and lead to the formation of a lateral periodontal abscess. The stream

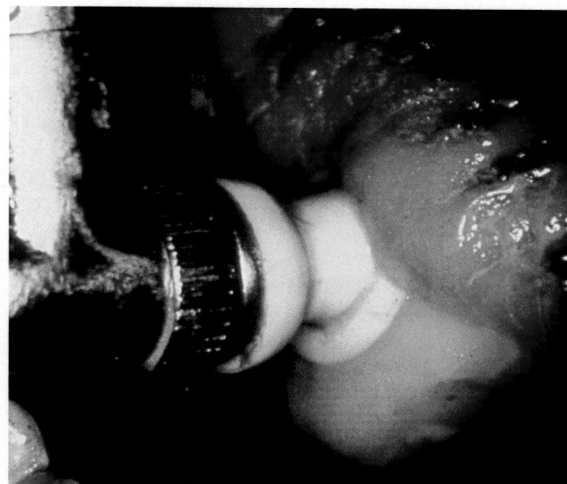

Fig. 9.19 Supragingival polishing Polishing smoothes the tooth surface and helps remove any remaining plaque and stained pellicle. It is good practice to check the adequacy of the periodontal debriding by applying a plaque-disclosing solution after polishing. Any residual dental deposits can then be identified and removed.

of fluid is directed subgingivally using a blunt-ended needle, 'lachrymal' catheter or a Water Pik device.

Periodontal surgery

Periodontal surgery includes gingivectomy (gingivoplasty), various flap techniques and osseous surgery. The main objective of periodontal surgery is to contribute to the preservation of the periodontium by facilitating plaque removal and plaque control. Periodontal surgery can help achieve this by:

1. Creating accessibility for professional scaling and root planing
2. Establishing a gingival morphology that facilitates plaque control by homecare regimes.

   Periodontal surgery is never first-line treatment for periodontitis. Cause-related treatment, as described in this chapter, is always the first step in managing periodontitis. The effect of the cause-related therapy must be evaluated. If a client cannot maintain good dental hygiene for their pet then, in the interest of the wellbeing of the animal, there is no indication for periodontal surgery.

   In lieu of the fact that periodontal surgery is rarely indicated in veterinary dentistry (clients cannot maintain adequate oral hygiene), periodontal surgery will not be covered in this book, with the exception of gingivoplasty.

Gingivoplasty. Gingivoplasty is the removal of gingival pockets by excision of the gingiva, or recontouring the gingiva to its proper anatomical form. It is indicated for the management of gingival hyperplasia. In this situation

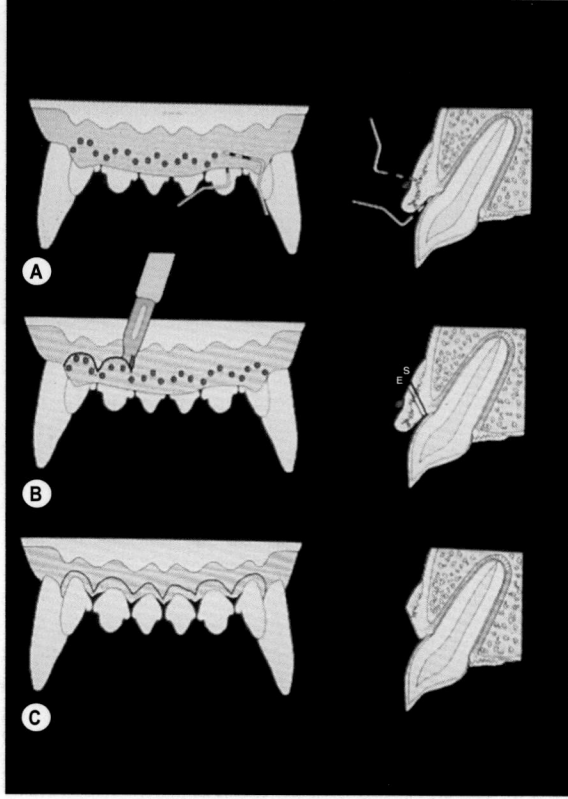

Fig. 9.20 Gingivoplasty procedure for management of gingival hyperplasia (A) Using the periodontal probe to measure and mark pocket depth. (B) Making the bevelled incision with a scalpel blade (S) or electrosurgery (E). (C) The end result – the scalloped border of the normal gingiva has been recreated.

the excessive gingival tissue should be excised, leaving a normal depth of healthy gingiva.

The procedure for gingivoplasty is as follows (Fig. 9.20):

1. Pocket depths are measured with a graduated periodontal probe or by means of pocket-marking forceps. The probe is withdrawn from the pocket and held against the outer surface of the gingiva to show the depth of the pocket. The tip of the probe is then turned horizontally and used to produce a bleeding point at the level of the bottom of the pocket. When pocket-marking forceps are used, the probing beak of the instrument is placed parallel to the long axis of the tooth. When the bottom of the pocket has been reached, the forceps are closed to pierce the gingiva thus producing a bleeding point on the outer surface of the soft tissue. The process is repeated along the whole circumference of the pocket producing bleeding points at several location points around each tooth.

2. A beveled incision, using either a scalpel blade (No. 11 or 15) or electrosurgery, is made, joining the bleeding points and recreating the scalloped edge of the normal gingival anatomy. The beveled incision is directed towards the base of the pocket or to a level slightly coronal to the apical extension of the junctional epithelium. When using electrosurgery the operator should allow for a 1 mm slough postoperatively. The electrode should be activated at the minimal effective setting in cut mode and stroked across the gingiva at the required angle. The cut surface should be pink and not bleeding if the setting is correct. Blanched tissue indicates that the setting is too high and should be reduced. To avoid overheating the tooth, the electrode should not be applied to the gingiva around the same tooth for more than 5 s.

3. The incised tissues are carefully removed by means of a curette or a scaler. Remaining tissue tags are easily removed with a curette or a pair of scissors.

4. Hemorrhage is controlled with gauze swabs and digital pressure. The crown and exposed root surfaces are carefully scaled and polished.

The postoperative phase is uncomfortable and analgesics are indicated for the first few days. It is vital that plaque is not allowed to form on the tooth surfaces, as this will interfere with healing. These animals are unlikely to accept toothbrushing immediately postoperatively, so chemical plaque control is indicated. A useful protocol is twice-daily application of chlorhexidine gluconate gel on a piece of gauze for the first week, then once-daily in combination with toothbrushing for the second week. Meticulous plaque control by means of daily toothbrushing and removing any predisposing causes, e.g. epanutin or ciclosporin administration, are necessary to prevent recurrence.

The healing of a gingivoplasty wound is similar to that of a simple soft-tissue wound except that there is a tooth in the centre of the wound. During the inflammatory phase of healing the underlying alveolar bone is slightly resorbed. Superficially, healing is complete when the epithelium reaches the tooth. This epithelium, however, is thin and non-keratinized and there is no normal epithelial attachment to the tooth. The maturation phase in the healing of a gingivoplasty wound takes much longer than in a simple soft-tissue wound. The normal gingival anatomy (epithelial attachment, gingival sulcus, keratinized oral gingival epithelium) slowly reforms and the connective tissue matures. Optimal plaque control is required for healing. Regeneration of the lost bone does not usually occur during the maturation phase.

CHRONIC GINGIVOSTOMATITIS

Chronic gingivostomatitis (CGS) describes a clinical syndrome characterized by focal or diffuse chronic inflammation of the gingivae and oral mucosa. It occurs in dogs, but is predominantly seen in cats (Gaskell and Gruffydd-Jones 1977; Johnessee and Hurvitz 1983; Williams and Aller 1992). Commonly described clinical findings in cats with CGS include elevated serum globulins, predominantly hypergammaglobulinemia (Zetner et al. 1989; White et al. 1992) and a submucosal inflammatory infiltrate consisting of plasma cells, lymphocytes, macrophages and neutrophils (Johnessee and Hurvitz 1983; Reindel et al. 1987; Hennet 1997). The elevated serum globulins in affected cats and the nature of the submucosal inflammatory infiltrate have led a number of authors to suggest that there may be an immunologic basis for the condition (Johnessee and Hurvitz 1983; Williams and Aller 1992; Sato et al. 1996). To date, no underlying intrinsic immunologic abnormality in cats affected by CGS has been identified; however, the condition may still be immune-mediated. Clinical studies have implicated the potential involvement of various viral agents, calicivirus in particular (Thompson et al. 1984; Knowles et al. 1989, 1991; Yamamoto et al. 1989; Gruffydd-Jones 1991; Tenorio et al. 1991; Waters et al. 1993) as well as Gram-negative anaerobic bacterial species (Love et al. 1989; Sims et al. 1990). However, attempts to reproduce the disease using these putative infective etiologic agents have been unsuccessful.

The most common sign of feline immunodeficiency virus (FIV) infection is oral inflammation. However, most cats with CGS test negative for FIV, but it needs to be excluded. Feline leukemia virus (FeLV) also needs to be excluded in the initial work-up. The role of feline calicivirus (FCV) in the development of CGS is unclear. FCV has been isolated from up to 100% of CGS cases, compared with up to 25% in a healthy population, indicating that the carrier state may be a prerequisite for the induction of chronic stomatitis. However, FCV isolated from cats with CGS and then inoculated into specific pathogen-free cats produced signs of acute calicivirus infection but not CGS, suggesting that other factors contribute towards the development of the oral inflammation. The fact that CGS often resolves in FCV-positive cats after extraction of all or most teeth and the subsequent reduction in dental plaque suggests that other antigenic stimuli are involved in the pathogenesis of the condition. It is possible that it is the sum of the total antigenic stimulation from plaque bacteria and viruses that is significant in the development of CGS.

Clinical signs

CGS can present clinically as focal or diffuse inflammation. Patterns of clinical presentation have been identified as follows (Harvey 1990).

Gingivitis with stomatitis (Fig. 9.21)

The gingival inflammation extends past the mucogingival junction onto the buccal and less often palatal/lingual

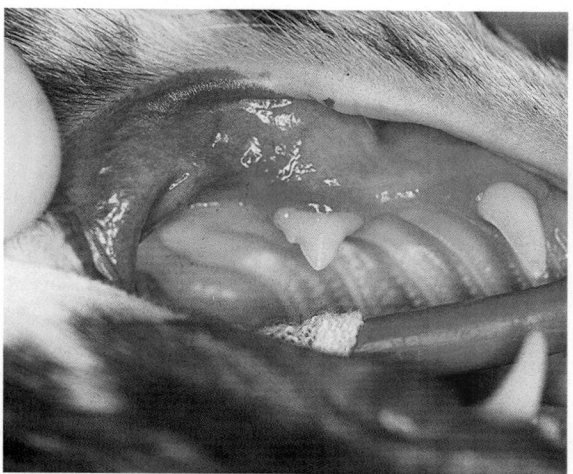

Fig. 9.21 Gingivitis with stomatitis The gingival inflammation extends past the mucogingival junction onto the buccal and less often palatal/lingual mucosa.

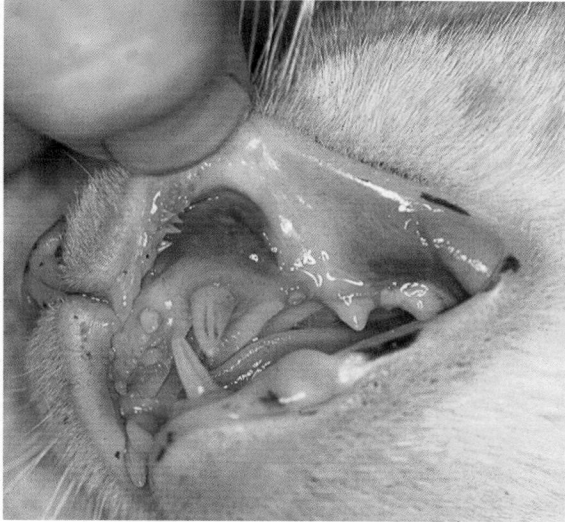

Fig. 9.22 Stomatitis with gingivitis The inflammatory reaction is more intense in the rest of the oral mucous membranes than in the actual gingivae. Affected cats are more likely to exhibit signs of oral discomfort than cats with predominantly gingivitis.

mucosa. Lesions are usually symmetrical and the premolar and molar regions are likely to be more inflamed than the incisor and canine regions.

Stomatitis with gingivitis (Fig. 9.22)

The inflammatory reaction is more intense in the rest of the oral mucous membranes than in the actual gingivae.

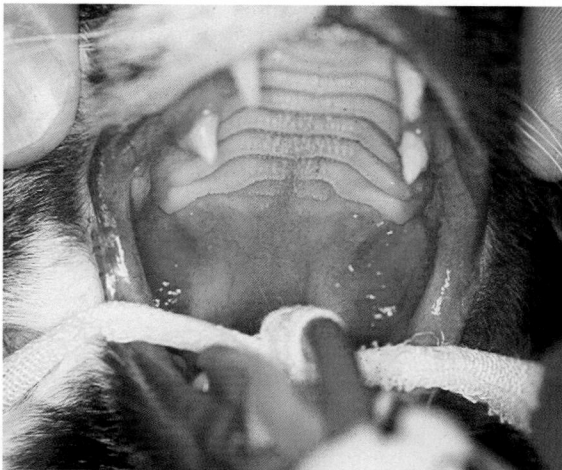

Fig. 9.23 'Faucitis' The term 'faucitis' is a misnomer. By definition the 'fauces' is the region *medial* to the palatoglossal folds. The inflammation which is commonly called 'faucitis' is largely confined to the palatoglossal folds and regions *lateral* to the folds. On close inspection, there is nearly always also evidence of gingivitis in the premolar and molar regions.

In particular, the palatoglossal folds are inflamed, but there may be extensive ulceration or granulation of the gingival and/or buccal mucosa. The mucosa of the hard palate or the tongue is rarely affected. Affected cats are more likely to exhibit signs of oral discomfort than cats with predominantly gingivitis.

Faucitis

The term 'faucitis' is a misnomer. By definition, the 'fauces' is the region *medial* to the palatoglossal folds. The inflammation which is commonly called 'faucitis' is largely confined to the palatoglossal folds and regions *lateral* to the folds (Fig. 9.23). On close inspection, there is nearly always also evidence of gingivitis in the premolar and molar regions.

Note that these are patterns of distribution rather than distinct diagnoses. There is often overlap, with a patient presenting with one or all of these patterns.

Diagnosis

Cats with chronic stomatitis require a thorough work-up prior to any treatment (Gorrel 2008). The purpose of the work-up is not to reach a diagnosis *per se*, but rather constitutes an attempt to identify possible underlying causes. The minimal work-up includes testing for FIV and FeLV, routine hematology and blood biochemistry; and a thorough oral and dental examination (including full-mouth radiographs to identify the presence of perio-dontitis, resorptive lesions, retained root remnants or other lesions). Systemic diseases, e.g. chronic renal failure and diabetes mellitus, which may predispose to the development of severe gingival inflammation in the presence of plaque, must be excluded before any treatment is initiated. Additional investigations include testing for FCV and biopsy for microscopic examination of the affected tissue.

I do not routinely test for FCV. It is only if the cat does not respond to extraction of all or most teeth that I determine FCV status. Only cats that test positive (virtually 100%) will be treated with interferon therapy. Biopsy and histopathologic examination of affected tissue are only performed if the lesions are asymmetric. The reason for the biopsy is then not primarily to diagnose CGS but to exclude other pathology, e.g. squamous cell carcinoma, which can mimic CGS clinically.

Treatment options

Historically, the intractable nature of the disease, in combination with a poor understanding of the etiopathogenesis of CGS, has resulted in the widespread use of empirical symptomatic treatment regimens (Hennet 1997; Harley et al. 1999).

The current treatment recommendations for cats with CGS include a combination of periodontal therapy and a homecare regimen whereby plaque accumulation is kept to a minimum. In some cats, this may result in a reduction in inflammation. Unfortunately, most cats will not cooperate adequately with homecare measures and plaque reforms beyond a critical level. These cats need extraction of premolar and molar teeth. In some cats, all teeth may require removal (Fig. 9.24). The extraction of premolar and molar teeth (Hennet 1997) has given the most dependable results, with up to 80% of cats being clinically cured or significantly improved. The 20% that are non-responsive to extraction can be treated with antiseptics, intermittent antibiotics or interferon.

FCV isolation should always be performed prior to using interferon and also to monitor viral status as a consequence of treatment. Interferon should only be used in FCV-positive cats where extraction of at least all premolars and molars has not led to a cure. Using interferon without surgical treatment (extraction) has not been shown to have any benefit.

In summary, cats with chronic gingivostomatitis are usually extremely uncomfortable. Every attempt should be made to identify and eliminate or treat any underlying cause for the intense oral inflammation. Full mouth radiographs are a mandatory component of the diagnostic work-up. In cats where an underlying cause, i.e. systemic or oral disease, is identified and treated, the oral inflammation will generally resolve (Gorrel 2008). In cats where no underlying cause can be identified for the intense oral

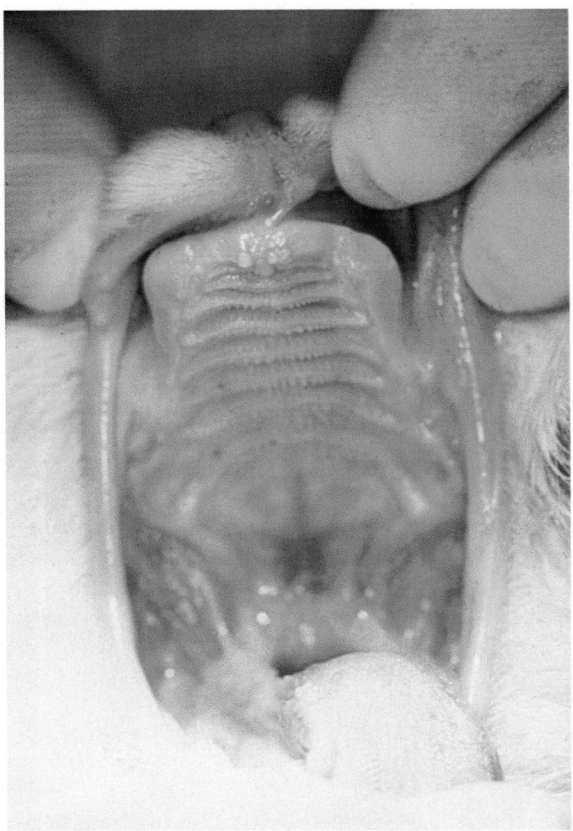

Fig. 9.24 Outcome of a radical extraction procedure At 1 month after radical extraction (all teeth except two upper incisors), the mucous membranes of the oral cavity are no longer inflamed. The two incisors were retained at the request of the owner who felt uncomfortable about her cat loosing all its teeth. This cat still eats a hard diet, but does require assistance with grooming.

inflammation, then extraction of teeth (initially all premolars and molars – but all teeth may need removal) is the treatment of choice. If CGS still persists after radical tooth extraction and the cat is positive for FCV, then interferon treatment should be instituted.

Chronic gingivostomatitis in dogs

CGS is less common in dogs than in cats. It is thought to be an inappropriate response to oral antigens, namely plaque bacteria present on the tooth surfaces. While underlying vesiculobullous disease, e.g. pemphigus and pemphigoid or discoid lupus erythematosus; cannot be excluded, it is essential to have plaque control before these can be investigated.

In the dog, I approach CGS as follows:

1. Hematology and biochemistry screens to exclude systemic diseases, e.g. endocrine or renal disorders, which may predispose to the development of severe gingival inflammation in the presence of plaque.
2. Meticulous oral examination to identify a possible reason for the intense inflammatory response, e.g. retained root remnants, periodontitis, other dental pathology.
3. Periodontal therapy (scaling and polishing) and treatment of pathologic lesion, i.e. extract root remnants, extract teeth affected by periodontitis.
4. Daily homecare (mechanical and chemical plaque control) is instituted.
5. Assess the response to treatment.

In the great majority of cases, the above approach results in complete cure. In some cases, the owner is not able to maintain adequate plaque control and selective extraction (removal of teeth that the owner cannot keep clean, usually the posterior teeth) is then performed. This is usually sufficient to achieve healthy oral mucosa. In rare cases, e.g. an aggressive dog that will not allow homecare, all teeth may need to be extracted.

Healthy oral mucosa is maintained with daily toothbrushing and adjunctive chlorhexidine rinsing as required. As long as adequate plaque control is maintained, the prognosis is excellent. However, if the owner becomes lax with plaque control then the gingivostomatitis will return within a few weeks. It is crucial that the owner understands this.

SUMMARY FOR TREATMENT OF GINGIVOSTOMATITIS

◆ Cats and dogs with chronic gingivostomatitis are usually extremely uncomfortable.
◆ Every attempt should be made to identify and eliminate or treat any underlying cause for the intense oral inflammation.
◆ Radiographs are a mandatory component of the diagnostic work-up.
◆ Initial treatment consists of a combination of periodontal therapy, any required remedial treatment (usually extraction of diseased teeth) and homecare. Corticosteroid and/or antibiotic therapy may also be required.
◆ In cases where homecare is inadequate, or in idiopathic (no underlying systemic or dental cause can be identified) cases, extraction of teeth is the treatment of choice.
◆ In cats that do not respond to extraction and are FCV-positive, interferon treatment is indicated.

REFERENCES

Allen, D.L., Kerr, D.A., 1965. Tissue response in the guinea pig to sterile and non-sterile calculus. Journal of Periodontology 36, 121–126.

DeBowes, L.J., Mosier, D., Logan, E., et al., 1996. Association of periodontal disease and histologic lesions in multiple organs from 45 dogs. Journal of Veterinary Dentistry 13 (2), 57–60.

Egelberg, J., 1965. Local effects of diet on plaque formation and gingivitis development in dogs. 2. Effect of frequency of meals and tube feeding. Odontolisk Revy 16, 50–60.

Engebretson, S.P., Lamster, I.B., Herrera-Abrev, M., et al., 1999. The influence of interleukin gene polymorphism on expression of interleukin-1β and tumor necrosis factor-α in periodontal tissue and gingival crevicular fluid. Journal of Periodontology 70, 567–573.

Gaskell, R.M., Gruffydd-Jones, T.J., 1977. Intractable feline stomatitis. Veterinary Annual 17, 195–199.

Gorrel, C., 2008. Chronic gingivostomatitis. In: Saunders Solutions in Veterinary Practice – Small Animal Dentistry. Saunders/Elsevier, Philadelphia, pp. 77–104.

Gruffydd-Jones, T.J., 1991. Gingivitis and stomatitis. In: August, J.R. (Ed.), Consultations in Feline Internal Medicine. WB Saunders, Philadelphia, pp. 387–402.

Hamp, S.E., Olsson, S., Farso-Madsen, K., et al., 1984. A macroscopic and radiologic investigation of dental diseases in dogs. Veterinary Radiology 25, 86–92.

Harley, R., Gruffydd-Jones, T.J., Day, M.J., 1999. Clinical and immunological findings in feline chronic gingivostomatitis. In: Proceedings of the 11th British Veterinary Dental Association's Annual Scientific Meeting, Birmingham, UK.

Harvey, C.E., 1990. Feline oral pathology, diagnosis and management. In: Crossley, D.A., Penman, S. (Eds.), Manual of Veterinary Dentistry. BSAVA, Cheltenham, pp. 129–138.

Hennet, P.R., 1997. Chronic gingivostomatitis in cats: long term follow-up of 30 cases treated by dental extractions. Journal of Veterinary Dentistry 14 (1), 15–21.

Hennet, P.R., Harvey, C.E., 1991. Anaerobes in periodontal disease in the dog: a review. Journal of Veterinary Dentistry 8 (2), 18–21.

Johnessee, J.S., Hurvitz, A.I., 1983. Feline plasma cell gingivitis-pharyngitis. Journal of the American Animal Hospital Association 19, 179–181.

Kinane, D.F., Lindhe, J., 1997. Pathogenesis of periodontitis. In: Lindhe, J., Karring, T., Lang, N.P. (Eds.), Clinical Periodontology and Implant Dentistry. Munksgaard, Copenhagen, pp. 189–225.

Knowles, J.O., Gaskell, R.M., Gaskell, C.J., et al., 1989. Prevalence of feline calicivirus, feline leukaemia virus and antibodies to FIV in cats with chronic stomatitis. Veterinary Record 124, 336–338.

Knowles, J.O., McArdle, F., Dawson, S., et al., 1991. Studies on the role of feline calicivirus in chronic stomatitis in cats. Veterinary Microbiology 27, 205–219.

Kornman, K.S., Crane, A., Wang, H.Y., et al., 1997. The interleukin 1 genotype as a severity factor in adult periodontal disease. Journal of Clinical Periodontology 24 (1), 72–77.

Listgarten, M.A., Ellegaard, B., 1973. Electron microscopic evidence of a cellular attachment between junctional epithelium and dental calculus. Journal of Periodontal Research 8, 143–150.

Löe, H., Theilade, E., Jensen, S.B., 1965. Experimental gingivitis in man. Journal of Periodontology 36, 177–187.

Loesche, W.J., 1979. Clinical and microbiological aspects of chemotherapeutic agents used according to the specific plaque hypothesis. Journal of Dental Research 58, 2404–2414.

Love, D.N., Johnson, J.L., Moore, L.V., 1989. Bacteroides species from the oral cavity and oral associated diseases of cats. Veterinary Microbiology 19 (3), 275–281.

Love, D.N., Vekselstein, R., Collings, S., 1990. The obligative and facultatively anaerobic bacterial flora of the normal feline gingival margin. Veterinary Microbiology 22 (2–3), 267–275.

Mallonee, D.H., Harvey, C.E., Venner, M., et al., 1988. Bacteriology of periodontal disease in the cat. Archives of Oral Biology 33 (9), 677–683.

Mombelli, A., Nyman, S., Bragger, U., et al., 1995. Clinical and microbiological changes associated with an altered subgingival environment induced by periodontal pocket reduction. Journal of Clinical Periodontology 22 (10), 780–787.

Nyman, S., Sarhed, G., Ericsson, I., et al., 1986. Role of 'diseased' root cementum in healing following treatment of periodontal disease. An experimental study in the dog. Journal of Periodontal Research 21 (5), 496–503.

Nyman, S., Westfelt, E., Sarhed, G., et al., 1988. Role of 'diseased' root cementum in healing following treatment of periodontal disease. A clinical study. Journal of Clinical Periodontology 15 (7), 464–468.

Reichart, P.A., Durr, U.M., Triadan, H., et al., 1984. Periodontal disease in the domestic cat: a histopathologic study. Journal of Periodontal Research 19 (1), 67–75.

Reindel, J.F., Trapp, A.L., Armstrong, P.J., et al., 1987. Recurrent plasmacytic stomatitis-pharyngitis in a cat with esophagitis, fibrosing gastritis and gastric nematodiasis. Journal of the American Veterinary Medical Association 190 (1), 65–67.

Sato, R., Inanami, O., Tanaka, Y., et al., 1996. Oral administration of bovine lactoferrin for treatment of intractable stomatitis in feline immunodeficiency virus (FlV)-positive and FlV-negative cats. American Journal of Veterinary Research 57 (10), 1443–1446.

Sims, T.J., Moncla, B.J., Page, R.C., 1990. Serum antibody response to antigens of oral Gram-negative bacteria in cats with plasma cell gingivitis-stomatitis. Journal of Dental Research 69 (3), 877–882.

Socransky, S.S., Haffajee, A.D., Smith, D.L., et al., 1987. Difficulties encountered in the search for the etiologic agents of destructive periodontal disease. Journal of Clinical Periodontology 14 (10), 588–593.

Tenorio, A.T., Franti, C.E., Madewell, B.R., et al., 1991. Chronic oral infection of cats and their relationship to persistent oral carriage of feline calici, immunodeficiency, or leukaemia viruses. Veterinary Immunology and Immunopathology 29 (1–2), 1–14.

Theilade, E., 1986. The non-specific theory in microbial etiology of inflammatory periodontal diseases. Journal of Clinical Periodontology 13 (10), 905–911.

Theilade, E., Wright, W.H., Jensen, S.B., et al., 1966. Experimental gingivitis in man. II. A longitudinal clinical and bacteriological investigation. Journal of Periodontal Research 1, 1–13.

Thoden van Velzen, S.K., Abraham-Inpijn, L., Moorer, W.R., 1984. Plaque and systemic disease: a reappraisal of the focal infection concept. Journal of Clinical Periodontology 11 (4), 209–220.

Thompson, R.R., Wilcox, G.E., Clark, W.T., Jansen, K.L., 1984. Association of calicivirus infection with chronic gingivitis and pharyngitis in cats. Journal of Small Animal Practice 25, 207–210.

Waerhaug, J., 1956. Effect of rough surfaces upon gingival tissues. Journal of Dental Research 35, 323–325.

Waters, L., Hopper, C.D., Gruffydd-Jones, T.J., et al., 1993. Chronic gingivitis in a colony of cats infected with feline immunodeficiency virus and feline calicivirus. Veterinary Record 132 (14), 340–342.

White, S.D., Rosychuk, R.A., Reinke, S.I., et al., 1992. Plasma cell stomatitis-pharyngitis in cats: 40 cases (1973–1991). Journal of the American Veterinary Medical Association 200 (9), 1377–1380.

Williams, C.A., Aller, M.S., 1992. Gingivitis/stomatitis in cats. In: Harvey, C.E. (Ed.), Feline Dentistry. Veterinary Clinics of North America: Small Animal Practice. WB Saunders, Philadelphia, pp. 1361–1383.

Yamamoto, J.K., Hansen, H., Ho, E.W., et al., 1989. Epidemiologic and clinical aspects of feline immunodeficiency virus infection in cats from the continental United States and Canada and possible mode of transmission. Journal of the American Veterinary Medical Association 194 (2), 213–220.

Zetner, K., Kampfer, P., Lutz, H., Harvey, C., 1989. Comparative immunological and virological studies of chronic oral diseases in cats. Weiner Tierarztliche Monatsschrift 76, 303–308.

FURTHER READING

Gorrel, C., 2008. Periodontal disease. In: Saunders Solutions in Veterinary Practice – Small Animal Dentistry. Saunders/Elsevier, Philadelphia, pp. 31–76.

Gorrel, C., 2008. Chronic gingivostomatitis. In: Saunders Solutions in Veterinary Practice – Small Animal Dentistry. Saunders/Elsevier, Philadelphia, pp. 77–104.

Chapter 10

Preventive dentistry

INTRODUCTION

Oral and dental conditions generally cause distress and many cause debilitating pain to the affected animal. Most owners do not routinely examine their pet's mouth and diseases are generally not diagnosed until late in the disease process, when the animal is showing obvious signs of oral discomfort or pain.

Prevention is always preferable to treatment and many oral and dental conditions are readily amenable to preventive measures. Common conditions that can be prevented (totally or partially) include:

- Periodontal disease
- Caries
- Excessive wear
- Tooth fracture
- Certain types of malocclusion.

PERIODONTAL DISEASE

The epidemiology, etiology, pathogenesis and treatment of periodontal disease are detailed in Chapter 9. This chapter will deal with preventive measures that should be encouraged for every dog and cat.

Prevention (and treatment) of periodontal disease have two components:

1. Maintenance of oral hygiene
2. Professional periodontal therapy.

Maintenance of oral hygiene is performed by the pet owner in the home of the animal. It is also called homecare. The goal of homecare is to remove, or at least reduce, the accumulation of dental plaque on the tooth surfaces, i.e. plaque control. The prevention and long-term control of periodontal disease requires adequate plaque control by means of homecare strategies.

Professional periodontal therapy is performed under general anesthesia and includes:

- Supra- and subgingival scaling
- Root planing
- Tooth polishing
- Subgingival lavage
- Extraction of unsalvageable teeth
- Periodontal surgery in specific situations.

The benefit of any professional periodontal therapy is short lived unless maintained by effective homecare. In fact, if no homecare is instituted after professional periodontal therapy, then plaque will rapidly reform and disease will progress. It has been shown that, if no homecare is instituted by 3 months after periodontal therapy, gingivitis scores are equivalent to those recorded prior to therapy (Gorrel and Bierer 1999).

Maintenance of oral hygiene

Client education

The cause (dental plaque) and effects (discomfort, pain, chronic focus of infection, loss of teeth, possibility of systemic complications) of periodontal disease must be thoroughly explained to the pet owner (Box 10.1). The owner must be made aware that homecare is the most essential component in both preventing and treating periodontal disease. The responsibility of maintaining oral hygiene, i.e. keeping plaque accumulation to a level compatible with periodontal health, rests with the owner of the pet. Once instituted, homecare regimens need

- Start toothbrushing as early in life as possible as prevention of disease development is the goal. The primary teeth will be exfoliated and replaced by the permanent dentition. Consequently, the benefit of introducing toothbrushing at a young age will not benefit the primary teeth, but the procedure will be accepted at the time the permanent teeth erupt. Moreover, it is far easier to train puppies and kittens to accept dental toothbrushing than middle-aged or older animals.
- Make the animal comfortable and approach from the side rather than in front.
- Start with just a few teeth (premolars and molars rather than incisors since retracting the lips is usually readily accepted, while many animals do not like having their nose lifted) and gradually increase the number of teeth cleaned each time until the whole mouth can be cleaned in a single session.
- Initially, the mouth does not need to be opened. Concentrate on brushing the buccal surfaces of the teeth, especially at the gingival margin.
- When the animal is comfortable with having the buccal surfaces of all its teeth brushed, an attempt should be made to open the mouth and carefully brush the palatal and lingual surfaces of the teeth. If this is not accepted, there is every reason to continue with daily brushing of the buccal surfaces. However, gingivitis will occur on the palatal and lingual surfaces if these are not brushed (Ingham and Gorrel 2001) and periodontitis may occur at these sites.
- Offer a reward at the end of the procedure, e.g. a game or a walk.
- Include toothbrushing as part of the daily grooming routine. Homecare is more likely to be acceptable to an older pet if it is introduced as an extension of a pre-existing routine, e.g. evening meal, walk, grooming. The owner is also more likely to remember a consistent routine.
- Owners can sit small dogs and cats on their lap while brushing, at the same time cuddling them to reduce their apprehension; alternatively, one person cuddles and restrains while a second performs the toothbrushing. Some animals may better accept the use of a 'grooming table' type situation.

continuous monitoring and reinforcement. The veterinary nurse can play a vital role in educating clients, checking compliance and reinforcing the need for homecare.

However, the owner must realize that, even with homecare, most animals will still need to have their teeth cleaned professionally at intervals. The intervals between

professional cleaning need to be determined for each animal. With good homecare, the intervals between professional cleaning can be greatly extended. It is useful to draw an analogy to the situation in humans, i.e. most of us do brush our teeth daily but still require dental examinations and professional periodontal therapy (at a minimum scaling and polishing) at regular intervals.

Toothbrushing

Toothbrushing is known to be the single most effective means of removing plaque. Studies have shown that in dogs with both experimentally induced gingivitis (Tromp et al. 1986) and naturally occurring gingivitis (Gorrel and Rawlings 1996a) daily toothbrushing is effective in returning the gingivae to health. In a 4-year study using the Beagle dog (Lindhe et al. 1975), it was shown that with no oral hygiene plaque accumulated rapidly along the gingival margin, with gingivitis developing within a few weeks. Dogs that were fed an identical diet under identical conditions but that were subjected to daily toothbrushing developed no clinical signs of gingivitis. In the group which were not receiving daily toothbrushing, gingivitis progressed to periodontitis in most individuals.

Toothbrushing is the 'gold standard' for plaque control. Every effort should be made to get every pet owner to commit to brushing their pet's teeth on a daily basis. The success of toothbrushing depends on pet cooperation and owner motivation and technical ability. Toothbrushing should be introduced gradually and as early in the animal's life as possible. Adult cats are generally less amenable to the introduction of toothbrushing than adult dogs, but with patience and persistence many will accept some degree of homecare. In contrast, kittens often accept toothbrushing more readily than puppies.

Toothbrushes. There are innumerable brush head and handle designs and sizes of human and veterinary toothbrushes available, but there is insufficient evidence to clearly recommend any particular one. The choice of brush should be based on the effectiveness of plaque control in the hands of each individual. In general, a soft to medium texture nylon filament brush of a suitable size for the intended pet seems to be the most comfortable.

A flannel cloth folded over a finger or a rubber 'finger brush' may be more comfortable for animals and owners, but is less effective (removes less plaque) than a nylon filament brush. The use of a finger brush or cloth during the training phase is useful, but every attempt should be made to get the animal to accept a proper toothbrush.

Toothpaste. The use of non-foaming tasty pet toothpaste is recommended, but not critical. It is the mechanical action of brushing which removes the plaque. Therefore, brushing with a toothbrush moistened with water will still do the job. However, the use of pet toothpaste is recommended as it tastes nice and the pet will therefore usually allow the owner to brush for longer, thus removing more plaque. The paste should be pressed down into the bristles to maintain it on the brush or the animal will just lick it off.

The use of a human toothpaste is not recommended, mainly because of the high fluoride content, which may lead to acute, but more likely chronic, toxicity problems as our pets do not rinse and spit but will swallow the toothpaste (Gorrel 1994).

Frequency of toothbrushing. In a study of experimental gingivitis in laboratory dogs, brushing once-daily was effective in returning the gingivae to health, while brushing three times or once a week was not effective (Tromp et al. 1986). Another study has shown that brushing every other day was not sufficient to maintain clinically healthy gingivae in dogs (Gorrel and Rawlings 1996a). Brushing twice-daily with a human's hard nylon filament brush resulted in traumatic gingival lesions in the dog (Sangnes 1976).

In the only published toothbrushing study involving cats, teeth brushed either daily or twice-daily on one side of the mouth had 95% less calculus, and teeth brushed once-weekly had 76% less calculus, than unbrushed teeth at the end of an 18-week trial period (Richardson 1965). Unfortunately, gingivitis was not scored in this study.

Based on the above studies, the current clinical recommendation should be daily toothbrushing to establish and maintain clinically healthy gingivae for the whole life of the animal. With the increasing life expectancy of

dogs and cats, preventive medicine becomes increasingly important.

Brushing technique. There is no one correct method of brushing; the objective is to remove plaque effectively without damaging either teeth or gingivae. A particular method must be dictated by individual preference and dexterity and the variable dentogingival morphology occurring with different stages of disease. In most instances, a combination of roll and miniscrub technique will achieve the objective. The teeth and gingival margin are brushed in a circular or side-to-side motion. The brush is angled at a 45° angle to the tooth surfaces, so that the bristles enter the gingival sulcus (Fig. 10.1). The circling motion should ensure that all cracks and crevices in and around the teeth are cleaned.

Dental diets and dental hygiene chews

The use of products (dental diets, hygiene chews and biscuits) aimed at encouraging chewing activity and which are designed with textural properties that maximize self-cleaning are beneficial in reducing the accumulation of dental deposits and, consequently, the degree of gingivitis that develops. *None of the products in this category is as effective as daily toothbrushing. Consequently, their use cannot achieve or maintain clinically healthy gingivae in the absence of toothbrushing.*

Periodontal disease has been linked with aspects of diet. Several studies have investigated the local effect of diet on

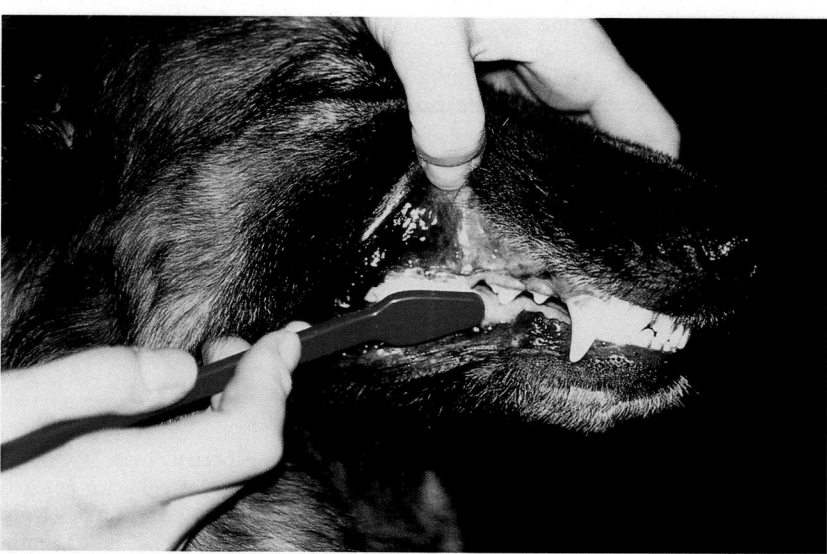

Fig. 10.1 Toothbrushing technique Subgingival plaque is a consequence of supragingival plaque migrating in an apical direction. To remove plaque from the gingival sulcus, the toothbrush is angled at 45° to the tooth surface, which allows the bristles to enter the sulcus. Even with optimal technique, toothbrushing will not clean more than 1–2 mm below the gingival margin. Consequently, the best way to prevent plaque accumulating in the sulcus is meticulous supragingival plaque control.

plaque formation and development of gingivitis in the dog (Egelberg 1965a,b). A coarse diet may reduce plaque accumulation on some teeth and on some tooth surfaces. Although consumption of soft foods may promote plaque accumulation, the general belief that dry foods provide significant oral cleansing should be regarded with skepticism. In fact, one study reported that feeding a canned food performed similarly to feeding a dry food in the degree of plaque and calculus accumulation (Boyce and Logan 1994). In a large epidemiologic survey, dogs consuming dry food did not consistently demonstrate improved periodontal health when compared with dogs eating moist foods (Harvey et al. 1996).

Specifically designed dental diets (Jensen et al. 1995; Logan et al. 2002) and dental hygiene chews (Gorrel and Rawlings 1996b; Gorrel et al. 1998, 1999; Gorrel and Bierer 1999; Ingham et al. 2002) with enhanced textural characteristics have been shown to significantly reduce accumulation of dental deposits and the degree of gingivitis, in both long- and short-term studies. It is not known whether this reduced degree of gingivitis is sufficient to prevent the development of periodontitis. Further studies of longer duration are required.

While every attempt should be made to ensure that daily toothbrushing is performed by the owner, the reduction of accumulation of dental deposits (plaque and calculus), thus reducing the severity of gingivitis by dietary means, is a useful adjunctive measure and is highly recommended to pet owners. In selecting an appropriate dental diet or dental hygiene chews, I would recommend using either a product that has been shown to be effective in peer-reviewed publications or a product that has been awarded a Veterinary Oral Health Council (VOHC®) Seal of Acceptance. The VOHC® Seal of Acceptance system identifies products that meet pre-set standards for prevention of accumulation of dental plaque and calculus (tartar). It is a product effectiveness recognition system, with no regulatory function, and is limited to considering products designed to control plaque and calculus.

Chemical plaque control

In addition to mechanical plaque control, chemical plaque control does have a role in treating periodontitis. These are not indicated to prevent or treat gingivitis. The prudent use of antibiotics and antiseptics in periodontal disease is detailed in Chapter 3.

CARIES

Caries occurs in dogs. It has not been described in cats. The etiology, pathogenesis and clinical feature of caries are detailed in Chapter 8.

In simple terms, caries occurs when plaque bacteria use fermentable carbohydrate (notably sugar) from the diet as a source of energy. The fermentation by-products are acidic and demineralize the enamel. Caries can thus be prevented by removing the bacteria (toothbrushing) in combination with removing their substrate (sugar and other easily fermentable carbohydrate). Dogs should not be fed human biscuits and confectionary, as they are high in sugar.

EXCESSIVE WEAR

Attrition (wear of tooth surfaces that are in contact with one another) and abrasion (wear of tooth surfaces that are not in contact with one another) are detailed in Chapter 8.

Excessive attrition can occur under certain circumstances – stone chewing is a common cause. Another common cause is playing with a ball on a sandy surface. The ball becomes wet and covered with sand or grit and, as the animal bites on the ball, the teeth are worn excessively. Prevention in such circumstances is restricting access to stones and playing with a ball in an environment where the ball does not become covered in abrasive material.

Loss of teeth (due to disease or trauma) and malocclusion may also predispose to excessive attrition. If extensive extractions are required, the resultant occlusion must be evaluated and preventive measures instituted as appropriate.

In humans, the most common cause of abrasion is incorrect use of a toothbrush. Other causes include the ingestion of solids or liquids that are highly acidic, or the regurgitation or vomiting of acids from the stomach that enhance the tissue destruction caused by incorrect brushing technique. In the dog, the most common cause of abrasion is cage biting. The result of the progressive loss of tooth substance is fracture (generally with pulpal exposure) of the weakened tooth. Every effort should be made to rid the animal of this habit. If this cannot be achieved, then the animal should not be caged.

TOOTH FRACTURE

Tooth fracture is dealt with in detail in Chapters 8 and 12. The incidence of tooth fracture, especially in dogs, can be reduced by preventing certain types of behavior (owner and pet). The owner should be discouraged from behavior such as throwing stones for the dog to collect, or reprimanding during training by hitting the animal across the face. As already mentioned in the previous section, circumstances and/or behavior that predisposes to excessive tooth wear and weakening of the teeth should be avoided. Chewing on hard bones or toys should not be encouraged. Endodontic treatment of fractured teeth is a large proportion of the clinical case load at my referral practice and a large number of the dogs referred for treatment fractured one or several teeth by biting on hard bones or toys. Softer bones should also be avoided. These will be chewed and swallowed, often causing digestive problems, or become impacted on or between teeth.

MALOCCLUSION

Malocclusion is common and may cause pain/discomfort and severe oral pathology. Occlusal evaluation is part of the basic oral examination of a conscious animal. To make an evaluation, the practitioner needs to be able to identify normal occlusion for the species and breed and have an understanding of the etiology and pathogenesis of malocclusion. Occlusion and malocclusion are detailed in Chapter 5. In general, the treatment of malocclusion is best left to a veterinarian with special skills in dentistry, namely expertise in endodontics and orthodontics. It is possible to prevent development of some types of malocclusion. General practitioners are encouraged to implement these measures.

Prevention of malocclusion

Preventive measures, which can be performed in a general practice, include:

- Extraction of persistent primary teeth
- Interceptive orthodontics
- A removable orthodontic device.

Extraction of persistent primary teeth

Persistent primary teeth should be extracted as soon as possible to prevent malocclusion. The golden rule is that the primary and permanent tooth of the same type should not be present at the same time. Extraction of persistent primary teeth should not be delayed past 12–14 weeks of age. The procedure for extracting primary teeth is found in Chapter 13.

Interceptive orthodontics

Interceptive orthodontics is used to describe the practice of extracting maloccluding primary teeth before eruption of their permanent counterparts. It will prevent dental interlock-induced malocclusion from developing. If the developing malocclusion is of skeletal origin, the value of interceptive orthodontics is negligible since the permanent teeth will form the same incorrect interlock. However,

it may still be indicated to prevent discomfort. Further treatment, once the permanent occlusion has formed, will be required.

Primary teeth involved in malocclusion should be extracted as early as possible, i.e. at 6–8 weeks of age. This will allow the maxilla and mandible to develop to their full genetic potential independently before the permanent dental interlock forms.

A removable orthodontic device

Lingually displaced mandibular canine teeth are a relatively common orthodontic problem in dogs. This malocclusion may be due to a dental abnormality, a skeletal abnormality, or a combination of both. The palatal contact of the mandibular canine crown tips frequently causes discomfort and pain, and may lead to palatal mucosal ulceration, infection and formation of a permanent oronasal communication. In properly selected cases (young dogs, no major jaw discrepancies), the use of a removable orthodontic appliance ('rubber toy' technique) has been proven successful in correcting the malocclusion within 4 weeks in most cases (Verhaert 1999). The technique also encourages development of a strong bond between owner and animal during the course of the treatment.

As with any technique, correct diagnosis is critical for success of treatment. No major jaw discrepancies should be present. The diastema between the 3rd incisor and canine tooth in the upper jaw should be wide enough to accommodate the mandibular canine tooth in its corrected position. In other words, the only orthodontic movement required is lateral movement of the mandibular canines, and there needs to be enough space available between the 3rd incisor and canine in the upper jaw for them to fit into their correct position.

The most appropriate objects to use are toys with a round or oval shape. The size is important. The correct size of toy sits in between and just behind the canine teeth, and is larger than the distance between the mandibular canine teeth (Fig. 10.2). The toy thus applies primarily lateral pressure to the teeth while the dog plays. A toy that is too small will be held more caudally in the mouth and thus exert no lateral force on the canine teeth. Too large a toy might cause intrusion rather than lateral tipping. In dogs that prefer to hold a toy between the carnassial teeth rather than the canine teeth, a very large toy may be needed. It needs to be so large that it cannot be fitted between the carnassial teeth. Rostral as well as lateral tipping of the mandibular canines occurs with a toy this large.

The composition and consistency of the toy are important. It should be of hard rubber that slightly deforms on chewing. If the toy is too soft, it is unlikely to create enough pressure for lateral tipping of the mandibular canines. If it is too hard, the result is tooth damage due to

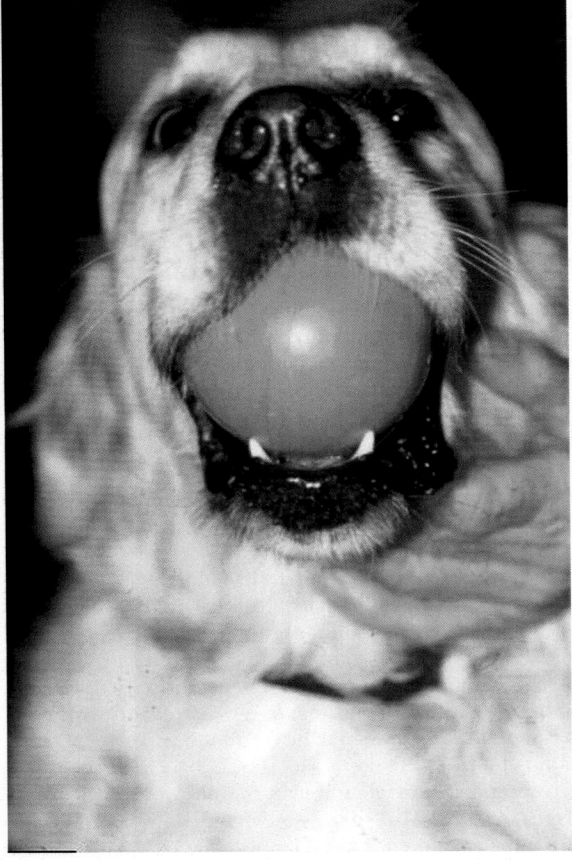

Fig. 10.2 A removable orthodontic device To achieve primarily lateral pressure to the canine teeth while the dog plays, the correct size of toy is critical. As depicted in this photograph, the toy needs to be larger than the distance between the mandibular canine teeth and when the dog holds it in its mouth the toy should sit in between and just behind the canine teeth. A toy that is too small will be held more caudally in the mouth and thus exert no lateral force on the canine teeth. Too large a toy might cause intrusion rather than lateral tipping.

abrasion. The toy should have a smooth surface to avoid excessive abrasion.

Active play for 15 min, three times per day is the recommended minimum. Longer and more frequent episodes are preferable and the owner should be recommended to play with the dog as often as possible and to take away all other toys. Assuming a 1-week learning phase, two additional weeks are needed before any benefit is likely to be seen. Occlusion is checked after 3 weeks of treatment and then monthly as necessary. If no movement is seen after 3 weeks, other treatment methods should be considered.

It is advisable to obtain full pre- and post-treatment impressions and radiographs to assess outcome. However, many owners are unwilling to have their dogs anesthetized just for this. As a compromise, hard wax bite wafers can be used to record crown tip positions in most conscious dogs. Photographs (rostral, left and right view) should always be taken to record the extent of the malocclusion prior to treatment.

Once the mandibular canines are in their correct position, the established canine dental interlock should prevent relapse. However, continued playing with the toy for several months is recommended. It appears that there is little risk of overcorrection (labioversion) of the canine teeth.

The technique works in teeth that are still erupting as well as in fully erupted teeth. However, the time required for correction is longer when the teeth are fully erupted.

SUMMARY

- There is no magic bullet that we can feed our pets to prevent periodontal disease: daily toothbrushing remains the single most effective method of restoring inflamed gingivae to health and of then maintaining clinically healthy gingivae.
- Compliance may be an issue for some people. Compliance failure has not been critically investigated in veterinary dentistry; however, it is not difficult to imagine that many factors may prevent owners from brushing their pets' teeth. Such factors include lack of skill, questionable perceived benefit, unpleasantness of the procedure and lifestyle (lack of time).
- One study evaluated compliance in a period of 6–21 months following periodontal therapy and homecare instruction (Miller and Harvey 1994). This study reported that 53% of clients surveyed were satisfactorily compliant. However, the report was based on a telephone survey and clinical effectiveness of compliance was not assessed.
- Our experience is that a combination of client education, continuous reinforcement and individually determined recalls to check efficacy yields surprisingly good compliance.
- Caries in dogs is prevented by toothbrushing and avoiding treats containing sugars.
- Attrition, abrasion and tooth fracture are prevented by modifying play behaviors or the animal's environment.
- Malocclusion can be prevented by extraction of persistent primary teeth, interceptive orthodontics and by the use of appropriate removable orthodontic devices.

REFERENCES

Boyce, E.N., Logan, E.I., 1994. Oral health assessment in dogs: study design and results. Journal of Veterinary Dentistry 11 (2), 64–74.

Egelberg, J., 1965a. Local effects of diet on plaque formation and gingivitis development in dogs. III. Effect of frequency of meals and tube feeding. Odontologisk Revy 16, 50–60.

Egelberg, J., 1965b. Local effects of diet on plaque formation and gingivitis development in dogs. I. Effect of hard and soft diets. Odontologisk Revy 16, 31–41.

Gorrel, C., 1994. The effects of fluoride and its possible uses in veterinary dentistry. Proceedings of the World Veterinary Dental Congress, Philadelphia, USA.

Gorrel, C., Bierer, T., 1999. Long term effects of a dental hygiene chew on the periodontal health of dogs. Journal of Veterinary Dentistry 16 (3), 109–113.

Gorrel, C., Rawlings, J.M., 1996a. The role of tooth-brushing and diet in the maintenance of periodontal health in dogs. Journal of Veterinary Dentistry 13 (3), 139–143.

Gorrel, C., Rawlings, J.M., 1996b. The role of a 'dental hygiene chew' in maintaining periodontal health in dogs. Journal of Veterinary Dentistry 13 (1), 31–34.

Gorrel, C., Inskeep, G., Inskeep, T., 1998. Benefits of a 'dental hygiene chew' on the periodontal health of cats. Journal of Veterinary Dentistry 15 (3), 135–138.

Gorrel, C., Warrick, J., Bierer, T., 1999. Effect of a new dental hygiene chew on periodontal health in dogs. Journal of Veterinary Dentistry 16 (2), 77–81.

Harvey, C.E., Shofer, F.S., Laster, L., 1996. Correlation of diet, other chewing activities and periodontal disease in North American client-owned dogs. Journal of Veterinary Dentistry 13 (3), 101–105.

Ingham, K.E., Gorrel, C., 2001. Effect of long-term intermittent periodontal care on canine periodontal disease. Journal of Small Animal Practice 42 (2), 67–70.

Ingham, K.E., Gorrel, C., Bierer, T.L., 2002. Effect of a dental chew on dental substrates and gingivitis in cats. Journal of Veterinary Dentistry 19 (4), 201–204.

Jensen, L., Logan, E.I., Finney, O., et al., 1995. Reduction in accumulation of plaque, stain and calculus in dogs by dietary means. Journal of Veterinary Dentistry 12 (4), 161–163.

Lindhe, J., Hamp, S.-E., Löe, H., 1975. Plaque induced periodontal disease in beagle dogs. A 4-year clinical, roentgenographical and histometrical study. Journal of Periodontal Research 10, 243–255.

Logan, E.I., Finney, O., Hefferren, J., 2002. Effects of a dental food on plaque accumulation and gingival health in dogs. Journal of Veterinary Dentistry 19 (1), 15–18.

Miller, B.R., Harvey, C.E., 1994. Compliance with oral hygiene recommendations following periodontal treatment in client-owned dogs. Journal of Veterinary Dentistry 11 (1), 18–19.

Richardson, R.L., 1965. Effect of administering antibiotics, removing the major salivary glands and toothbrushing on dental calculi formation in the cat. Archives of Oral Biology 10, 245–253.

Sangnes, G., 1976. A pilot study on the effect of toothbrushing on the gingiva of a beagle dog. Scandinavian Journal of Dental Research 84, 106–108.

Tromp, J.A., van Rijn, L.J., Jansen, J., 1986. Experimental gingivitis and frequency of tooth-brushing in the beagle dog model. Clinical findings. Journal of Clinical Periodontology 13, 190–194.

Verhaert, L., 1999. A removable orthodontic device for the treatment of lingually displaced mandibular canine teeth in young dogs. Journal of Veterinary Dentistry 16 (2), 69–75.

Chapter 11

Resorptive lesions

INTRODUCTION

Resorption of teeth is common in domestic cats. Tooth resorption has also been shown to occur in feral (Verstraete et al. 1996; Clarke and Cameron 1997) and wild cats (Berger et al. 1996; Levin 1996). It has also been reported in dogs (Arnbjerg 1996) and in the chinchilla (Crossley et al. 1997). This chapter, however, will deal exclusively with tooth resorption in cats.

Resorptive lesions (RLs) occur as a result of an external root resorption, where the hard tissues of the root surfaces are destroyed by the activity of multinucleated cells called odontoclasts. The destroyed root surface is replaced by cementum-like or bone-like tissue. The process starts in cementum and progresses to involve the dentine, where it spreads along the dentine tubules and eventually comes to involve the dentine of the crown as well as the root. The peripulpal dentine is relatively resistant to resorption and the pulp thus only becomes involved late in the disease. The process extends through the crown dentine, eventually reaching the enamel. The enamel is either resorbed or it fractures off and a cavity becomes clinically evident (Figs 11.1, 11.2A).

In the absence of routine radiography, the lesions are first noted clinically when they become evident in the crown, often as cavities at the cemento-enamel junction (CEJ). Figure 11.2B depicts the radiographic appearance of the clinical lesion seen in Figure 11.2A. *The first clinical manifestation of a RL is thus a late-stage lesion.* In many cases, the progressive dentine destruction with RLs weakens and undermines the crown to such an extent that minor trauma, e.g. during chewing, causes the crown to fracture off, leaving the root in the alveolar bone. The resorbing root remnants are usually covered by intact gingiva (Fig. 11.3). However, in some cases the overlying gingiva may be inflamed (Fig. 11.4).

Because the first clinically detectable lesion is often seen at the CEJ, the disease has also been described as feline neck lesions, cervical line lesions or feline caries. However, RLs should not be confused with dental caries. Early caries is a passive inorganic demineralization of the enamel, while odontoclastic resorption occurs as an active progressive destruction of the dental tissues by clastic cells.

RESORPTION OF HARD TISSUE

Hard tissues (bone, cementum, dentine) are normally protected from resorption by their surface layer of cells (Lindskog and Hammarström 1980; Verstraete et al. 1998). Root resorption is classified as:

1. Internal
2. External.

Internal root resorption occurs when the integrity of the odontoblast layer is broached. It thus starts on the pulpal surface and extends towards the external aspect of the tooth. Internal root resorption is usually a consequence of pulpal inflammation.

External root resorption may follow any damage to the protective periodontal ligament (PDL) and cementoblast layer. It thus starts on the external root surface and progresses within the tooth. External root resorption (Andreasen 1988) is classified as:

- Surface
- Replacement
- Inflammatory.

Surface resorption is self-limiting and reversible. It is thought that minor trauma caused by unintentional biting

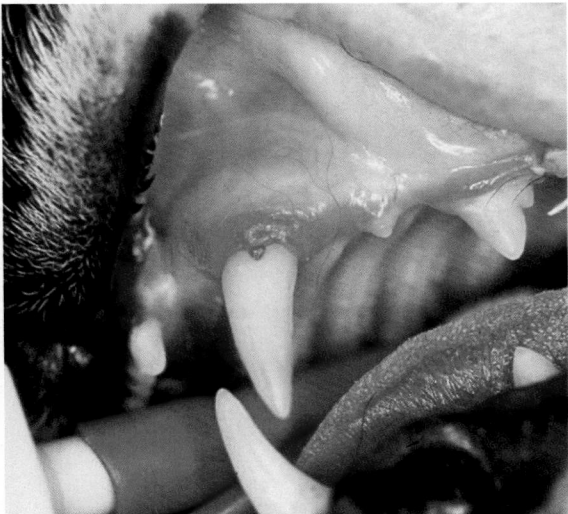

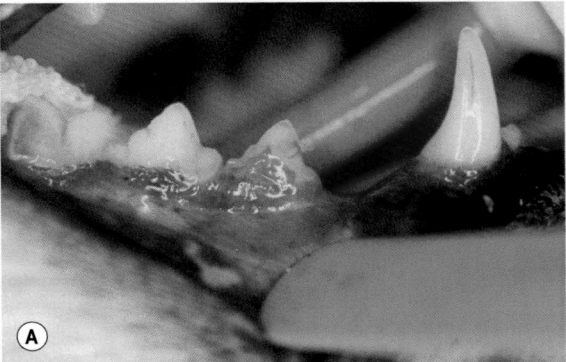

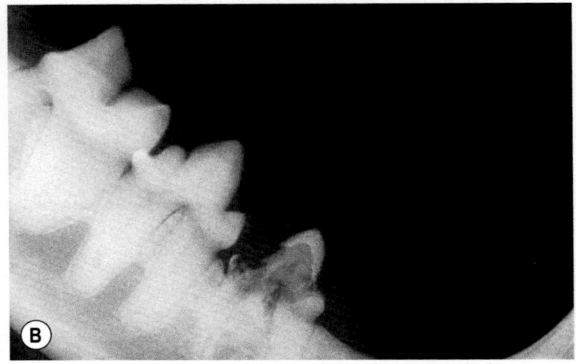

Fig. 11.1 Clinical appearance of feline resorptive lesions The lesions are first noticed clinically when they become evident in the crown, often as a cavity at the cemento-enamel junction. The process has extended into the crown dentine and come to involve the enamel, which has either resorbed or fractured off to reveal a small cavity filled with granulation-like tissue, at the buccal aspect of the gingival margin of the upper canine. Contrary to common belief, this is a late-stage lesion.

Fig. 11.2 Clinical and radiographic appearance of resorptive lesions (A) Clinical appearance. The lower right 3rd premolar tooth has an extensive cavity at the cemento-enamel junction. The destroyed dentine and enamel have been replaced by connective tissue. Again, this is a late-stage lesion. (B) Radiographic appearance. The radiographic appearance of the right 3rd mandibular premolar tooth depicted in (A). Both roots show evidence of extensive resorption, i.e. loss of distinct periodontal ligament space, replacement of tooth substance by bone-like material, and most of the crown dentine is destroyed. This tooth requires treatment.

on hard objects, bruxism, etc. can cause localized damage to the PDL and cementoblast layer and trigger this type of resorption. The denuded root surface attracts clastic cells, which will resorb the cementum for as long as osteoclast-activating factors are released at the site of injury – usually a few days. When the resorption stops, cells from the PDL will proliferate and populate the resorbed area resulting in deposition of reparative dental tissue (Lindskog et al. 1983, 1987). The majority of human teeth show signs of active or healed surface resorptions.

Replacement resorption results in replacement of the dental hard tissue by bone. The etiology of replacement resorption appears to be related to the absence of a vital PDL cover on the root surface (Andreasen 1985). It is assumed that damaged PDL is repopulated with progenitor cells from adjacent bone marrow. These cells establish themselves on the resorbed root surface and bone will thus be formed directly upon the dental hard tissues (Andreasen and Kristerson 1981). This results in fusion between bone and tooth, i.e. ankylosis. Replacement resorption can thus be seen as a form of healing: the bone has accepted the dental hard tissue as part of itself and the tooth becomes involved in the normal skeletal turnover, i.e. during subsequent remodeling of bone both dental hard tissue and bone will be resorbed (Hammarström et al. 1989).

Inflammatory root resorption is a consequence of inflammation in the adjacent tissues. There are two main forms, namely peripheral inflammatory root resorption (PIRR) and external inflammatory root resorption (EIRR).

In PIRR, the osteoclast-activating factors, which keep the resorptive process going, are provided by an inflammatory lesion in the adjacent periodontal tissues (Andreasen 1985; Gold and Hasselgren 1992; Ne et al. 1999). PIRR occurs immediately apical to the marginal tissues and is thus often situated cervically. It has therefore also been termed cervical root resorption.

EIRR, on the other hand, receives its stimulus for continued resorption from an infected necrotic pulp (Andreasen 1985). This type of root resorption is a complication that can follow dental trauma. It begins as a

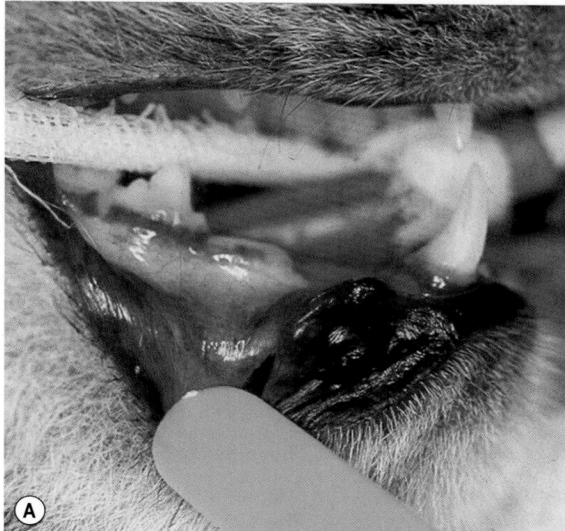

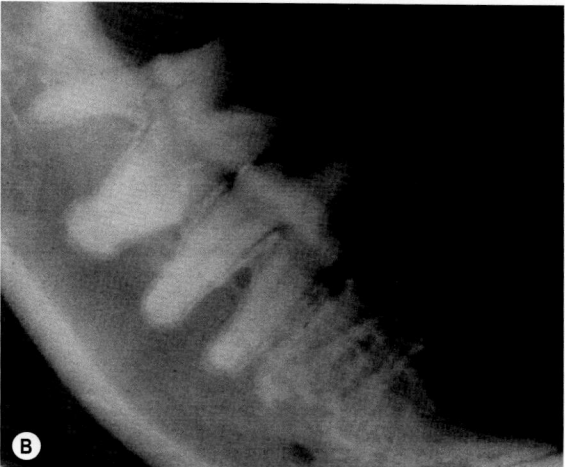

Fig. 11.3 **Missing tooth with gingival overgrowth** (A) Clinical appearance. The right mandibular 3rd premolar is absent on clinical examination. The overlying gingiva is not inflamed. (B) Radiographic appearance. The roots are retained in the alveolar bone. The roots are showing evidence of ongoing resorption. The only treatment required is clinical and radiographic monitoring, i.e. there is no indication to extract the retained roots.

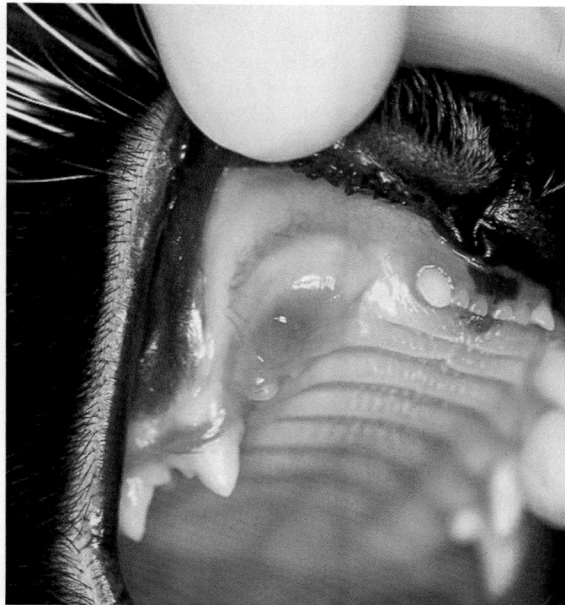

Fig. 11.4 **Missing tooth with gingival inflammation** In this patient, the progressive dentine destruction has weakened and undermined the crown of the right maxillary canine tooth to such an extent that minor trauma, e.g. during chewing, has caused it to fracture, leaving the root in the alveolar bone. The gingiva overlying the retained root remnant is inflamed. The retained root remnant needs to be extracted.

surface resorption due to damage to the periodontal ligament and cementoblast layer in conjunction with the traumatic injury. However, the pulp is also damaged by the trauma and becomes necrotic. As the surface resorption approaches the dentine, necrotic and possible infected pulp matter is released into the PDL from the thus exposed dentine tubules. The pulp products will then maintain an inflammatory process in the adjacent periodontal tissues that in turn will trigger the continuance of the resorption.

The RLs seen so commonly in cats are external and either fit into the PIRR category or fit into the replacement resorption category. In other words, the RLs seen in cats are either inflammatory or non-inflammatory (replacement) in origin. In the literature, with the exception of one study (DuPont and DeBowes 2002) a distinction is not made between RLs of inflammatory origin and those that are truly idiopathic. This makes it difficult to draw meaningful conclusions.

EPIDEMIOLOGY

Prevalence rates ranging from 28.5% to 67.0% have been reported and the incidence increases with increasing age (Coles 1990; van Wessum et al. 1992; Verstraete et al. 1996; Lund et al. 1998; Lommer and Verstraete 2000; Ingham et al. 2001). Differences in breed susceptibility have also been suggested in some studies, but differences in the mean age among different breed groups make comparisons of significance suspect.

The large variation in prevalence rates can be explained by the different populations of cats studied (random vs dental vs mixed) and by the different methods used to diagnose RLs (clinical vs radiographic). The incidence was generally higher in the studies where the cats examined were presented for dental examination or treatment than in the studies looking at random or mixed (i.e. presented for dental or other problem) populations of cats. However, in an Australian study looking at a mixed population of cats, 52% of cats were affected with a mean of 3.2 lesions per affected cat (Coles 1990).

All types of teeth in the feline dentition may be affected by RLs, but lesions seem more common in certain teeth (Ingham et al. 2001). The manifest lesions can often be diagnosed clinically by visual and tactile examination. As already mentioned, they commonly present as a cavity at the CEJ of the tooth. Studies which included radiography (Lindskog and Hammarström 1980; Verstraete et al. 1998; Ingham et al. 2001) have demonstrated that the resorption can occur anywhere on the root surfaces, i.e. not only at the CEJ. Clinical methods will only detect lesions that involve the crown, while radiography will also detect lesions confined to the root. Thus, the prevalence of RLs in studies that include radiography is higher.

In a study (Ingham et al. 2001) which investigated the incidence of RLs in a clinically healthy population of 228 cats (mean age was 4.92 years), using a combination of clinical examination and radiography, it was found that the overall prevalence rate was 29%. The mandibular 3rd premolars (307, 407) were the most commonly affected teeth and the pattern of RL development was symmetrical in most cats. The risk of having RLs was found to increase with increasing age and cats with clinically missing teeth were more likely to have RLs. Neutering, sex, age at neutering or mean whole mouth gingivitis index did not affect the prevalence of RLs.

ETIOLOGY AND PATHOGENESIS

While the ongoing or established resorptive process has been detailed (Hopewell-Smith 1930; Okuda and Harvey 1992; Shigeyana et al. 1996), the *etiology of many RLs is not clear*.

As previously described, it seems likely that at least two different types of resorption with different etiologies are currently diagnosed as the same condition. This is supported by the findings of a study (DuPont and DeBowes 2002) investigating the radiographic appearance of cat teeth with RLs. In the study 543 teeth with RLs were examined radiographically and two types of roots were identified. Type 1 roots had a normal root radiodensity and an intact PDL space (Fig. 11.5), whereas Type 2 roots were

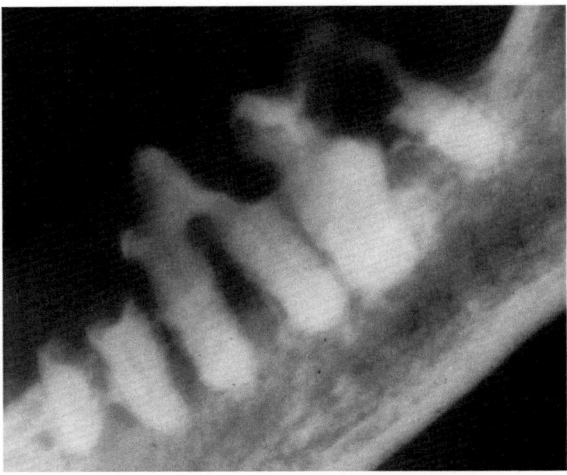

Fig. 11.5 Type 1 roots The periodontal ligament space is clearly evident and the root radiodensity is normal.

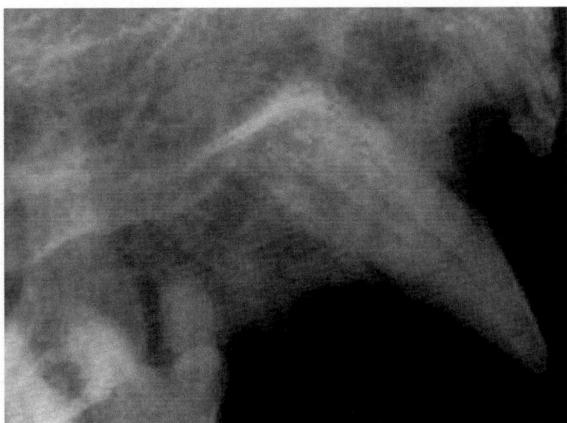

Fig. 11.6 Type 2 roots The periodontal ligament space is not obvious and the tooth root is radiolucent.

radiolucent and lacked a clear PDL space (Fig. 11.6). Of the 543 teeth that were examined, 268 (49.4%) were Type 1 and 275 (50.6%) were Type 2. Periodontitis was present in 72% of teeth with Type 1 roots, but only in 15.6% of teeth with Type 2 roots. Based on these findings it seems possible that Type 1 resorption is inflammatory and associated with periodontal disease while Type 2 roots are truly idiopathic.

It had been assumed that RLs represented a PIRR type of lesion and were associated with periodontal disease (Hopewell-Smith 1930; Reichart et al. 1984; Gold and Hasselgren 1992; Okuda and Harvey 1992). Studies have shown that the histologic lesion is a non-inflammatory replacement resorption, resulting in ankylosis (Gorrel and

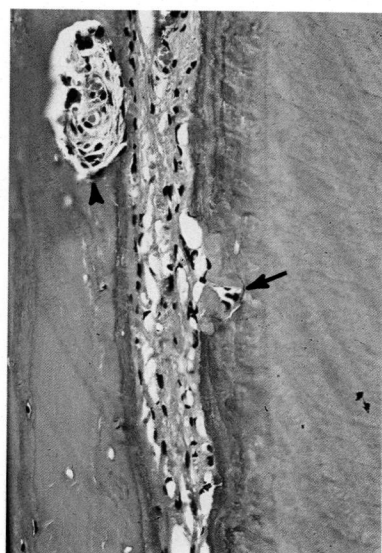

Fig. 11.7 Healing surface resorption There is a shallow localized resorption cavity (arrow) in the cementum. The lesion is showing evidence of healing, i.e. it is filled with reparative cementum-like tissue. There is also resorption in adjacent alveolar bone (arrowhead). The periodontal ligament is not inflamed, but it is atypical with a lack of horizontal fibers. See Fig. 11.10A for comparison with normal periodontal ligament (H&E ×100).

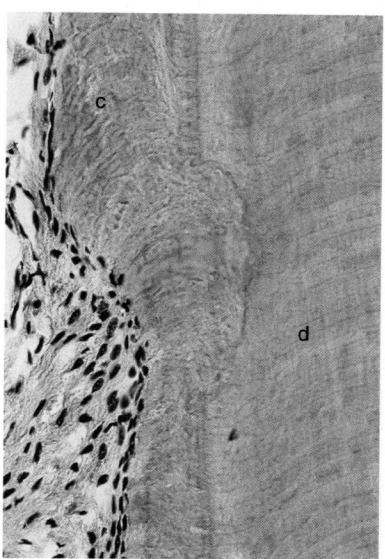

Fig. 11.8 Healed surface resorption The slide depicts a healed root resorption. The process had penetrated through the cementum (c) and into the dentine (d) and the defect is now filled with reparative cementum (H&E ×100).

Larsson 2002), and that the gingivitis index did not affect the prevalence of RLs (Ingham et al. 2001). These findings indicate that, while a PIRR type of lesion does exist, it is not the only type of root resorption. In fact, a non-inflammatory replacement resorption is equally common. The cause of the PIRR-type lesions is inflammation of adjacent tissue, i.e. periodontitis, while the cause of the non-inflammatory replacement resorption is as yet unknown, i.e. truly idiopathic.

In a study investigating the histologic features of the early lesion (Gorrel and Larsson 2002), it was found that surface RLs in the root cementum were common. The level along the root at which the lesions were identified varied, but they were always below the level of the alveolar crest, and were not associated with inflammation in the adjacent PDL. Therefore, in conflict with some data in the literature (Coles 1990; van Wessum et al. 1992), this study found no evidence to support the hypothesis that resorption starts at the CEJ or in the cervical part of the root.

Surface RLs of the root cementum in some teeth showed evidence of healing (Figs 11.7, 11.8). Whenever dentine was involved in the resorptive process, there was also evidence of ankylosis (Fig. 11.9). There was no inflammation of the PDL associated with the resorption cavities. However, the PDL in teeth affected by resorption (with

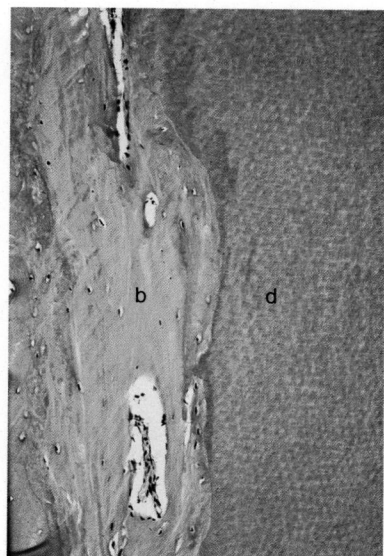

Fig. 11.9 Root resorption and ankylosis Cementum and dentine (d) resorption has been repaired by bone-like tissue (b) forming a bridge with adjacent alveolar bone. The tooth and bone are thus fused at this point. Whenever dentine is involved in the resorptive process, ankylosis is likely to follow (H&E ×50).

or without ankylosis) was atypical. The PDL of teeth unaffected by resorption is depicted in Figure 11.10A. In teeth affected by resorption without ankylosis, the PDL was narrower than normal and lacked distinctive fiber bundles (Figs 11.7, 11.10B). The PDL in teeth with resorption and ankylosis was a loose vascular connective tissue (Fig. 11.10C). The authors concluded that further studies are necessary to determine exactly what causes the high incidence of this type of 'idiopathic' feline external root resorption. However, they suggest several etiopathogenic explanatory models (Fig. 11.11), as follows.

First, that all cats suffer from surface root cementum resorption but cats that develop RLs fail to heal such lesions. The failure to heal could be a result of an inherent cementum defect. It could also be age related, i.e. that as a cat ages the healing process becomes slower than the resorptive process and the balance between the two processes changes and the surface resorption reaches the dentine. Once this occurs, RL formation and ankylosis become inevitable.

Alternatively, cats that develop RLs may suffer from defects in the protective properties of the PDL and cementoblast layer. This hypothesis is indirectly supported by the observed anatomic differences of the PDL in teeth with root resorption compared with unaffected teeth. These anatomic differences may also give rise to a suspicion that the affected teeth in cats which develop RLs are subject to suboptimal mechanical forces or are non-functional, resulting in lack of the stimulus required to maintain the functional integrity of the PDL. It is known that hypofunction (King and Hughes 1999) or reduced masticatory stimulation (Andersson et al. 1985) may result in tooth ankylosis.

Another line of research investigated calcium homeostasis in cats with or without RLs (Reiter and Mendoza 2002). In fact, a link between raised circulating levels of 25-hydroxy-vitamin D and odontoclastic RLs has been reported (Reiter and Mendoza 2002). This study concluded that chronic excess intake of vitamin D may play an important role in the development of odontoclastic RLs. Later studies (Zhang et al. 2006; Booij-Vrieling 2009; Girard et al. 2010) did not identify raised circulating levels of 25-hydroxy-vitamin D in cats with tooth resorption and conclude that increased serum vitamin D levels as a causative factor for root resorption could not be supported.

In summary, some of the RLs seen in cats are associated with inflammation of adjacent tissue, usually periodontitis, but a large number of lesions are idiopathic.

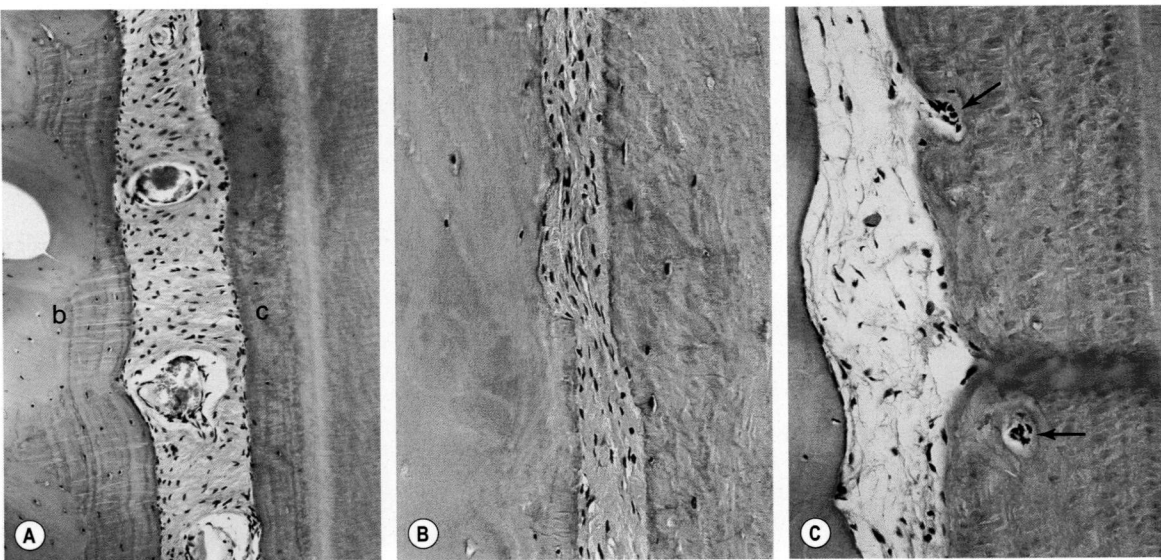

Fig. 11.10 Appearance of the periodontal ligament (PDL) (A) Normal PDL in teeth that were unaffected by resorptive lesions. The PDL fills the space between the alveolar bone (b) and the cementum (c). The fibers are aligned horizontally and obliquely. This appearance is characteristic of functioning PDL (H&E ×25). (B) Atypical PDL in teeth affected by resorption without ankylosis. The ligament space is narrower than normal and the fibers are aligned in a vertical direction, rather than the normal horizontal and oblique orientation (H&E ×100). (C) Atypical PDL in teeth affected by resorption and ankylosis. The section depicts a region distant from the ankylosis. The PDL does not have the normal fibrous architecture. Instead, it has a loosely vascular and edematous appearance. The loose vascular appearance of the PDL is presumably a 'functional adaptation' to the loss of tooth mobility due to the ankylosis. Note the localized resorption channels (arrows) in the cementum (H&E ×100).

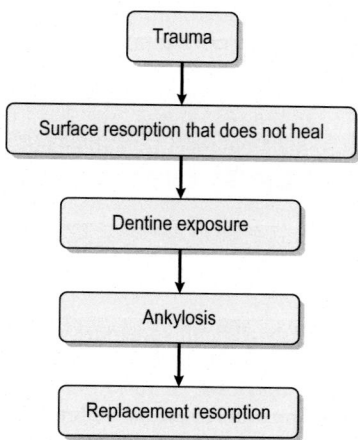

Fig. 11.11 Possible etiopathogenic models for 'idiopathic' feline external root resorption First, that all cats suffer from surface root cementum resorption but cats that develop resorptive lesions (RLs) fail to heal such lesions. The failure to heal could be a result of an inherent cementum defect. It could also be age related, i.e. that as a cat ages the healing process becomes slower than the resorptive process and the balance between the two processes changes and the surface resorption reaches the dentine. Once this occurs, RL formation and ankylosis become inevitable. Alternatively, cats that develop RLs may suffer from defects in the protective properties of the PDL and cementoblast layer.

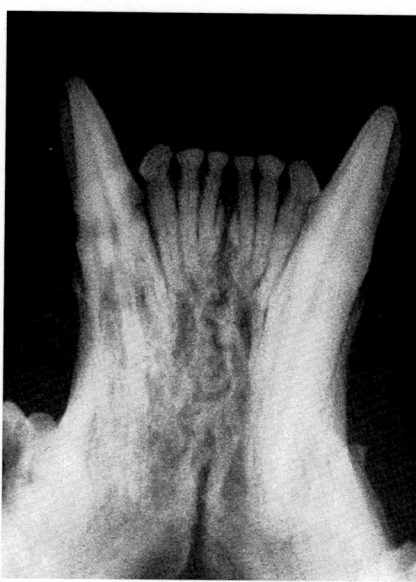

Fig. 11.12 Value of radiography for diagnosis and treatment selection Radiography will identify lesions that are localized to the root surfaces within the alveolar bone, which would not be detected by clinical methods. Consequently, radiography is required for diagnosis of RL. Moreover, it is only with the aid of radiography that the extent of the resorption can be evaluated. In the radiograph shown, the left lower canine has a resorbing root, where the process has not yet extended into the crown dentine. In fact, there was no clinical evidence of RL. The left lower canine could thus be treated conservatively. In contrast, in the right lower canine tooth, the process has progressed to involve the crown and most of the root has been resorbed and replaced by bone-like tissue. Extraction is not possible and coronal amputation becomes the treatment of choice.

DIAGNOSIS

Radiography is required for diagnosis of RLs. The lesions can be detected by means of a combination of:

- Visual inspection
- Tactile examination with a dental explorer
- Radiography.

Visual inspection and tactile examination with a dental explorer will only identify end-stage lesions, i.e. when the process is involving the crown and has resulted in an obvious cavity (Figs 11.1, 11.2A). Radiography will identify lesions that are localized to the root surfaces within the alveolar bone (Fig. 11.12), which would not be detected by clinical methods. Moreover, it is only with the aid of radiography that the appearance and extent of a resorptive process can be identified (Figs 11.2B, 11.12). Selection of the best treatment option thus depends on radiography. In fact, a series of full mouth radiographs (the technique is covered in Ch. 7) is recommended for all cats presented for dental therapy. If taking a series of full mouth radiographs is not possible, e.g. because of financial restrictions, then take one view of each mandibular premolar/molar region. The mandibular 3rd premolars are the most commonly affected teeth. If radiographs show resorption of these teeth, then a full mouth series must be taken. A study (Heaton et al. 2004) has shown that in nine out of 10 cats with RLs the disease would be identified in these two views. It was recommended that this technique be used as a rapid screening test.

TREATMENT

The aim of any treatment is to relieve pain, prevent progression of pathology and restore function. It remains a matter of debate as to whether RLs cause discomfort or pain to the affected individual. Based on the fact that pulpal inflammation occurs late in the disease process, it seems likely that lesions that are limited to the root surfaces and do not communicate with the oral environment are asymptomatic. However, once dentine destruction has progressed to such an extent that the process invades the pulp and/or a communication with the oral cavity has been established (when the enamel has been resorbed or it has fractured off to reveal the dentine to the oral cavity), then discomfort and/or pain are likely as the pulp becomes inflamed. Some cats may show clinical signs indicating oral discomfort or pain, e.g. changes in food preferences (soft rather than hard diet), reduced food intake, but many cats do not.

To date, there is no known treatment which prevents development and/or progression of the idiopathic type of RL. It seems unlikely that such treatment can be developed without knowledge of the cause of the pathology. Currently, the suggested methods of managing RLs are:

• Conservative management
• Tooth extraction
• Coronal amputation.

In the past restoration of the tooth surface has incorrectly been recommended for the treatment of accessible lesions which extend into the dentine and do not involve pulp tissue. Several studies have shown that tooth resorption continues and the restorations are lost (Hopewell-Smith 1930; Okuda and Harvey 1992; Shigeyana et al. 1996). Consequently, the use of restoration of feline RLs as a major treatment technique cannot be recommended.

Conservative management

Conservative management consists of monitoring the lesions clinically and radiographically. This approach is recommended for lesions that are not evident on clinical examination, i.e. only seen radiographically and there is no evidence of discomfort or pain. As most lesions are only diagnosed when pathology is extensive, conservative management is rarely indicated in the general practice situation.

In most cases, extraction or coronal amputation of an affected tooth is indicated. With extraction, the whole tooth is removed. This is the gold standard. However, when the root has been extensively resorbed it is often not possible to extract all tooth substance (Fig. 11.12) and coronal amputation is indicated. Preoperative radiographs are mandatory to allow selection of the appropriate treatment option.

Extraction

Teeth with RLs are notoriously difficult to extract as the root is resorbing and being replaced by bone-like tissue. Moreover, there are areas of ankylosis, i.e. fusion of bone and tooth substance, along the root surface. In addition to preoperative radiographs to detect the lesions and determine appropriate treatment, postoperative radiographs to ensure that the whole tooth has been removed are required. The details of the technique for extracting feline teeth are covered in Chapter 13.

Coronal amputation

As already mentioned, when the root has been extensively resorbed it is often not possible to extract all tooth substance. Coronal amputation is then indicated. The indications for and outcome of coronal amputation have been well documented (DuPont 1995) and the procedure is recommended, but needs radiographic monitoring at regular intervals postoperatively to ensure that the root is resorbing and that healing is uneventful.

The technique for coronal amputation (Fig. 11.13) involves raising a gingival flap both buccally and palatally/lingually to expose the margin of the alveolar bone. The crown of the affected tooth is amputated using a round bur. A small amount of root tissue is also removed with the bur, just enough to ensure that the intentionally retained root(s) are apical to the alveolar crest. The gingival flap is replaced and sutured in place.

SUMMARY

◆ External root resorption is common in the cat.
◆ Root resorption is either inflammatory in origin (periodontal disease) or idiopathic.
◆ The lesions are progressive.
◆ Diagnosis requires radiography.
◆ The purpose of the treatment is the relief of discomfort or pain. In most instances, extraction of

the tooth or coronal amputation remain the preferable treatment options.
◆ Successful extraction and uncomplicated healing needs clinical and radiographic monitoring.

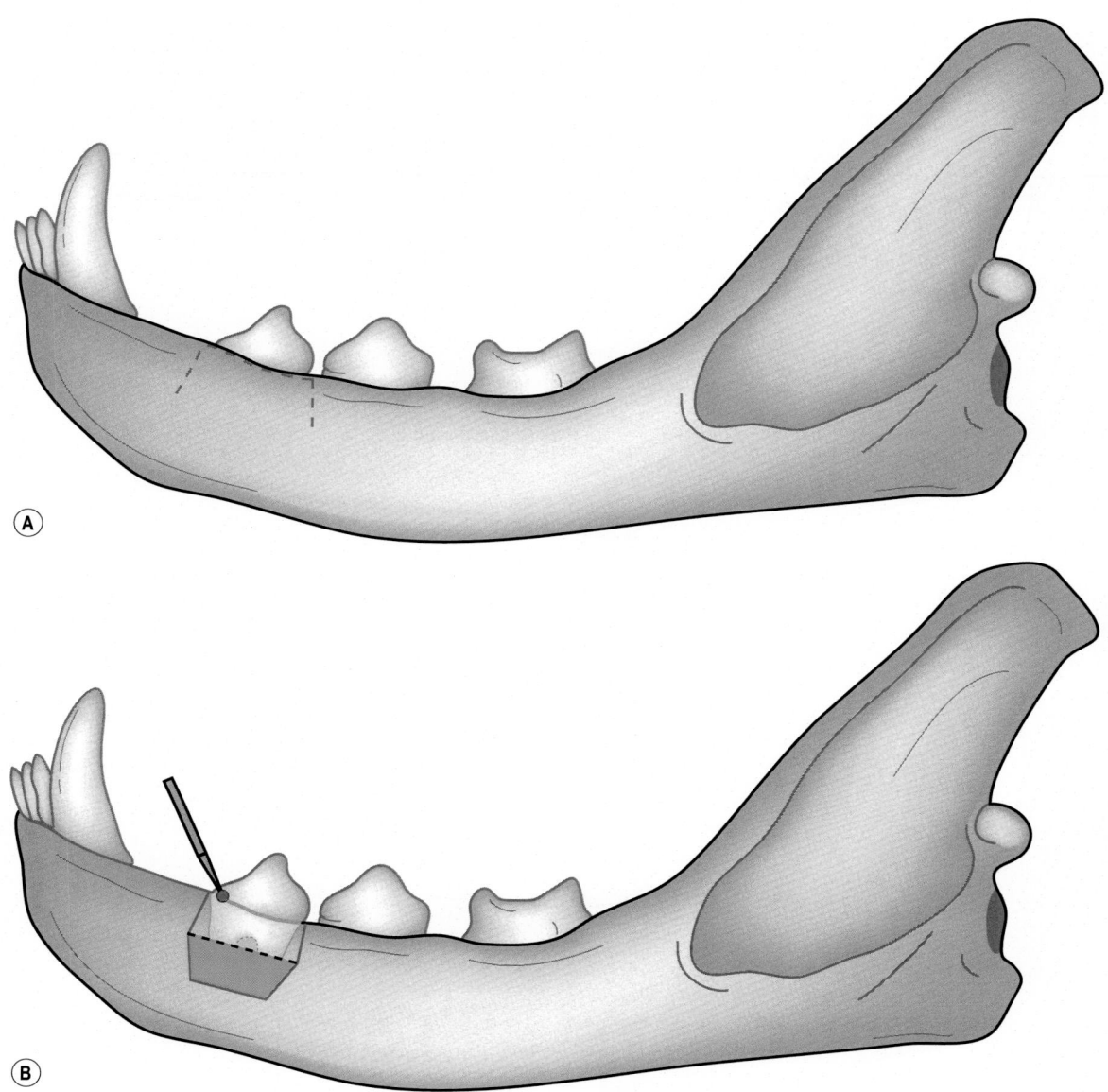

Fig. 11.13 Coronal amputation (A) Raising a gingival flap. Two short releasing incisions (one placed mesial to, and the other distal to, the tooth) extending to, or just past, the mucogingival junction facilitate raising the flap. (B) Raising a gingival flap and amputating the crown. A periosteal elevator is used to raise a full-thickness gingival flap. The flap is reflected to expose the buccal alveolar bone plate. The crown of the affected tooth is amputated using a small round bur.

Continued

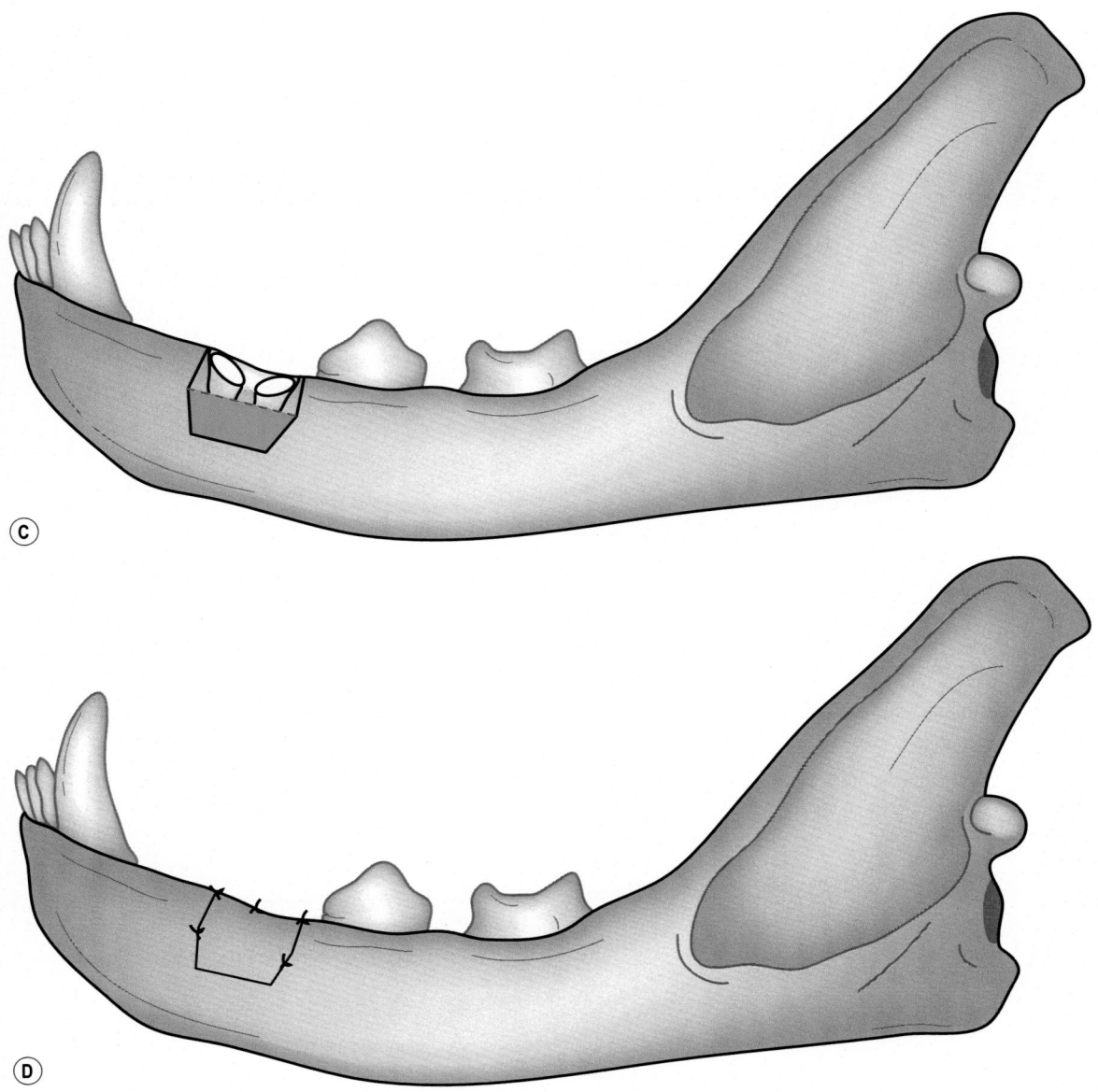

Fig. 11.13, cont'd (C) Removing root substance. A small amount of root tissue is also removed with the bur, just enough to ensure that the intentionally retained root(s) are apical to the alveolar crest. (D) Replacing the flap. The gingival flap is replaced, ensuring that there is no tension, and sutured in place. If there is tension, the releasing incisions can be extended and the flap freed past the mucogingival junction.

REFERENCES

Andersson, L., Lindskog, S., Blomlöf, L., et al., 1985. Effect of masticatory stimulation on dentoalveolar ankylosis after experimental tooth replantation. Endodontics and Dental Traumatology 1, 13–16.

Andreasen, J.O., 1985. External root resorption: its implications in dental traumatology, paedodontics, periodontics, orthodontics and endodontics. International Endodontic Journal 18, 109–118.

Andreasen, J.O., 1988. Review of root resorption systems and models. Etiology of root resorption and the homeostatic mechanisms of the periodontal ligament. In: Davidovitch, Z. (Ed.), Proceedings of the International Conference on the Biological Mechanisms of Tooth Eruption and Root Resorption. Ebesco Media, Birmingham, pp. 9–21.

Andreasen, J.O., Kristerson, L., 1981. The effect of limited drying or removal of the periodontal ligament. Periodontal healing after replantation of mature incisors in monkeys. Acta Odontologica Scandinavica 39, 1–13.

Arnbjerg, J., 1996. Idiopathic dental root replacement resorption in old dogs. Journal of Veterinary Dentistry 13 (3), 97–99.

Berger, M., Schawalder, P., Stich, H., et al., 1996. Feline dental resorptive lesions in captive and wild leopards and lions. Journal of Veterinary Dentistry 13 (1), 13–21.

Booij-Vrieling, H.E., 2009. Tooth resorption in cats: contribution of vitamin D and inflammation. PhD Thesis, Utrecht, the Netherlands.

Clarke, D.E., Cameron, A., 1997. Feline dental resorptive lesions in domestic and feral cats and the possible link with diet. In: Proceedings of the 5th World Veterinary Dental Congress. Birmingham, UK, pp. 33–34.

Coles, S., 1990. The prevalence of buccal cervical root resorptions in Australian cats. Journal of Veterinary Dentistry 7 (4), 14–16.

Crossley, D., Dubielzig, R., Benson, K., 1997. Caries and odontoclastic resorptive lesions in a chinchilla (Chinchilla lanigera). Veterinary Record 141, 337–339.

DuPont, G.A., 1995. Crown amputation with intentional root retention for advanced feline resorptive lesions – a clinical study. Journal of Veterinary Dentistry 12 (1), 9–13.

DuPont, G.A., DeBowes, L.J., 2002. Comparison of periodontitis and root replacement in cat teeth with resorptive lesions. Journal of Veterinary Dentistry 19 (2), 71–75.

Girard, N., Servet, E., Hennet, P., et al., 2010. Tooth resorption and vitamin D3 status in cats fed premium dry diets. Journal of Veterinary Dentistry 27 (3), 142–147.

Gold, S.I., Hasselgren, G., 1992. Peripheral inflammatory root resorption. A review of the literature with case reports. Journal of Clinical Periodontology 19, 523–534.

Gorrel, C., Larsson, Å., 2002. Feline odontoclastic resorptive lesions: unveiling the early lesion. Journal of Small Animal Practice 43, 482–488.

Hammarström, L., Blomlöf, L., Lindskog, S., 1989. Dynamics of dentoalveolar ankylosis and associated root resorption. Endodontics and Dental Traumatology 5, 163–175.

Heaton, M., Wilkinson, J., Gorrel, C., et al., 2004. A rapid screening technique for feline odontoclastic resorptive lesions. Journal of Small Animal Practice 45 (12), 598–601.

Hopewell-Smith, A., 1930. The process of osteolysis and odontolysis, or so-called 'absorption' of calcified tissues: a new and original investigation. The evidences in the cat. Dental Cosmos 72, 1036–1048.

Ingham, K.E., Gorrel, C., Blackburn, J.M., et al., 2001. Prevalence of odontoclastic resorptive lesions in a clinically healthy cat population. Journal of Small Animal Practice 42, 439–443.

King, G.N., Hughes, F.J., 1999. Effects of occlusal loading on ankylosis, bone and cementum formation during morphogenetic protein-2-stimulated periodontal regeneration in vivo. Journal of Periodontology 70, 1125–1135.

Levin, J., 1996. Tooth resorption in a Siberian tiger. In: Proceedings of the 10th Annual Veterinary Dental Forum, Houston, Texas, USA, pp. 212–214.

Lindskog, S., Hammarström, L., 1980. Evidence in favour of an anti-invasion factor in cementum or periodontal membrane. Scandinavian Journal of Dental Research 88, 161–163.

Lindskog, S., Blomlöf, L., Hammarström, L., 1983. Repair of periodontal tissues in vitro and in vivo. Journal of Clinical Periodontology 10, 188–205.

Lindskog, S., Blomlöf, L., Hammarström, L., 1987. Cellular colonization of denuded root surfaces in vivo: cell morphology in dentin resorption and cementum repair. Journal of Clinical Periodontology 14, 390–395.

Lommer, M.J., Verstraete, F.J.M., 2000. Prevalence of odontoclastic resorption lesions and periapical radiographic lucencies in cats: 265 cases (1995–1998). Journal of the American Veterinary Medical Association 217, 1866–1869.

Lund, E.M., Bohacek, L.K., Dahlke, J.L., et al., 1998. Prevalence and risk factors for odontoclastic resorptive lesions in cats. Journal of the American Veterinary Medical Association 212, 392–395.

Ne, R.F., Witherspoon, D.E., Gutmann, J.L., 1999. Tooth resorption. Quintessence International 30, 9–25.

Okuda, A., Harvey, C.E., 1992. Etiopathogenesis of feline dental resorptive lesions. Feline dentistry. Veterinary Clinics of North America: Small Animal Practice. WB Saunders, Philadelphia, pp. 1385–1404.

Reichart, P.A., Durr, U.-M., Triadan, H., et al., 1984. Periodontal disease in the domestic cat. Journal of Periodontal Research 19, 67–75.

Reiter, A., Mendoza, K.A., 2002. Feline odontoclastic resorptive lesions: an unsolved enigma in veterinary dentistry. Veterinary Clinics of North America: Small Animal Practice 32, 791–837.

Shigeyana, Y., Grove, T.K., Strayhorn, C., et al., 1996. Expression of adhesion molecules during tooth resorption in feline teeth: a model system for aggressive osteoclastic activity. Journal of Dental Research 75, 1650–1657.

van Wessum, R., Harvey, C.E., Hennet, P., 1992. Feline dental resorptive lesions. Prevalence patterns. Feline dentistry. Veterinary Clinics of North America: Small Animal Practice. WB Saunders, Philadelphia, pp. 1405–1416.

Verstraete, F.J.M., Aarde Van, R.J., Nieuwoudt, B.A., et al., 1996. The dental pathology of feral cats on Marion Island. Part II: periodontitis, external odontoclastic resorptive lesions and mandibular thickening. Journal of Comparative Pathology 115, 283–297.

Verstraete, F.J.M., Kass, P.H., Terpak, C.H., 1998. Diagnostic value of full mouth radiography in cats. American Journal of Veterinary Research 59, 692–695.

Zhang, G., Cupp, C., Kerr, W., 2006. Vitamin D status in cats with and without feline odontoclastic resorptive lesions. Compendium on Continuing Education for the Practising Veterinarian 28, 77.

FURTHER READING

Gorrel, C., 2008. Root resorption. In: Saunders Solutions in Veterinary Practice – Small Animal Dentistry. Saunders/Elsevier, Philadelphia, pp. 105–128.

Chapter 12

Emergencies

INTRODUCTION

The conditions which may be considered emergencies generally result from trauma to the face and oral cavity (Fig. 12.1). While they are not life-threatening, most cause discomfort and some cause severe pain and even systemic complications to the affected animal, so treatment should not be delayed. All practicing veterinarians will come across these conditions and need to be able to diagnose and provide first-line management and then refer to a specialist for treatment if indicated.

The basic principles of managing a severely traumatized animal are covered in other texts. It must always be remembered that there is a body attached to the head and, in the severely traumatized animal, dental and oral problems may not generally be the main initial consideration.

SOFT-TISSUE TRAUMA

The principles of wound management are the same as elsewhere in the body. Consequently, only lip injuries and management of oronasal fistulae will be dealt with in detail in this chapter.

The immediate priority is to control hemorrhage without compromising the blood supply to the damaged area. Most traumatic wounds will be contaminated. Early efforts should be made to reduce contamination. Particulate debris is best removed by gentle lavage with a balanced electrolyte solution. Antiseptic solutions should only be used in very dilute solutions. Larger fragments embedded in a wound can be removed manually during surgical exploration of the wound. Surgical drains left *in situ* may be useful in severely contaminated wounds. Surgical excision of necrotic tissue (debridement) is essential to promote early granulation. Following debridement, several options are available for closure of wounds. These are:

- Primary closure
- Delayed primary closure
- Healing by secondary intention
- Grafting techniques.

The choice of closure technique will depend on:

- Location of the wound
- Size of the wound
- Age of the wound
- Degree of contamination.

Lip injuries

The anatomy of the lip is particularly suited to grafting techniques. Advancement, rotation and transposition flaps (Fig. 12.2) all have their uses.

Degloving injury to the lower lip frequently occurs in cats involved in road traffic accidents. If the skin is viable, it can be pulled forward and sutured using the canine teeth as anchors. If the skin is not viable, then, after debridement, the exposed bone can be covered by creating an advancement flap, which is pulled forward and anchored to the canine teeth. It may be necessary to incise the commissures of the lips to mobilize a sufficiently large advancement flap. To close the commissures, the mucosa is sutured to the skin.

Injury to the anterior maxilla with loss of part of the rhinarium can also be repaired using advancement, rotation or transposition flap. Ensure patency of the nares.

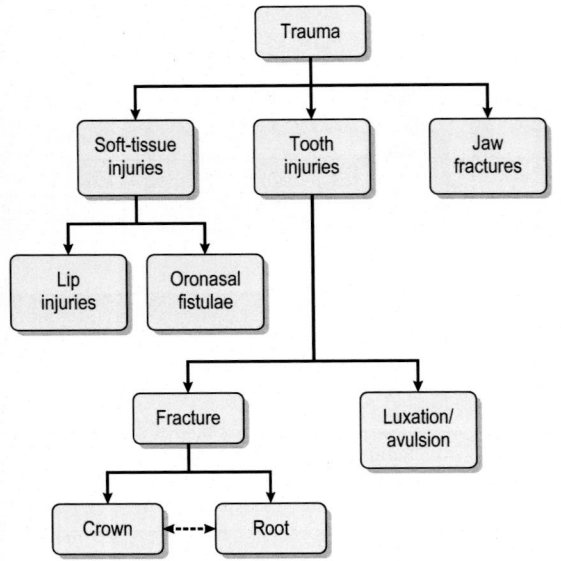

Fig. 12.1 Oral emergencies

Table 12.1 Recommendations for choice of repair option depending on type of defect

Type of defect	Repair options
Narrow	Unilateral pedicle flap rotated or transposed to cover defect
Large midline	Bilateral pedicle flaps (Langenbeck or Veau–Wardill) Overlapping double flap
Large rostral	Vestibular flap Palatal prosthesis
Circular or caudal	Hard palate rotational flap Soft palate advancement flap Split palatal U-flap Palatal prosthesis

There is a lot of spare tissue available to cover defects. Think 'large' when creating flaps and ensure that flaps are never sutured under tension.

Oronasal fistulae

An oronasal fistula is a pathologic communication between the oral cavity and the nasal chambers. The fistula is lined by epithelium and can therefore not heal over. The two most common locations are full thickness palate defects and communication between a maxillary tooth alveolus and the nasal chamber.

Hard palate

Acquired hard palate defects in dogs and cats may occur following:

- Road traffic accident
- Electrical shock
- Foreign body penetration
- Gunshot wounds
- Pressure necrosis.

Several methods of managing hard palate clefts (congenital and acquired) have been described.

The choice of technique will depend on:

- Location of the defect, i.e. rostral or caudal
- Size and shape of the defect
- Amount of tissue available for pedicle grafting procedures.

Small rostral defects not involving the nasal cavity but communicating into the incisal bone will not cause nasal regurgitation and do not need to be repaired. Table 12.1 shows recommendations for choice of technique for repair of different types of hard palate defects.

Principles of palate surgery

1. The flaps must be tension free. Large flaps should be raised to avoid tension and ensure overlap between the flap and adjacent healthy tissue.
2. The blood supply to the flap must be retained. When raising palatal flaps it is important to identify and preserve the palatine artery. This artery exits from the palatine bone 0.5–1.0 cm medial to the upper carnassial tooth (Fig. 12.3). Palatal flaps should be full thickness mucoperiosteum with the incisions located away from the palatine artery. For vestibular flaps, find a tissue plane that will leave most of the connective tissue attached to the mucosal flap.
3. Ensure that the epithelial margin of the defect is debrided.
4. Ensure that connective tissue surfaces or cut edges are sutured together, as intact epithelium will not heal to any other surface.
5. Suture lines should not lie over a defect if possible. The use of asymmetrical flaps may help avoid this.
6. Gastrostomy or pharyngostomy tubes are not necessary. Nasogastric tubes are preferable if the animal will not eat. Careful, gentle technique and planning the procedure so that there is no tension on the sutured edges is much more important in preventing dehiscence.

Repair options described for hard palate lesions are:

- Various pedicle grafting techniques
- The Langenbeck technique
- The Veau–Wardill technique

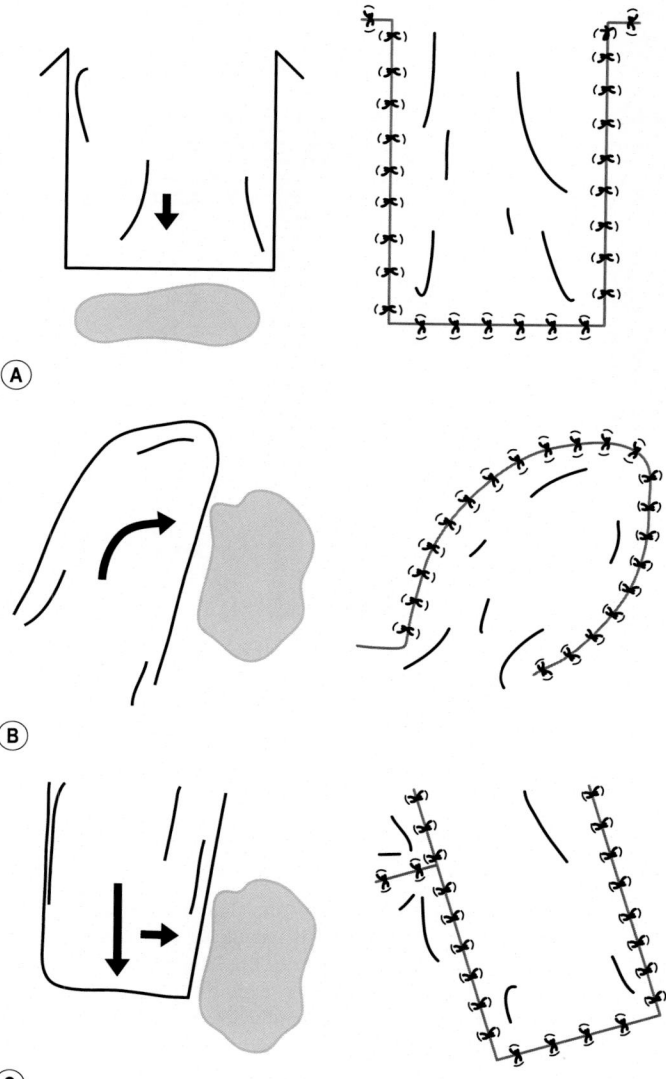

Fig. 12.2 Some useful grafting techniques
(A) Advancement flap. (B) Rotation flap.
(C) Transposition flap.

- Double overlapping double flap
- Split palatal U-flap
- Other techniques
- Silicone or acrylic prosthesis.

Various pedicle flaps. These techniques are unilateral pedicle grafts based on the major palatine artery. The flap is either rotated (Fig. 12.2B) or transposed (Fig. 12.2C) to cover the defect. It is essential to debride the epithelial margins of the defect with a scalpel blade and to ensure that the flap is sutured without tension. These techniques work well for narrow defects.

The Langenbeck technique. This technique is essentially a bilateral pedicle flap and is useful for large midline defects. The main disadvantage of the Langenbeck technique is that there is a tendency for breakdown and persistence of the cleft rostrally. It is outlined in Figure 12.4.

1. Debride the epithelial margins of the defect with a scalpel blade.
2. Incisions are made into the mucoperiosteum at the dental margin on either side of the defect. Be careful not to transect the palatine arteries.

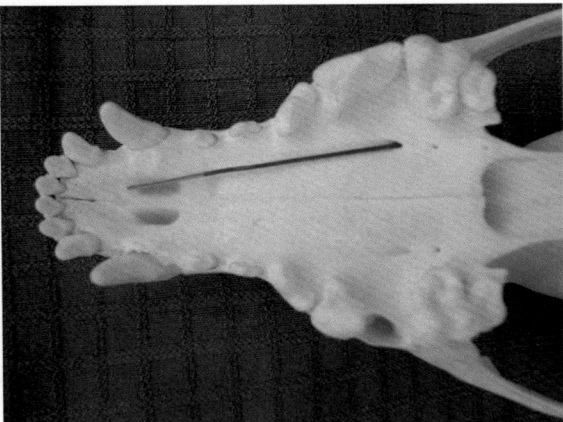

Fig. 12.3 The palatine artery This artery exits from the palatine bone 0.5–1.0 cm medial to the upper carnassial tooth. When raising palatal flaps, it is essential to preserve the palatine artery as it is the main blood supply to the flap.

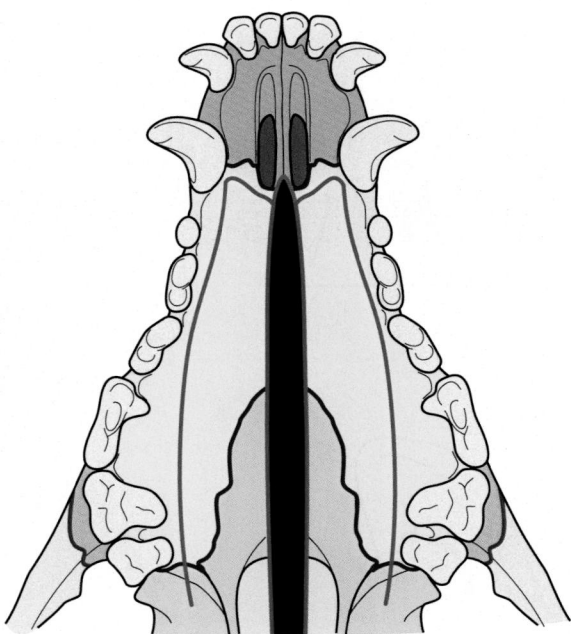

Fig. 12.5 The Veau–Wardill technique This technique is similar to the Langenbeck, except that rostral incisions extending from the dental margin to the midline bilaterally are also made. This allows caudal as well as lateral movement of the flaps and may reduce tension on closure. It is useful for the repair of large midline defects.

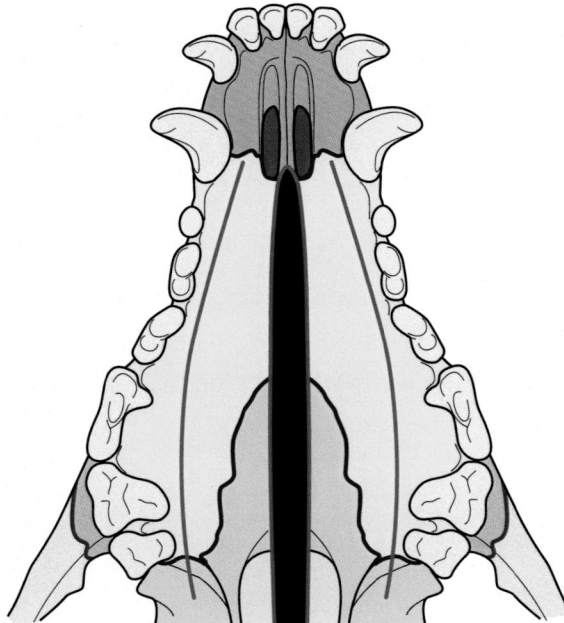

Fig. 12.4 The Langenbeck technique This bilateral pedicle flap is useful to repair large midline defects.

3. The mucoperiosteum is released from the palate with a periosteal elevator, thus raising two longitudinal strips of mucoperiosteum from the hard palate on either side of the defect.

4. The two strips of released mucoperiosteum are slid together and sutured at the midline, thus closing the cleft.

5. The exposed bone at the dental margin bilaterally is left to granulate and epithelialize.

The Veau–Wardill technique. This technique is also a bilateral pedicle flap and is useful for the repair of large midline defects. It is similar to the Langenbeck technique, except that rostral incisions extending from the dental margin to the midline bilaterally are also made (Fig. 12.5). This allows caudal as well as lateral movement of the flaps and this may help to reduce tension on closure.

The double overlapping flap technique. This technique is also called the upside down overlapping flap technique. It is useful for repair of large midline palatal defects. There is less risk of rostral breakdown using this technique. It is summarized in Figure 12.6.

1. Debride the epithelial margins of the defect with a scalpel blade.

2. Incisions are made in the mucoperiosteum at the defect on one side, and along the dental margin on the other side.

3. Flaps **a** and **b** (Figure 12.6) are raised using a periosteal elevator. Make sure that the palatine arteries are not transected.

4. Flap **a** is folded back on itself and sutured under flap **b** so that the connective tissue surfaces are in

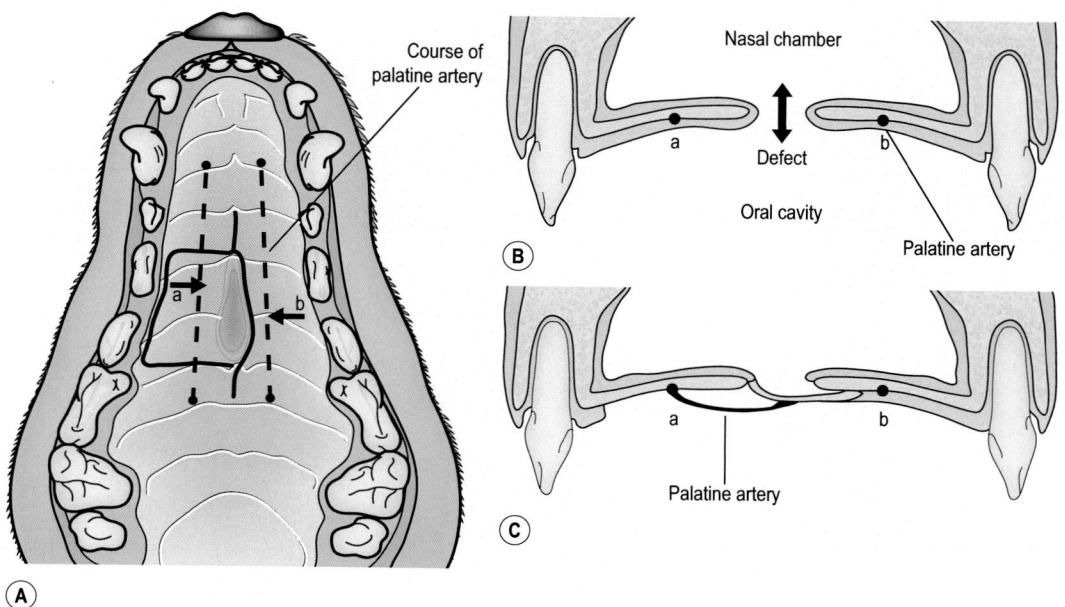

Fig. 12.6 The double overlapping flap technique (A–C) This technique is also called the upside down overlapping flap technique. It is useful for the repair of large midline defects.

contact. The sutures are preplaced in **a** mattress pattern. The epithelium of flap **a** will thus form the nasal epithelium and flap **b** will contribute the oral epithelium.

5. The exposed palatine bone is again left to granulate and epithelialize.

The split palatal U-flap technique. This technique is particularly useful for large caudal defects. The procedure is outlined in Figure 12.7.

1. Debride the epithelial margins of the defect with a scalpel blade.
2. Create a large U-shaped mucoperiosteal flap rostral to the defect using a periosteal elevator.
3. Incise along the midline of the raised flap to create two equally sized flaps.
4. Rotate flap **a** (Figure 12.7) 90° and transpose to cover the defect.
5. The medial aspect of flap **a** is sutured to the caudal aspect of the palatal defect and the tip of this flap is sutured to the lateral aspect of the palatal defect.
6. Flap **b** is rotated 90° and transposed anterior to flap **a**.
7. The medial aspect and tip of flap **b** are sutured to the edge of flap **a**.
8. The rostral aspect of the palate from which the flap was harvested is left to granulate.

Other techniques. For large, rostral defects a vestibular flap can be used. Holes are made in the flap to allow for teeth in the area, or teeth are extracted as required.

Alternatively, a **prosthesis of silicone or acrylic** can be custom-made. This technique requires a minimum of two anesthetic episodes.

Soft palate

Soft palate clefts are usually congenital rather than traumatic or acquired. Closure of soft palate defects should be a double layer repair (Fig. 12.8). Incisions are made along the medial margins of the palate on each side. Blunt-ended scissors are used to separate the palate tissue on each side into dorsal and ventral flaps. The two dorsal flaps are sutured in a simple interrupted pattern to form a complete nasal epithelium, and the two ventral flaps are sutured to form a complete oral epithelium. The palate is closed to just caudal to the tonsils.

Maxillary alveolus

The maxillary canine teeth are the most frequent sites of oronasal fistula formation and the premolars the least frequent. The three most common causes of oronasal fistula formation between a maxillary alveolus and the nasal chamber are:

1. Periodontitis
2. Periapical lesions
3. Iatrogenic.

An oronasal fistula in the region of the canine tooth is commonly the result of periodontitis, where the process perforates the medial bony wall of the dental alveolus.

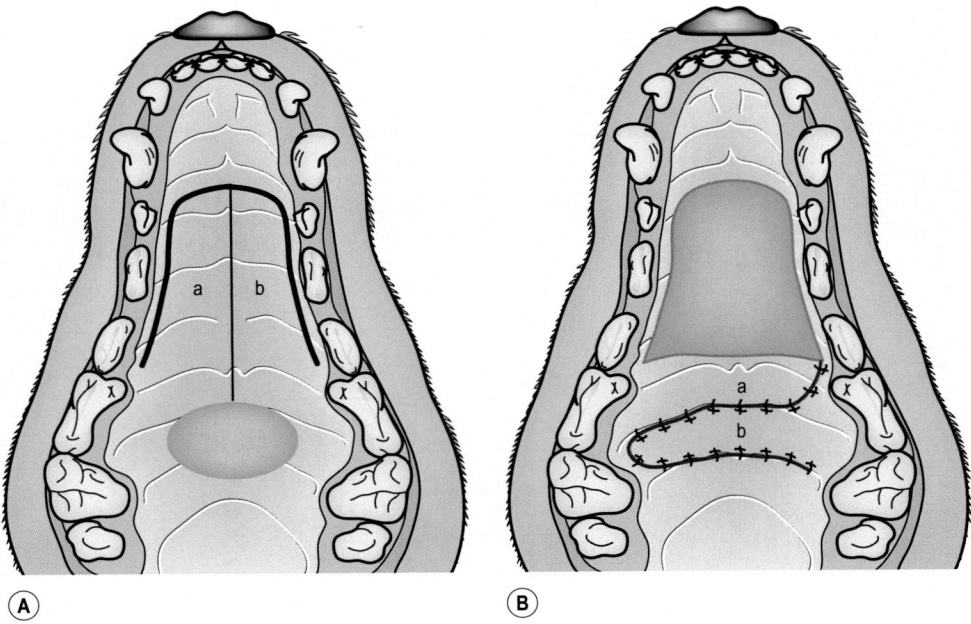

Fig. 12.7 The split palatal U-flap technique (A,B) This technique is particularly useful for large caudal defects.

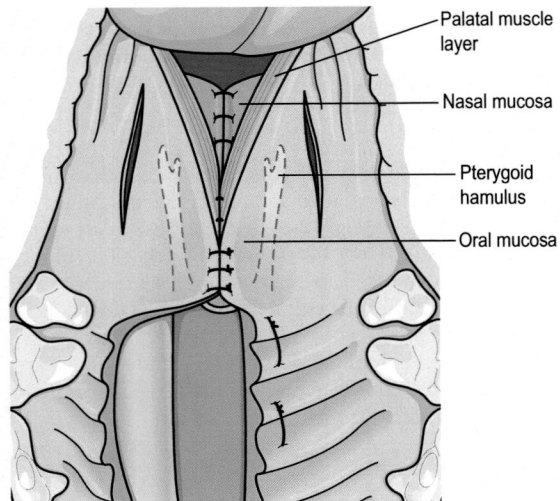

Palatal muscle layer

Nasal mucosa

Pterygoid hamulus

Oral mucosa

Fig. 12.8 Double layer soft palate repair Closure of soft palate defects should always be a double layer repair.

Periapical pathology of the maxillary canine teeth and premolars can also cause perforation of the medial wall of the alveolus, as can extraction of the maxillary canine tooth. Large fresh defects or long-standing defects causing clinical signs, i.e. nasal discharge, food impaction and chronic infection, should be surgically repaired. In the case of a long-standing, chronically infected lesion

preoperative, as well as postoperative, antibiotics are recommended. The choice of antibiotic should ideally be based on culture and sensitivity.

Single layer repair. The single layer repair is the surgery of choice. It works very well in most instances. The important step is to mobilize enough tissue to allow an absolutely tension-free repair. This usually requires extending the flap elevation beyond the buccal vestibule, i.e. the site at which the mucosa leaves the bone and reflects onto the interior of the cheek to become the buccal mucosa. Scarifying the edges of the defect to remove the epithelium is also essential for healing.

The procedure is outlined in Figure 12.9.

1. The epithelial attachment is cut on the labial side from the caudal aspect of the 1st premolar, along the buccal edge of the defect extending to the mesial aspect of the upper lateral incisor using a scalpel blade.
2. Vertical releasing incisions are made at the mesial aspect of the lateral incisor and the distal aspect of the 1st premolar.
3. A full thickness flap is raised using a periosteal elevator.
4. It is essential that the flap extends beyond the mucogingival line, i.e. the alveolar mucosa is released from the underlying alveolar bone.
5. Dissection of the alveolar mucosa continues until sufficient tissue has been mobilized to cover the defect. This may require extending the flap elevation to or beyond the height of the buccal vestibule.

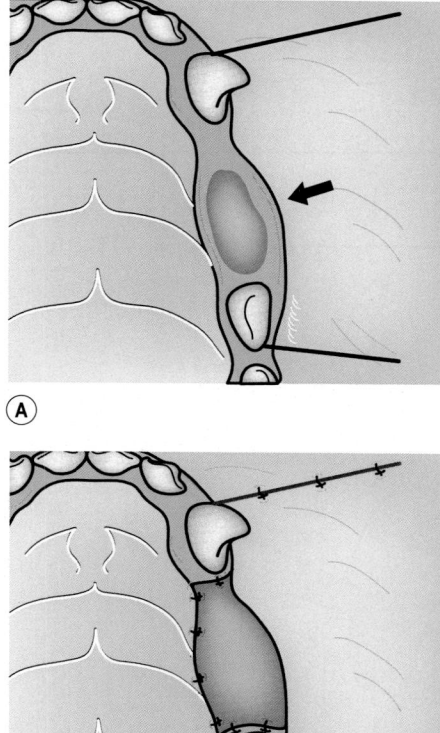

Fig. 12.9 Single layer oronasal fistula repair

6. Split the periosteum at the base of the flap to afford complete mobility of the flap.
7. The margins of the oronasal fistula are scarified.
8. The flap is advanced across the defect and sutured to the palatine mucosa using an absorbable suture material.
9. Soft food is recommended for 2 weeks postoperatively.

Double layer repair. If single layer repair fails or if the defect is large and of long standing, a double layer technique may be used (Fig. 12.10). This technique can be modified for gingival recession or alveolar bone loss (Fig. 12.11).

TRAUMATIC TOOTH INJURIES

Traumatic tooth injuries are common and may involve fracture of the tooth or damage to the periodontium. They

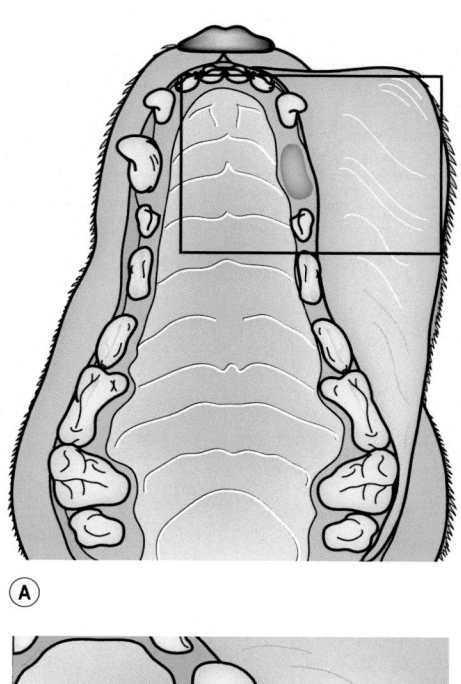

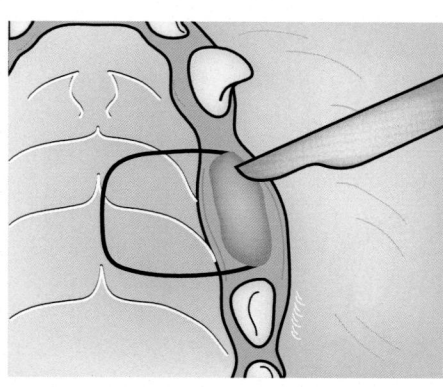

Fig. 12.10 Double layer oronasal fistula repair
(A) Oronasal fistula at the upper left canine site. The box indicates the area drawn in detail. (B) Raising the palatal flap and scarifying the lateral margin of the fistula.
Continued

are generally the result of a road traffic accident, blunt blow to the face or chewing on hard objects.

Teeth that have been affected by trauma often require endodontic treatment (see Appendix) if they are to be maintained.

Tooth fracture

Tooth fracture may affect the crown (Fig. 12.12), the crown and root (Fig. 12.13) or just the root (Fig. 12.14).

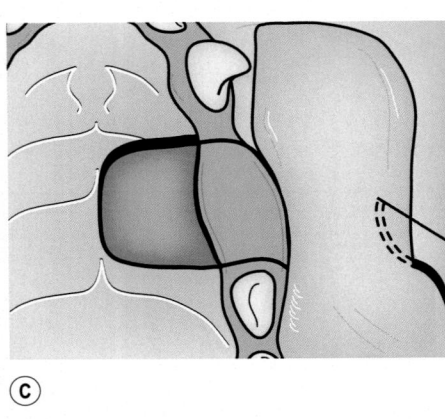

(C)

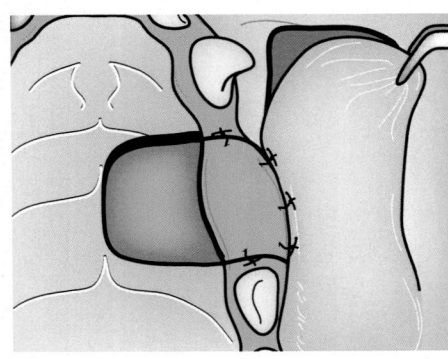

(D)

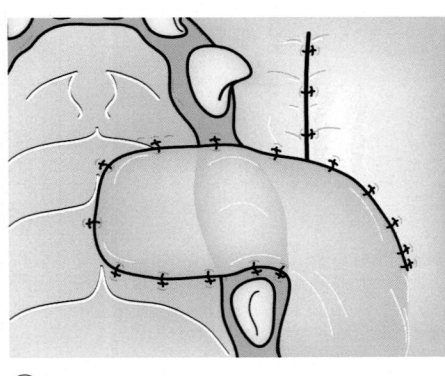

(E)

Fig. 12.10, cont'd (C) Laying the tension-free palatal flap and raising the mucosal finger flap. (D) The palatal flap is sutured in place. (E) The mucosal finger flap is rotated and sutured to the palatal mucosa.

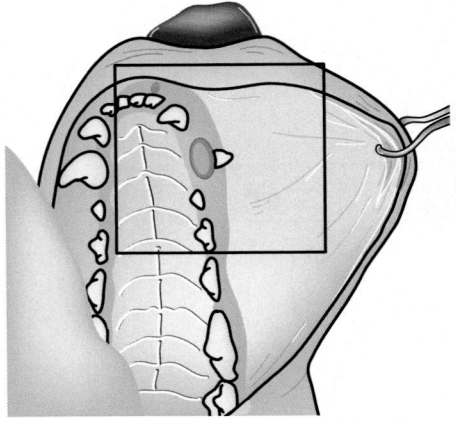

(A)

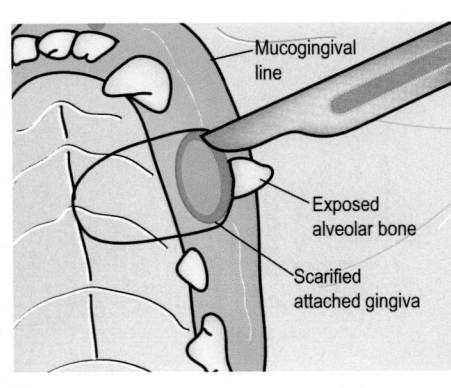

Mucogingival line

Exposed alveolar bone

Scarified attached gingiva

(B)

Fig. 12.11 Repair of oronasal fistula complicated by gingival recession beyond the mucogingival junction (A) Oronasal fistula at the upper left canine site. The box indicates the area drawn in detail. (B) Raising the palatal flap and scarifying the attached gingiva.

Crown

Crown fractures are classified as complicated if the fracture line exposes the pulp to the oral environment and as uncomplicated if they do not involve pulpal exposure. Crown fractures are obvious visually. However, at times it can be difficult to determine whether the pulp is exposed by the fracture line and general anesthesia for examination with a dental explorer and radiography are necessary.

Complicated crown fractures always need treatment. An exposed pulp will become inflamed and may eventually undergo necrosis. The inflammation can spread from the pulp to involve the periapical area (Fig. 12.15). A primary tooth with complicated crown fracture should be extracted

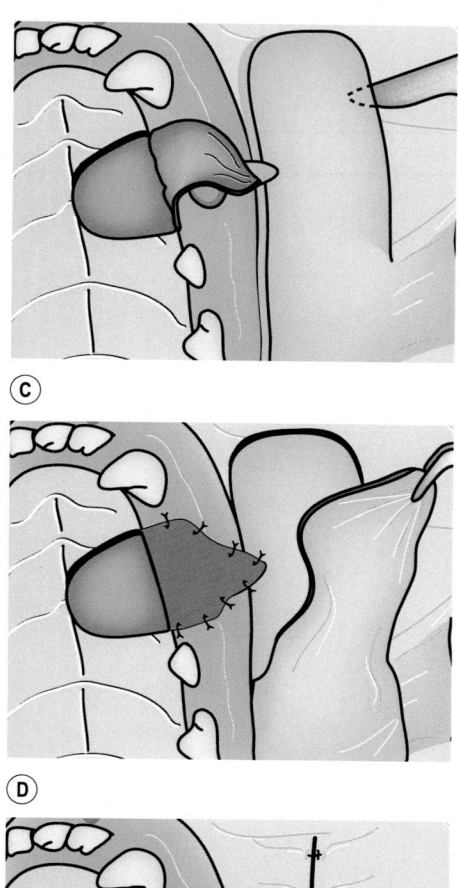

(C)

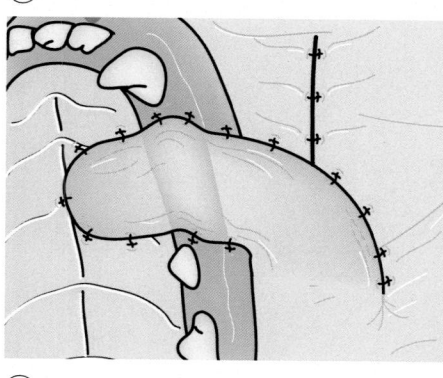

(D)

(E)

Fig. 12.11, cont'd (C) Laying the palatal flap and raising the mucosal finger flap. (D) The lifted palatal flap is sutured in place and the finger flap lifted. (E) The mucosal finger flap is rotated and sutured to the palatal mucosa.

to avoid damage to the adjacent developing permanent tooth. A permanent tooth, if unaffected by periodontal disease, can be treated by means of endodontic therapy. If the tooth has periodontitis or the fracture is too extensive, then extraction is the treatment of choice. In fact, with complicated crown fractures extraction is preferable to no treatment at all.

Immature permanent teeth are a special consideration in that viable pulp is necessary for apexogenesis (continued root growth and closure of the root apex). Thus, a specific endodontic procedure, namely partial pulpectomy and direct pulp capping, is indicated if the pulp is still vital. This procedure needs to be carried out as soon as possible after the injury, ideally within hours. The goal of this procedure is to maintain a living pulp and thus get continued tooth development. Once the tooth is mature (apex is closed and adequate dentine thickness of root walls) then the final endodontic therapy (pulpectomy and root filling) should be performed.

Immature teeth where the pulp is necrotic should generally be extracted. There is a specific endodontic technique called apexification which may be used to maintain immature teeth with pulp necrosis, but it is rarely indicated. It must be remembered that immature permanent teeth might well be present in the adult animal if trauma to the developing teeth caused pulp necrosis (Fig. 12.16).

Uncomplicated crown fractures may also require treatment as the exposed dentine tubules allow communication between the pulp and the oral environment and can thus result in inflammation or death of the pulp. An uncomplicated crown fracture usually requires minimal treatment, e.g. removal of sharp edges with a bur and sealing of the exposed dentine with a suitable liner or restorative material. However, such fractures do require monitoring (clinical examination and radiography) at regular intervals to ensure that the pulp remains vital. If pulp and periapical disease develop, the tooth requires either extraction or endodontic therapy.

Crown and root

Fractures that involve both the crown and root of a tooth are also classified as complicated or uncomplicated, depending on whether the pulp is exposed by the fracture line or not.

Treatment of crown and root fractures depends on how far below the gingival margin the fracture line extends. If the fracture line does not involve the pulp and does not extend more than 4–5 mm below the gingiva, restorative dentistry can be performed. If the pulp is exposed, endodontic therapy needs to be performed prior to restoration. If the fracture line extends more than 5 mm below the gingiva and its apical extension is below the margin of the alveolar bone, then the tooth should usually be extracted.

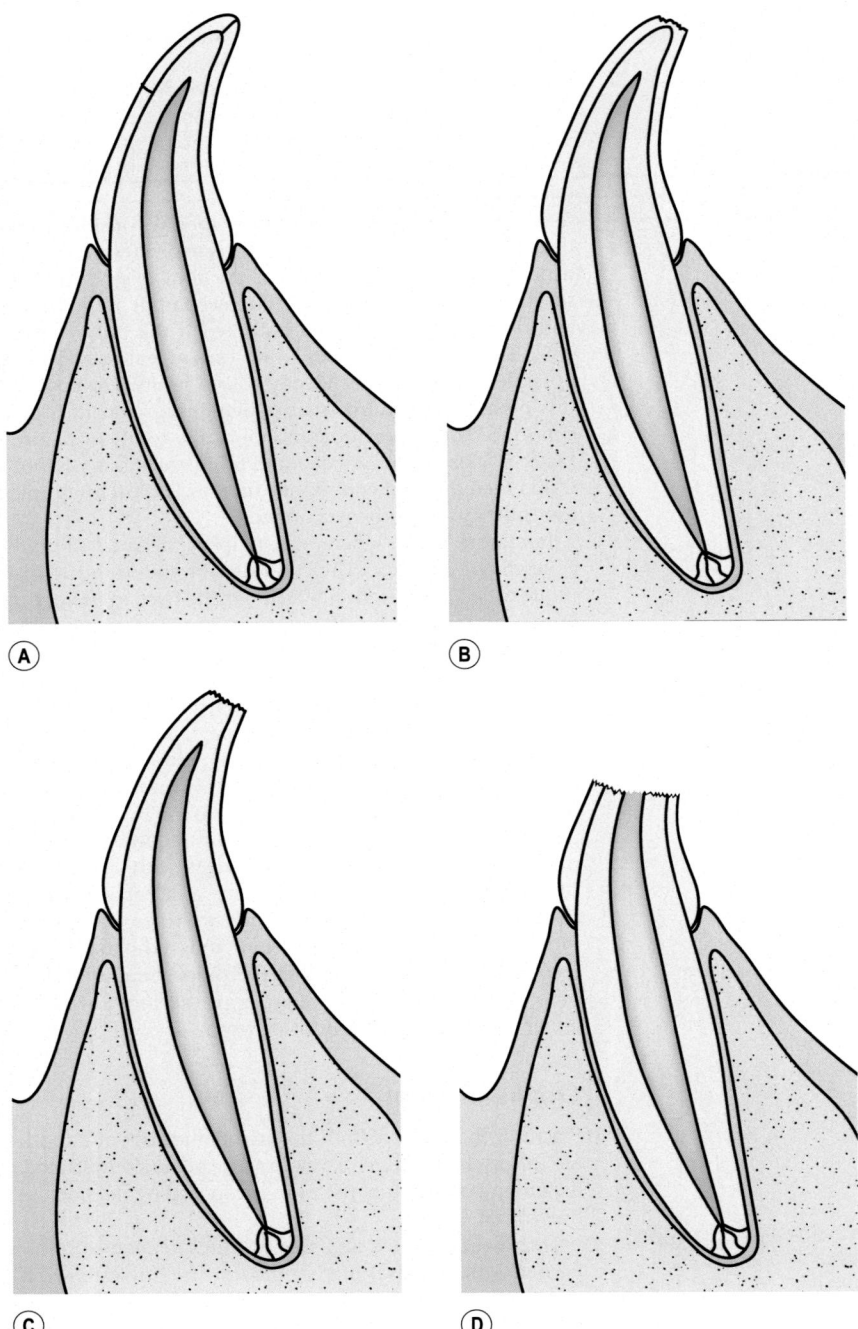

Fig. 12.12 Types of tooth crown injuries (A) Fracture lines in the enamel without loss of tooth substance. The fractures extend only to the dentino-enamel junction. They require no treatment, but the tooth should be monitored for signs of pulp and periapical disease. (B) Uncomplicated crown fracture affecting only the enamel. Treatment consists of smoothing off jagged edges. (C) Uncomplicated crown fracture exposing dentine. Restoration is indicated, especially if the fracture line is close to the pulp. (D) Complicated crown fracture, i.e. the pulp chamber is exposed. This is an indication for endodontic therapy.

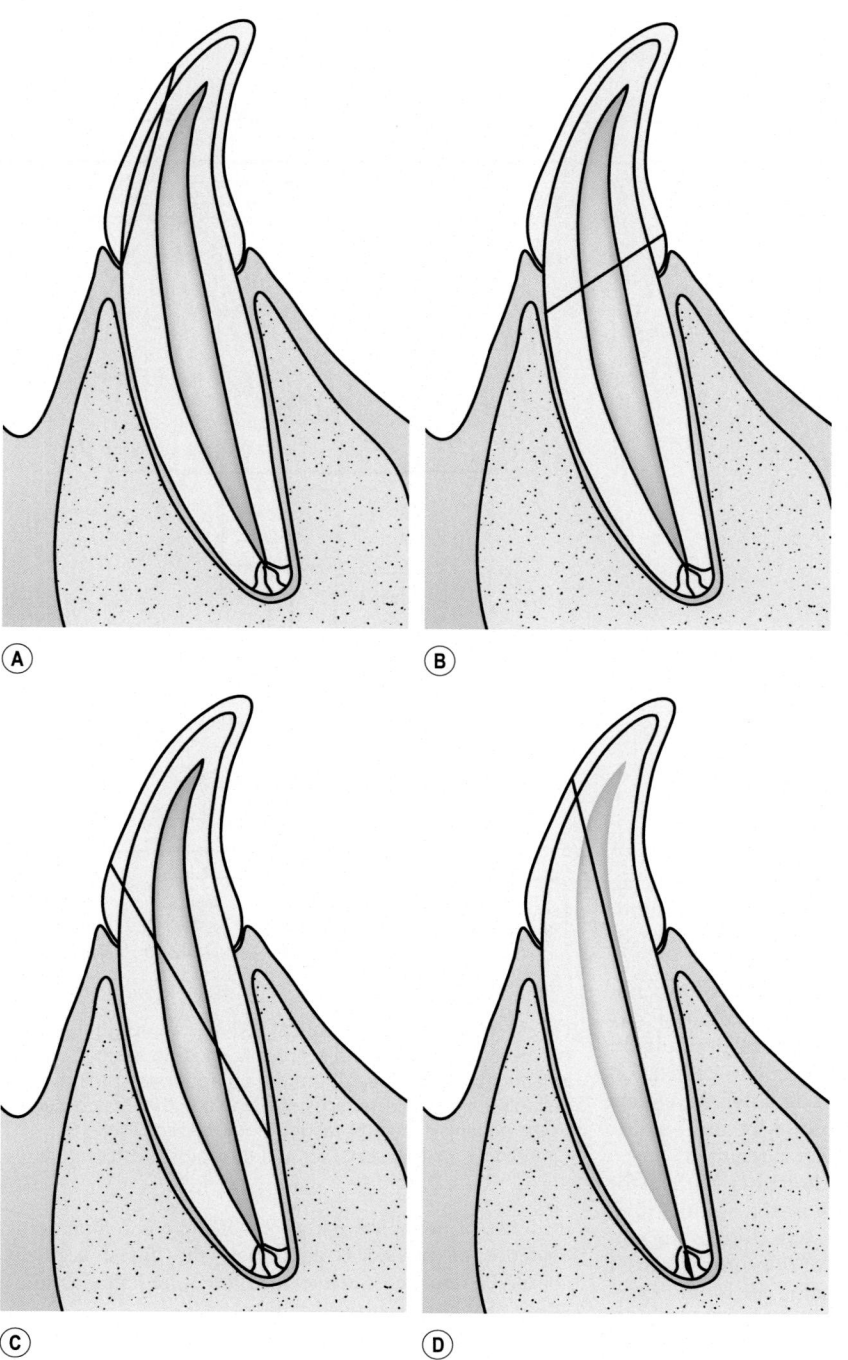

Fig. 12.13 Types of crown and root fractures (A) Uncomplicated crown and root fracture. (B) Complicated crown and root fracture. (C) Complicated crown and root fracture, which usually involves damage to the alveolar bone. (D) Long axis crown and root fracture. This is an absolute indication for extraction.

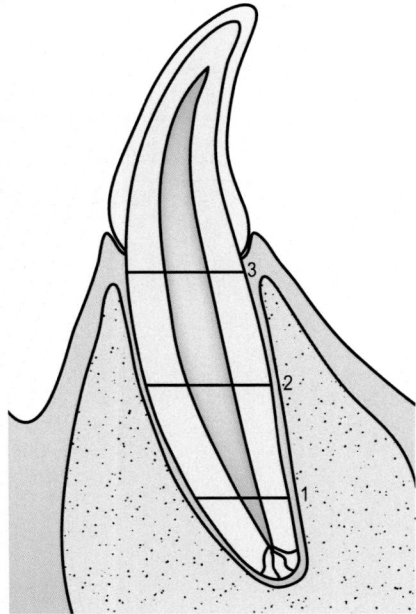

Fig. 12.14 Horizontal root fractures (1) Fracture of apical segment. (2) Midroot fracture. Both 1 and 2 will heal with immobilization. (3) Fracture of the coronal root close to the gingival margin. This fracture is unlikely to heal. If the root is to be retained, it needs endodontic treatment.

Root

Root fractures may be horizontal or oblique. In general, horizontal root fractures have the best prognosis. A tooth with a long axis fracture is an absolute indication for extraction.

Abnormal mobility, horizontal or vertical, of a periodontally sound tooth may lead you to suspect a root fracture. Definitive diagnosis of root fractures depends on radiography. The choice of correct treatment, i.e. fixation or extraction, is only possible based on a definitive diagnosis. Fixation is by means of ligature wire and acrylics. Radiographic monitoring of treatment is required.

The fracture level determines the choice of treatment for horizontal root fractures. A fracture in the apical region carries a better prognosis than a fracture close to the gingival margin. A horizontal fracture of the coronal part of the root is, in most cases, an indication for tooth extraction. Horizontal midroot and apical fractures will heal if the tooth is immobilized. Horizontal root fractures can heal by means of a dentino-cemental callus, connective tissue union, fibrous union, or an osteofibrous union (Fig. 12.17). If the pulp of the coronal fragment becomes necrotic, the fracture will not heal. Endodontic treatment of the coronal segment is then indicated. The apical segment may be left in place if there is no radiographic

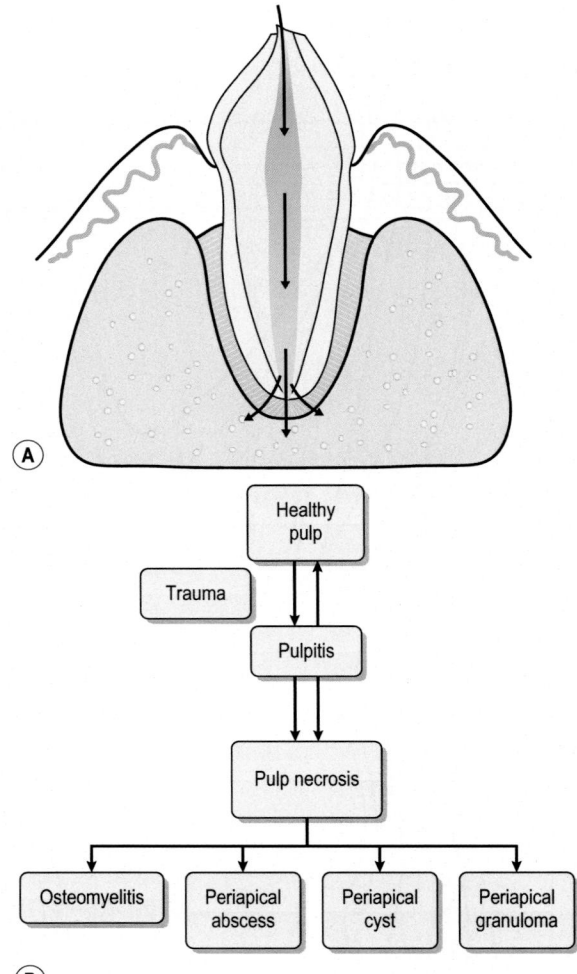

Fig. 12.15 Pulp and periapical disease An exposed pulp will become inflamed and eventually undergo necrosis. The inflammation can spread from the pulp to involve the periapical area (A). The types of pathology that may occur in the periapical area (B) range from localized reactions (granuloma, cyst, abscess) around the apex to osteomyelitis.

evidence of periapical pathology. If there is radiographic evidence of periapical pathology, the apical segment should be removed. Such teeth will require lifelong radiograph monitoring at regular intervals.

Endodontic treatment in general practice

Trauma to the teeth causing crown fracture and exposure of the pulp needs prompt endodontic treatment if the affected teeth are to be maintained. The principles and

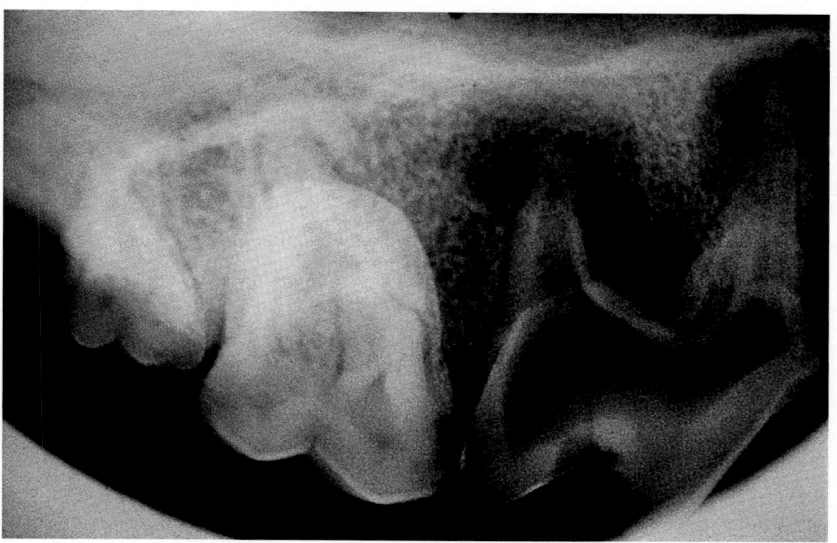

Fig. 12.16 Immature permanent maxillary 1st molar in an 11-year-old dog The trauma that caused the complicated tooth fracture with consequent pulp and periapical disease occurred when the animal was less than 1 year old.

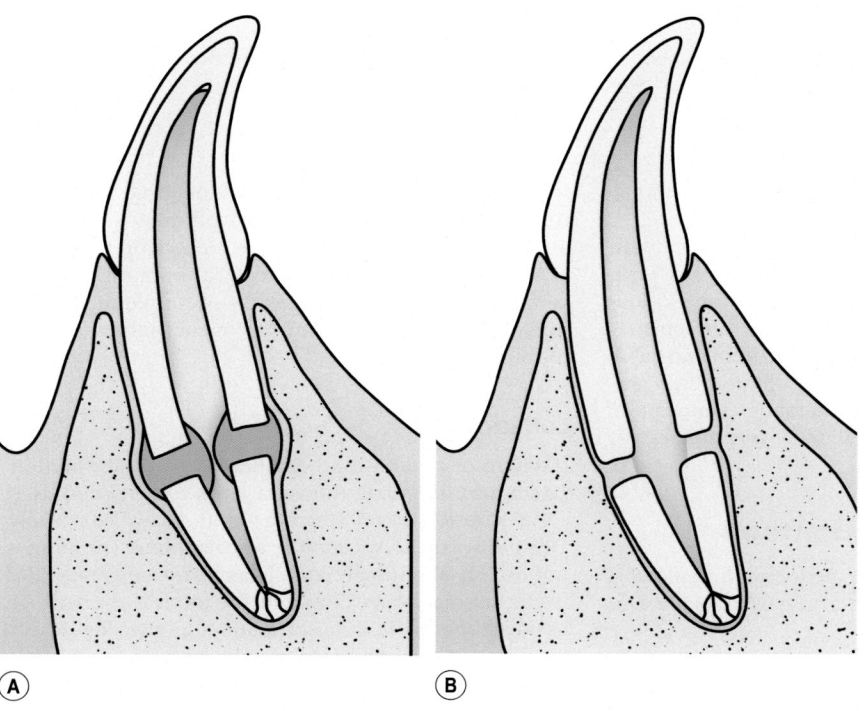

(A)   (B)

Fig. 12.17 Types of root fracture healing (A) Formation of a dentino-cemental callus. (B) Connective tissue union.

Continued

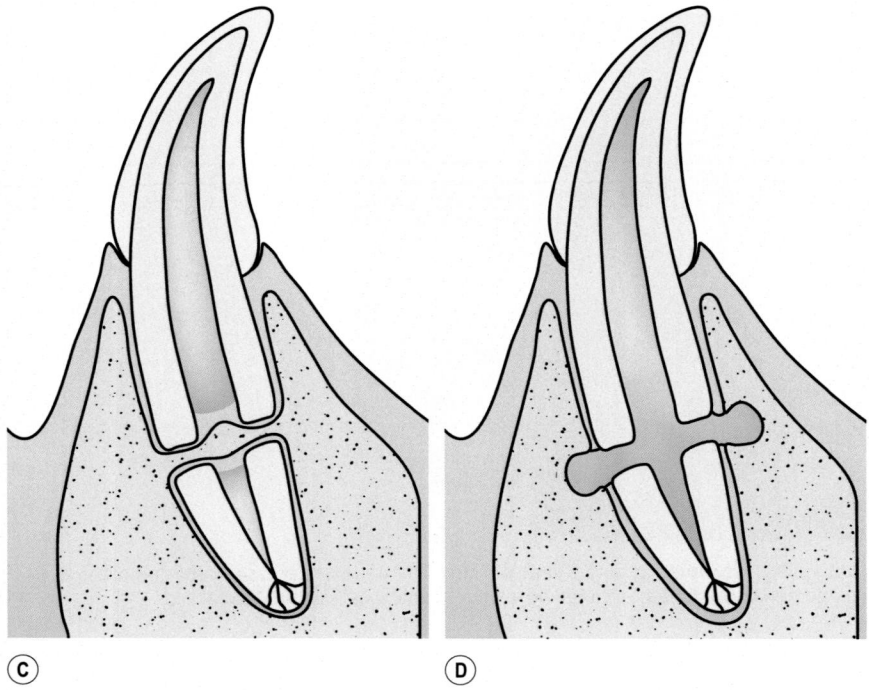

C   D

Fig. 12.17, cont'd (C) Union by connective tissue and bone. (D) Non-union: treatment of a non-union involves endodontic treatment of the coronal segment, removal of the apical segment and retrograde root filling.

the types of endodontic treatment possible are summarized in the Appendix.

Endodontics requires investment in equipment, instrumentation and material. The techniques are time-consuming, and require practice and a meticulous technique for a successful outcome. The consequences of failed endodontic treatment are both painful and debilitating for the affected animal. In my opinion, it is generally impractical to include endodontic treatment in general practice. Prompt referral to a specialist is my recommendation.

Damage to the periodontium

Trauma may cause injury to the periodontium allowing the tooth to subluxate, luxate or avulse from its alveolus (Fig. 12.18).

Subluxation

In a subluxation, the periodontium has been damaged so that the tooth is loosened in its alveolus. Tooth mobility is limited to increased horizontal movement. The tooth has not been displaced in a vertical direction. No treatment is indicated except soft food and no toys

for a week. Pulp vitality of the traumatized tooth does need to be monitored radiographically (radiograph at the time of diagnosis and then a check-up radiograph 6 months later), as pulp necrosis is the most common complication. If this happens, the tooth requires extraction or referral for endodontic treatment (pulpectomy and rootfilling).

Luxation

Luxation of a tooth can be either in a vertical direction, i.e. an intrusion or an extrusion, or in a lateral direction.

An intrusion occurs when the tooth is pushed apically. This pushes the tooth into the alveolar bone. The tooth is not usually abnormally mobile as it is firmly embedded in the alveolar bone. Clinically, the tooth is shorter than its neighbors as it is pushed into the alveolus. Radiographically, the periodontal membrane is narrower.

An extrusion occurs when the tooth is dislocated vertically from the alveolus. The tooth is mobile in both horizontal and vertical directions and appears longer than its neighbors. Radiographically, the periodontal space is increased.

A lateral tooth luxation (Fig. 12.19) occurs when the trauma pushes the crown in a palatal/lingual direction and

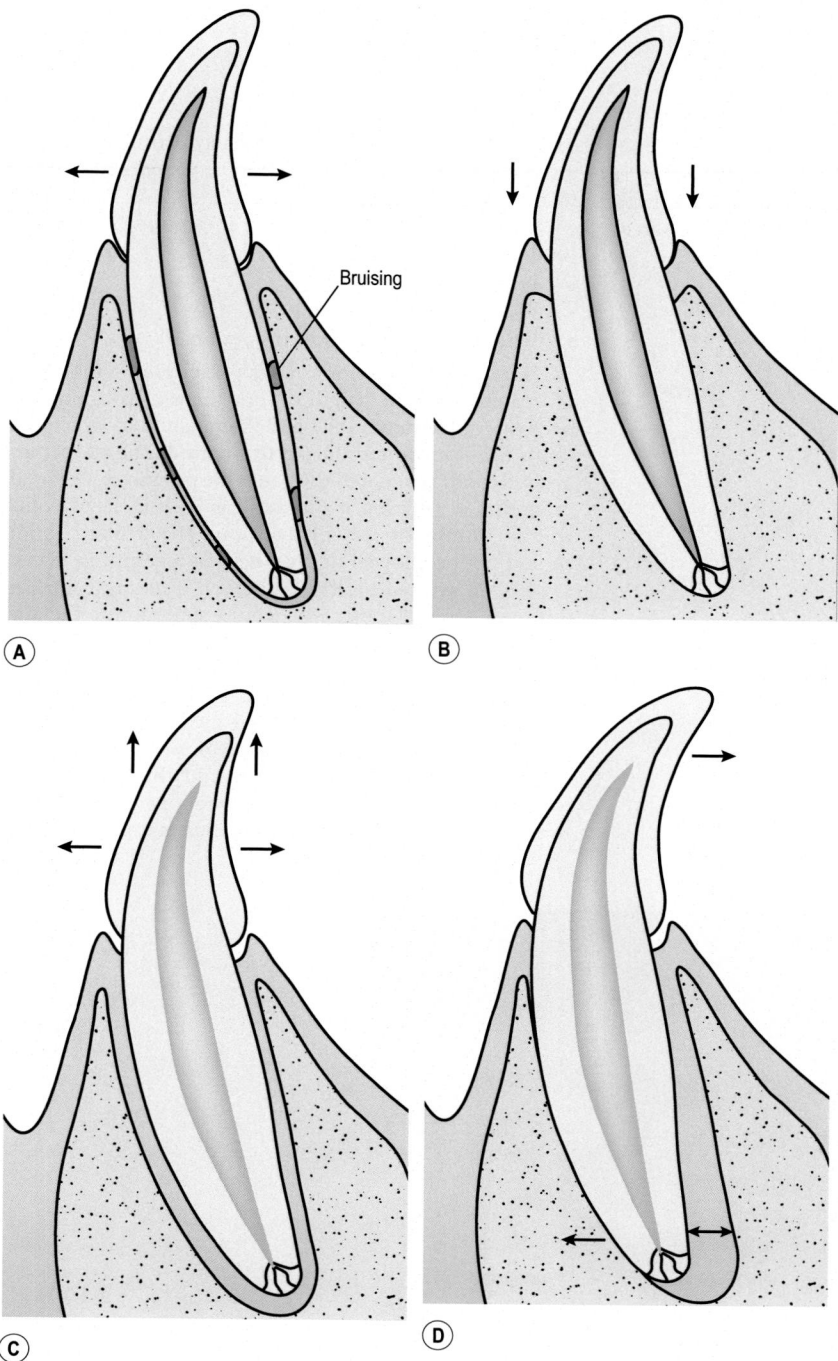

Bruising

Continued

Fig. 12.18 Subluxation, luxation and avulsion of teeth (A) Subluxation. The damage to the periodontium leads to loosening of the tooth. There is increased horizontal movement but the tooth has not been displaced in a vertical direction. (B) Intrusion. The tooth has been pushed apically. Clinically, the tooth is shorter than its neighbors, as it has been pushed into the alveolus. It is not mobile, being firmly embedded in bone. (C) Extrusion. The tooth is dislocated vertically from the alveolus. It is mobile in both horizontal and vertical directions, and appears longer than its neighbors. (D) Lateral luxation. This occurs when the trauma pushes the crown in one direction and the root in the opposite direction. Fracture of the labial/buccal or palatal/lingual alveolar bone plate allows the tooth to luxate rather than fracture.

the root in a labial/buccal direction or vice versa. This type of luxation is always associated with a fracture of the palatal/lingual or labial/buccal alveolar bone plate, which allows the tooth to luxate rather than fracture.

A luxated tooth needs repositioning and stabilizing (using ligature wire and acrylics) as soon as possible. Endodontic therapy of the affected tooth after healing is generally required. Repositioning and stabilizing can be performed in general practice but endodontics is rarely feasible and thus prompt referral to a clinician specializing in veterinary dentistry is indicated.

Avulsion

An avulsed tooth has been completely extruded from its alveolus. It needs to be replaced in its socket and fixed in its normal position.

Contraindications for replacing and fixating an avulsed tooth are:

- Primary tooth
- Periodontitis
- Extensive caries or resorptive lesion.

The two most important factors determining the result of treatment are the length of time the avulsed tooth has been out of its bony socket and the medium in which the tooth has been stored during this period. The sooner an avulsed tooth is replaced the better the prognosis. Optimal prognosis is achieved if the tooth is back in its alveolus within 30 min or less of avulsion. The avulsed tooth should not be allowed to dry. The best medium in which to store an avulsed tooth is saline, or, if not available, in milk. An avulsed tooth will require endodontic therapy after it has healed back in its alveolus.

Luxation and avulsion injuries require prompt replacement and fixation of the tooth in its original position in its alveolus. This can be achieved by the general practitioner. Teeth affected by these sorts of injury will invariably require endodontic treatment and thus need to be referred to a specialist. As already mentioned, endodontic treatment is time-consuming and requires experience and

Fig. 12.18, cont'd (E) Avulsion. The tooth has been totally removed from its alveolus by the trauma.

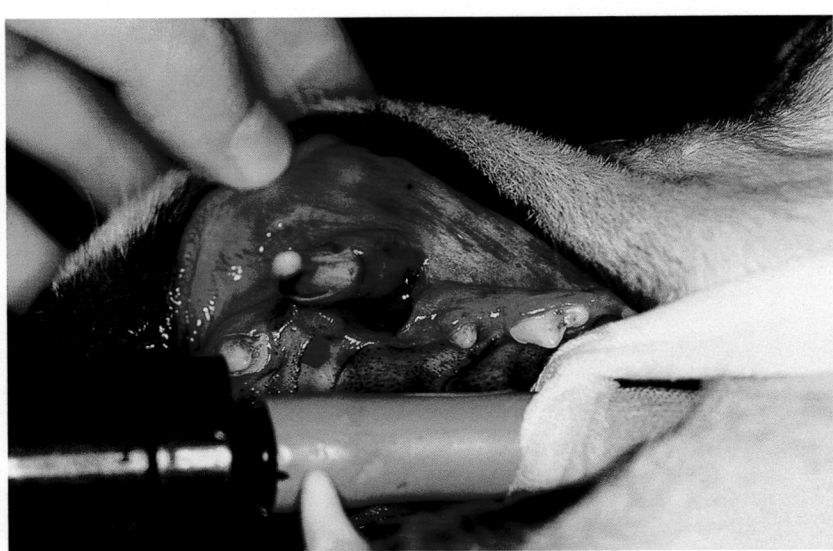

Fig. 12.19 Lateral tooth luxation The trauma (dog fight) has pushed the crown of the maxillary canine in a buccal direction and the root in a palatal direction.

special equipment and materials. It is not advisable to try to include it in general practice.

Procedure

Reimplantation

It is extremely important that the avulsed tooth is handled only by its crown. It is gently rinsed with sterile saline solution. If severely contaminated the tooth root can be gently cleaned with sterile gauze swabs moistened with saline. Be gentle! Handling of the tooth root should be kept to a minimum as it is essential not to remove the periodontal membrane from the root. A viable periodontal ligament is necessary for healing.

The tooth is then replaced in its bony socket without removing the blood clot from the alveolus. The tooth is just firmly placed in its bony socket and fixed in position.

Fixation

Luxated/avulsed teeth can be stabilized using wire secured with acrylic or composite (Fig. 12.20). It is essential that the stabilizing appliance does not interfere with occlusion nor touch the soft tissue. The animal must be able to close its mouth with the appliance in place.

The procedure (Fig. 12.21) for fixation of a luxated or avulsed canine tooth is as follows:

1. The teeth to be splinted are scaled and polished.
2. The area to be splinted is measured and an appropriate length of fine ligature wire cut.
3. The teeth are positioned in proper alignment; a wax plate is placed across the palate (to protect soft tissue while making the appliance and to ensure that the

finished appliance will not touch the palatal mucosa) and the ligature wire is woven in a figure-of-eight fashion across the palate. The figure-of-eight wire is tightened with a hemostat. The resulting knot can be placed at the distal or palatal aspect of the anchor canine.
4. The end is cut and the 'pigtail' tucked in.
5. The canine teeth are acid-etched.
6. An acrylic or composite splint is placed and polished smooth.

Aftercare

A water pick or curved-tip syringe is used to flush debris from between the splint, teeth and soft tissue. Post-operative antibiotics are recommended for the first few weeks.

The appliances are removed using pliers or a high-speed drill after 4–6 weeks. The tooth should at this stage be stable or very slightly mobile. Radiographs should be taken. If the tooth is still loose, then reimplantation has failed and the tooth should be extracted.

An avulsed tooth will always have an inflamed/necrotic pulp and the tooth must receive endodontic treatment (pulpectomy and root filling) 4–6 weeks after reimplantation or periapical pathology and tooth root resorption will occur. Luxated teeth often suffer pulp necrosis and should be checked clinically and radiographically at regular intervals. Signs of pulp pathology, e.g. tooth discoloration, or radiographic evidence of periapical pathology are indications for either endodontic treatment or extraction of an affected tooth.

JAW FRACTURE

Jaw fracture is common in small animal practice. Most are the result of road traffic accidents. However, disease processes such as periodontitis may cause such severe bone loss that spontaneous jaw fracture occurs (Fig. 12.22). The most common site for such spontaneous fracture is the mandibular premolar region and it is frequently bilateral. Rough extraction technique can result in iatrogenic fracture of an already weakened mandible (Fig. 12.23). Preoperative radiographs prior to tooth extraction are mandatory.

Traumatic jaw fracture is usually located in a dentate area involving alveolar sockets. Most are compound and many are open. The upper jaw consists of the premaxilla, maxilla and nasal bones. All of these are thin plates of bone surrounding an air-filled cavity and, therefore, fracture easily at the site of impact. The location of common mandibular fractures in the dog and cat is summarized in Figure 12.24. Mandibular fracture is more common in dogs and cats (Umphlet and Johnson 1988, 1990).

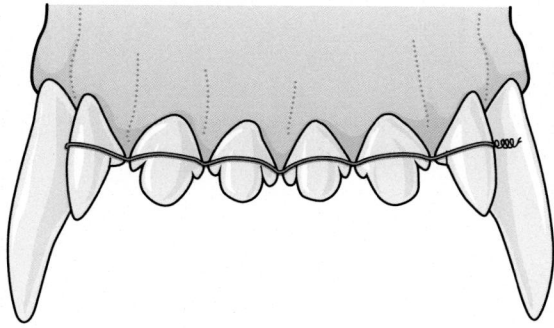

Fig. 12.20 Fixation of luxated/avulsed upper incisor The luxated/avulsed tooth has been repositioned. Fixation has been achieved using a figure-of-eight wire. This device can be further strengthened by applying acrylic or composite creating a stronger splint. It is essential that the device does not interfere with occlusion.

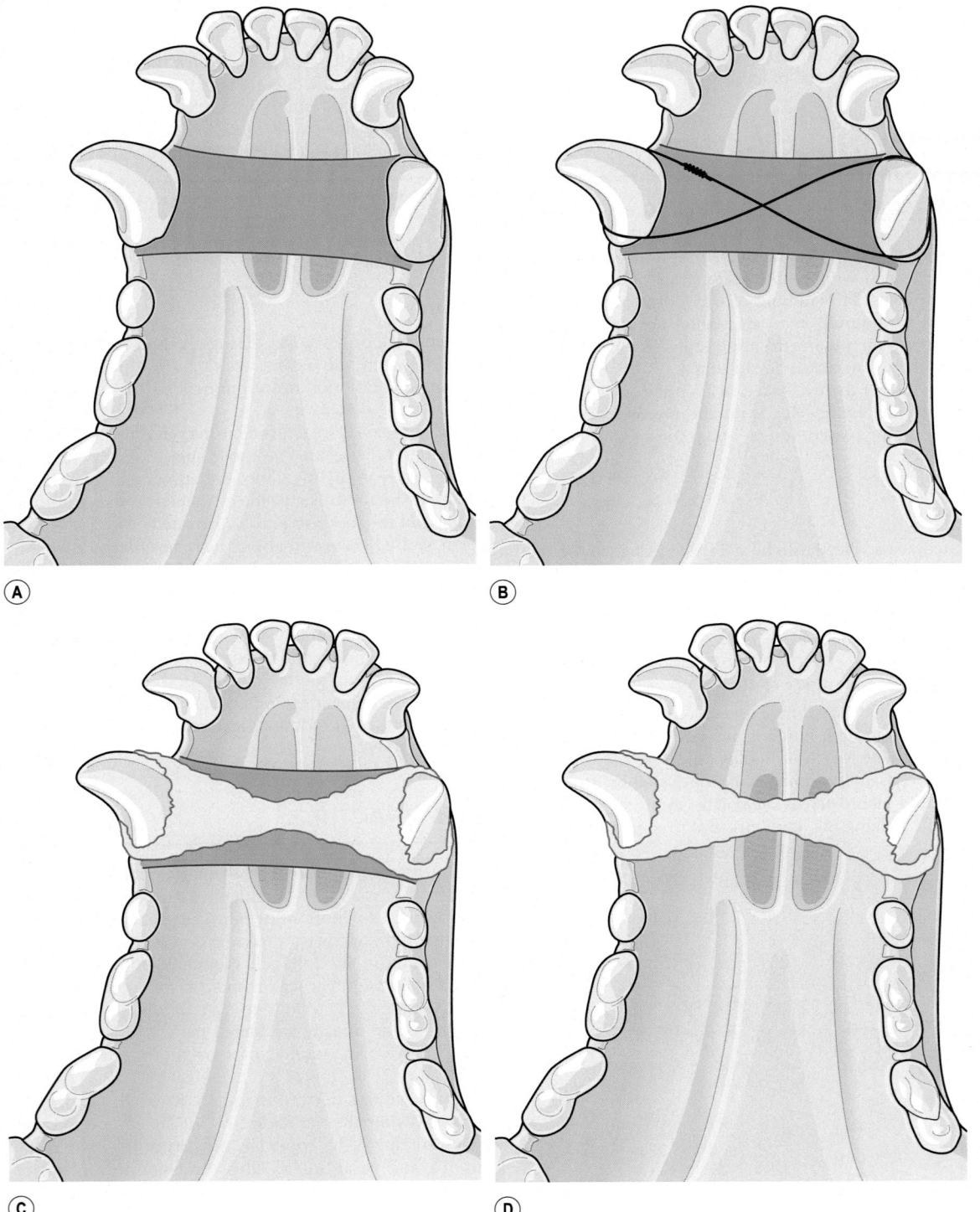

Fig. 12.21 Procedure for fixation of a luxated or avulsed upper canine tooth (A) The luxated/avulsed tooth has been repositioned. A wax plate is placed across the palate to protect the mucosa and to ensure that the finished appliance will not touch it. (B) The upper canines are stabilized using a figure-of-eight wire. (C) The wire is anchored in place with composite or acrylic. (D) The wax plate has been removed and occlusion has been checked. The appliance should not touch the palatal mucosa and the animal should be able to close its mouth without interference.

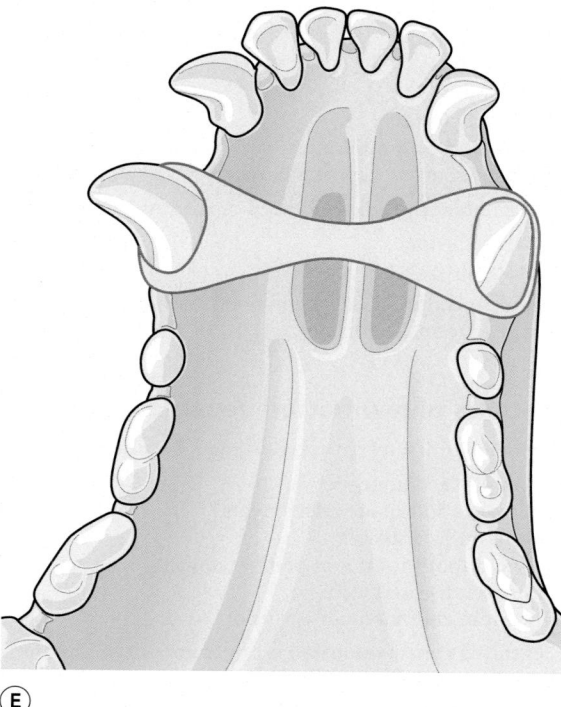

(E)

Fig. 12.21, cont'd (E) The composite/acrylic splint has been polished smooth for comfort and hygiene purposes.

Biomechanics of jaw fracture repair

Jaw opening is virtually passive (digastricus only), while jaw closure is active (pterygoids, masseter and temporalis). The pressures of occlusion tend to push the rostral end of the maxilla dorsally and the rostral end of the mandible ventrally. The caudal areas of these bones, embedded in muscle, are more stable. Hence, the occlusal surface of both the maxilla and the mandible is the tension side. The compression side of the maxilla is the nasal chamber and of the mandible is its ventral border (Fig. 12.25). A favorable fracture is depicted in Figure 12.26A and an unfavorable fracture is shown in Figure 12.26B.

Indications for repair

Many fractures do not need surgical fixation, particularly those where the fracture lines are contained within the areas of attachment of the masticatory muscles, as the muscles will effectively splint the fracture during healing.

Although many fractures of the upper jaw require only conservative treatment, others are more complex to manage. The upper jaw consists of relatively thin bone supporting the teeth and framing the nasal cavity. Rigid fixation of these thin plates of bone is rarely possible. An additional complication is that the nasal cavity may be exposed because of the fracture. There is often damage to intranasal structures that may reduce or prevent air movement through the nose for some time after the injury.

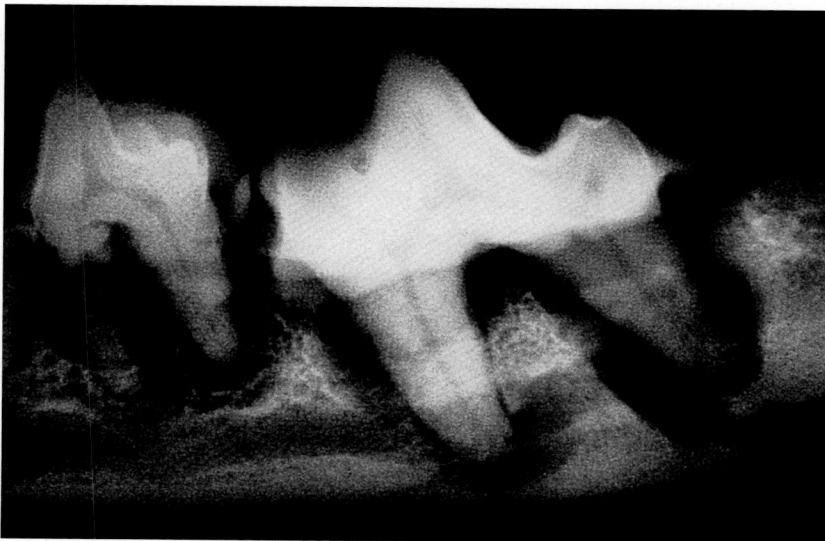

Fig. 12.22 Spontaneous jaw fracture due to advanced periodontitis

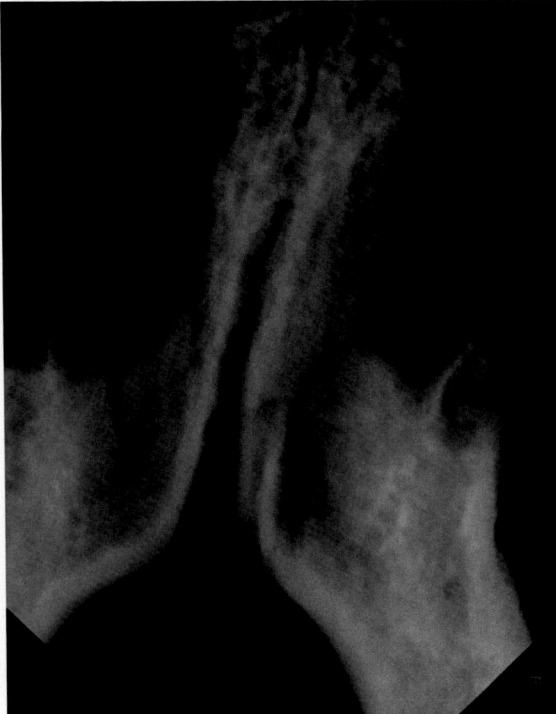

Fig. 12.23 Iatrogenic jaw fracture during extraction of lower canine teeth A complete fracture of the ventral mandible is obvious on the left. The fracture extends from the apical portion of the extraction socket to the ventral mandible and the fracture ends over-ride. There is also an incomplete fracture of the right alveolar bone. Iatrogenic fracture of the mandible is always a risk when extracting lower canines, especially if the reason for extraction is periodontitis. I generally make owners aware of the risk prior to surgery.

In general, maxillary fractures will need repair if they cause:

- Malocclusion
- Instability
- Facial deformity
- Oronasal communication
- Obstruction of the nasal cavity.

Mandibular fractures will need repair if they cause:

- Malocclusion
- Instability.

Stable fractures, if causing malocclusion, need repair to recreate a normal occlusion.

Principles of jaw fracture repair

The main guidelines for successful jaw fracture repair are:

- Simple technique
- Preserve soft-tissue attachments
- Minimum implants
- Avoid tooth roots and periapical areas
- Extract diseased teeth
- Restore and maintain occlusion.

Ensuring correct occlusion is of paramount importance. The presence of an endotracheal tube in the mouth makes this impossible. Intubation through a pharyngotomy incision (see Ch. 2) allows an accurate assessment of the occlusion. The tongue is folded down into the pharynx, leaving the mouth clear of obstructions.

Methods of jaw fracture repair

Jaw fracture repair techniques can be divided into two types: traditional (bone implants) and tooth-borne appliances.

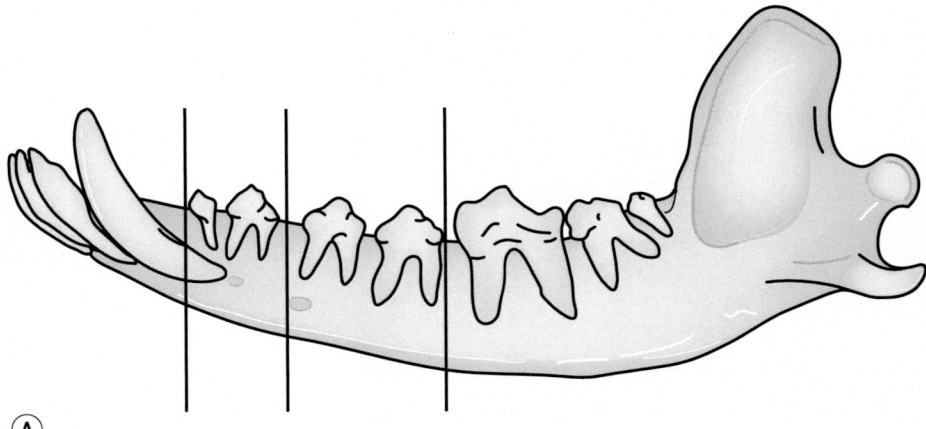

(A)

Fig. 12.24 Common locations for mandibular fractures (A) Dog.

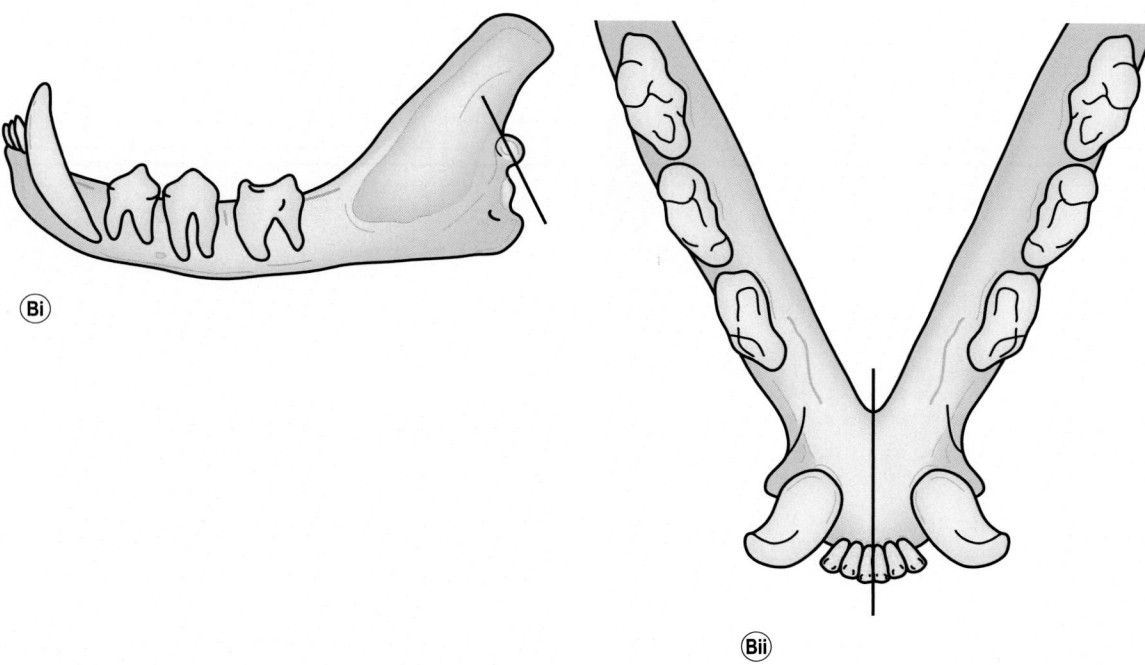

Fig. 12.24, cont'd (B) Cat.

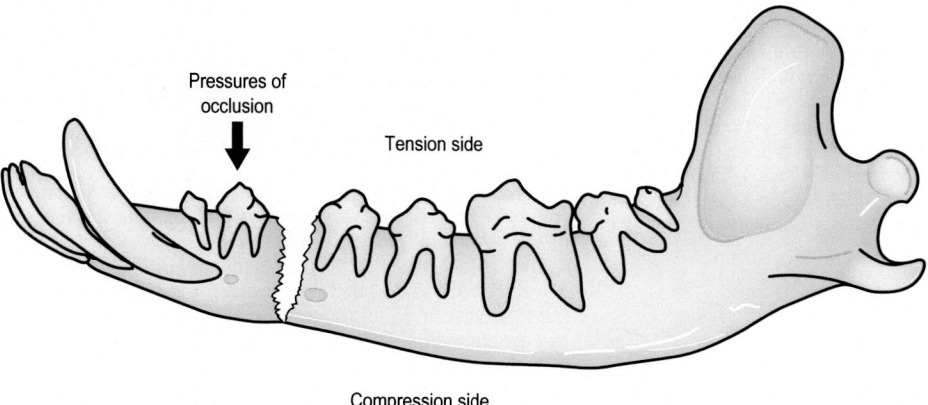

Pressures of occlusion

Tension side

Compression side

Fig. 12.25 The compression and tension sides of the mandible Repair methods that secure the tension side, thus favoring compression, allow optimal bone healing.

Some traditional orthopedic techniques, e.g. screwed plates and intramedullary pins, should not be used for jaw fracture repair. Because of the anatomy of the jaws, it is virtually impossible to place screwed plates without damage to teeth (Fig. 12.27) or anatomic structures. An intramedullary pin placed in the mandibular canal is cruel. *The mandibular canal is not a medullary cavity.* The mandibular canal contains the neurovascular supply to the jaw bone, teeth and adjacent soft tissue. Inserting a pin into this structure causes intense chronic pain and usually results in complications such as bone resorption, pulpitis, tooth loss, neuroma and poor fracture healing.

Other traditional orthopedic techniques, e.g. external fixator and orthopedic wiring, can be used in either jaw to

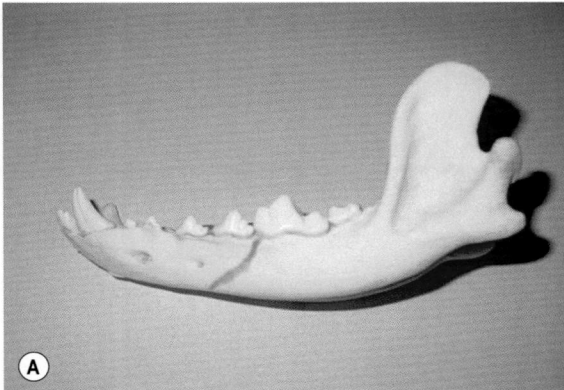

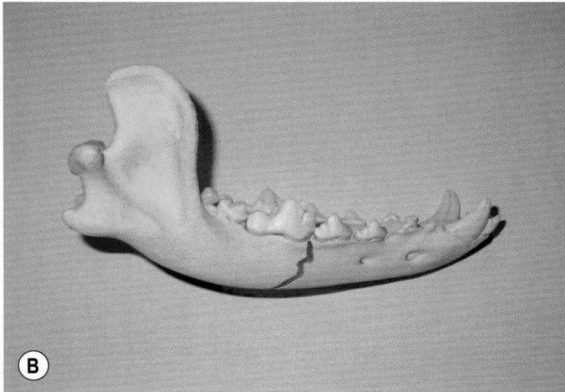

Fig. 12.26 A favorable and unfavorable fracture line (A) A favorable fracture line. The fracture runs from the occlusal aspect rostrally to the ventral mandible. This does not compromise the tension side as much and is therefore considered a favorable fracture line. (B) An unfavorable fracture line. The fracture runs from the occlusal aspect caudally to the ventral mandible. The tension side is thus totally unsecured and it is considered an unfavorable fracture line.

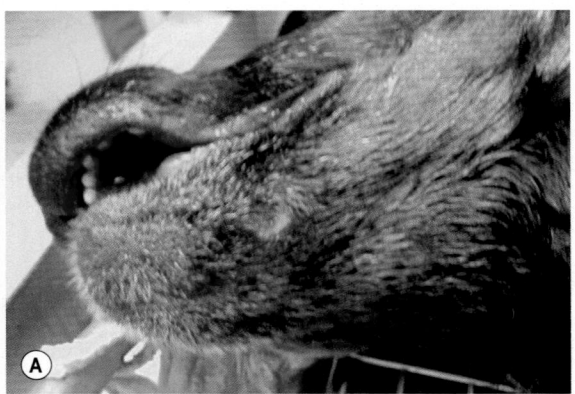

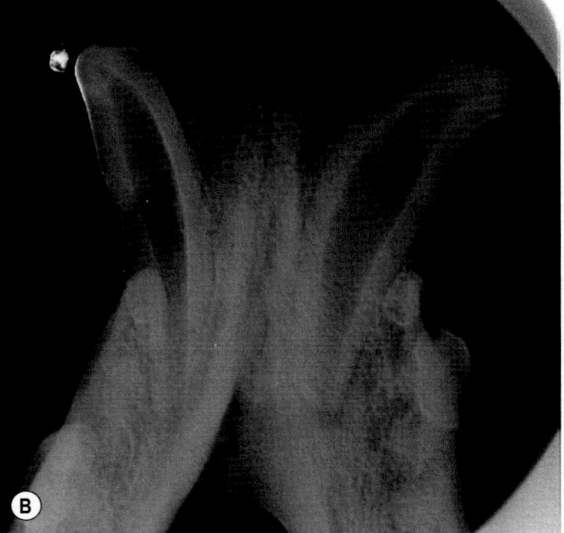

Fig. 12.27 Iatrogenic injuries as a result of jaw fracture repair The 6-year-old patient was presented with a swelling of the left rostral mandible and a draining fistula at the ventral border of the left rostral mandible. (A) Anamnesis revealed that the dog had been treated for a mandibular fracture when it was 9 months old. (B) A radiograph revealed immature canine teeth with incomplete closure of the apices. The stage of development of these teeth is compatible with a dog younger than 1 year of age. Consequently, pulpal inflammation and necrosis (which stops further tooth development) must have occurred at about 9 months of age. The pulpal inflammation and necrosis of 304 have spread to involve the periapical tissues as evidenced by the radiolucent zone around the apex of the root. The periosteal bone proliferation on the left is a consequence of the pulp and periapical disease of 304. There are also distinct circular lucencies midroot at 304 and 404. These are compatible with drill holes for a pin or screw to repair a mandibular fracture. The only possible treatment of such teeth is extraction.

achieve normal occlusion and fracture fixation as long as pin and wire placement is done under strict radiographic control to avoid damage to tooth roots and anatomic structures, e.g. mandibular canal.

Tooth-borne appliances use the teeth to maintain normal occlusion thus stabilizing the fracture and allowing healing. The appliances achieve interdental fixation by means of interdental wire and/or interdental acrylic splints.

To summarize, the most useful methods of jaw fracture repair available to the general practitioner are:

1. Traditional
   - External fixator
   - Wire

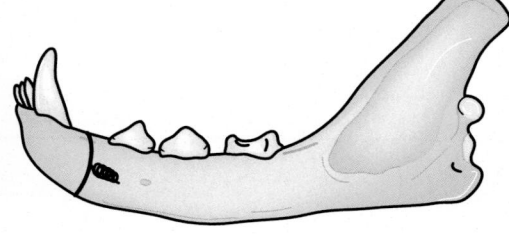

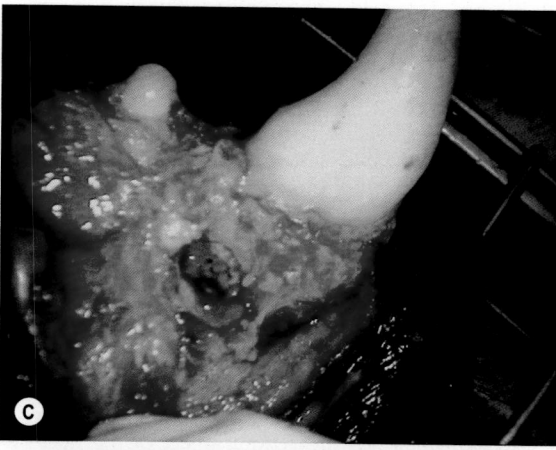

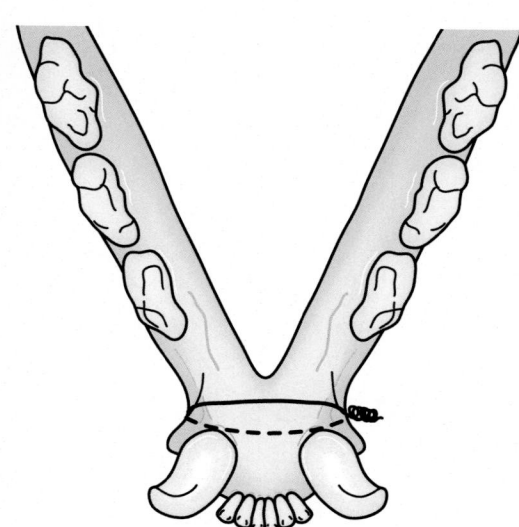

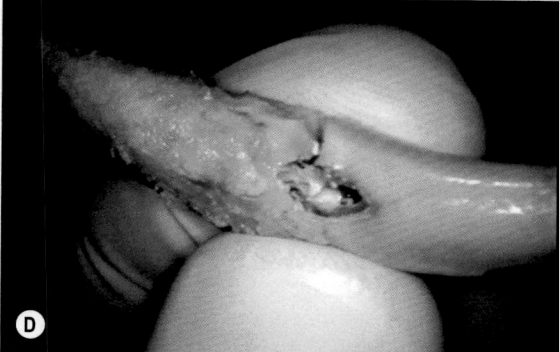

Fig. 12.27, cont'd (C) The appearance of 404 during extraction. (D) The extracted 304.

Fig. 12.28 Repair of a mandibular symphyseal fracture with cerclage wiring

2. Tooth-borne appliances
   - Intermaxillary fixation
   - Monomaxillary fixation, i.e. interdental fixation.

Intermaxillary fixation can be rigid and fixed, e.g. resin fixation of maxillary and mandibular canine teeth or semirigid and removable, e.g. tape muzzle.

Whatever technique is used to repair a jaw fracture, it is essential that occlusion is maintained. This means that pharyngotomy intubation (see Ch. 2) is required to allow optimal access to the oral cavity and assessment and maintenance occlusion.

Useful traditional orthopedic techniques

Orthopedic wiring. Interdental or interfragmentary cerclage/hemicerclage techniques or combinations of these are useful in repairing some jaw fractures. Primary fixation of large fragments of the premaxilla and maxilla can be achieved with wire sutures, tension wires, or intraosseous screws and wire. Pre- and intraoperative radiographs are required to avoid damage to tooth roots and periapical areas.

Most veterinarians will be familiar with the technique of a cerclage wire behind the canine teeth to stabilize fractures of the mandibular symphysis (Fig. 12.28). An adaptation, which avoids placing a knot in the oral cavity, thus reducing patient discomfort, is depicted in Figure 12.29. In the cat, nylon suture material can be used instead of wire. The fracture usually heals in 4–6 weeks. Healing is confirmed radiographically and the wire is then removed.

Cerclage/hemicerclage techniques can also be used for fixation of fractures of the horizontal ramus of the mandible. Depending on the forces involved 18–22 gauge wire should be used. These techniques should only be performed under strict radiographic control to avoid damage to tooth root and root apex areas. Pre and intraoperative radiographs must be taken.

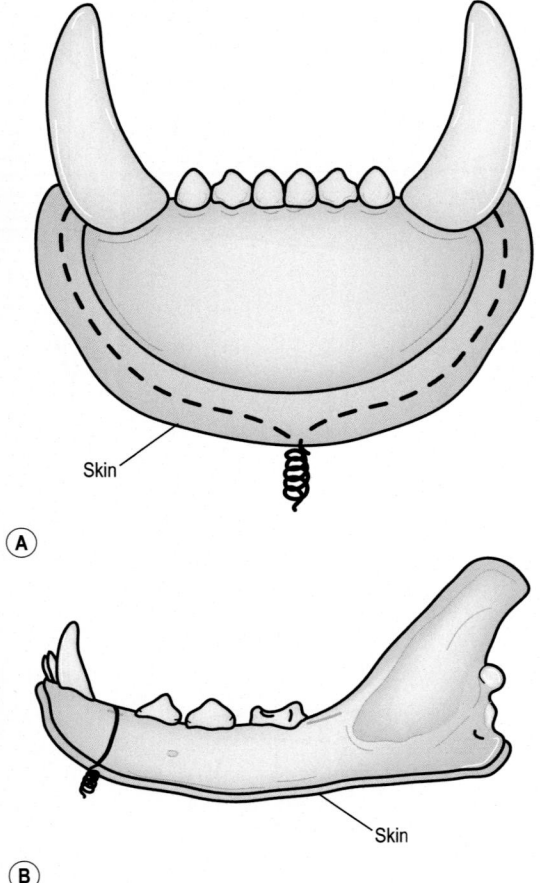

Skin

(A)

Skin

(B)

Fig. 12.29 Repair of a mandibular symphyseal fracture with surgical nylon (cat) or wire (dog or cat) The suture knot is tied (A) beneath the skin (wire) or (B) outside the oral cavity, on the skin (surgical nylon).

The principles of using these wiring techniques are:

- The wires must be perpendicular to the fracture line.
- Drilled holes must be at least 5 mm away from the fracture line.
- Drilled holes need to be angled slightly towards the fracture to improve tightening on the medial aspect of the bone.

Fractures of the horizontal ramus between the canine and 1st premolar (Fig. 12.30) can be repaired by placing a wire suture close to the buccal margin of the fracture. Holes for the wire should be drilled between the teeth roots. There is no need to raise a buccal flap to drill holes. The wire is tied over the mucosa. This will cause ulceration but it soon heals once the wire has been removed. To improve stability, it may be useful to place a wire tension band on the ventral aspect of the fracture. Access to the ventral border of the mandible is through a skin incision.

Fractures of the horizontal ramus caudal to the first molar (Fig. 12.31) can be repaired by using interdental cerclage wire in combination with a wire suture joining the bone fragments.

The use of intraosseous screws and wire in the mandible is not advised, as it is virtually impossible to place the screws without damaging the teeth.

External fixation. In the upper jaw, fixation can be provided by transverse pinning and an acrylic 'bumper' bar, which holds the pins in the correct alignment with respect to both the fracture lines and the occlusion of the teeth. The fragments are transfixed with pins and the ends of the pins are incorporated in an acrylic resin 'bumper' moulded around the nose. It is useful to use flexible plastic tubing or gutter tubing as a mould for the acrylic. Ensure that occlusion is normal before fixing the pins in that position with the acrylic bar. Once again, it is essential that the placing of the pins does not damage the teeth.

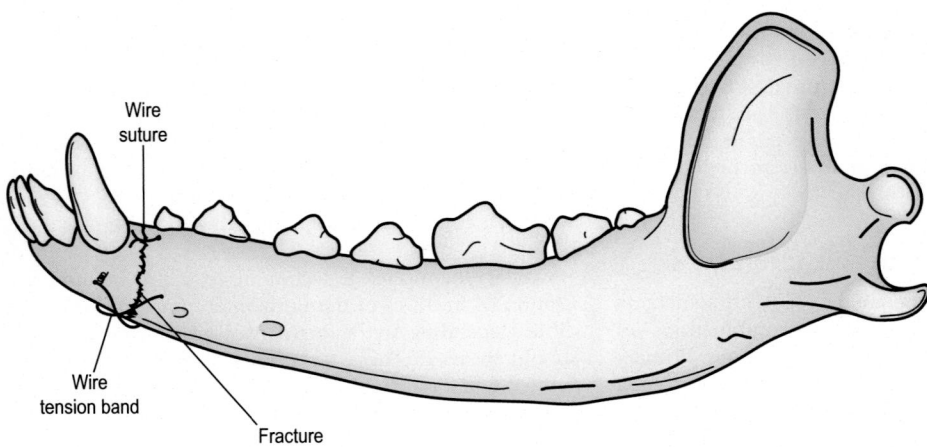

Wire suture

Wire tension band

Fracture

Fig. 12.30 Repair of fracture of the horizontal ramus of the mandible between the canine and the 1st premolar Radiography will reveal the state of the tooth roots and their exact location, so that they can be avoided.

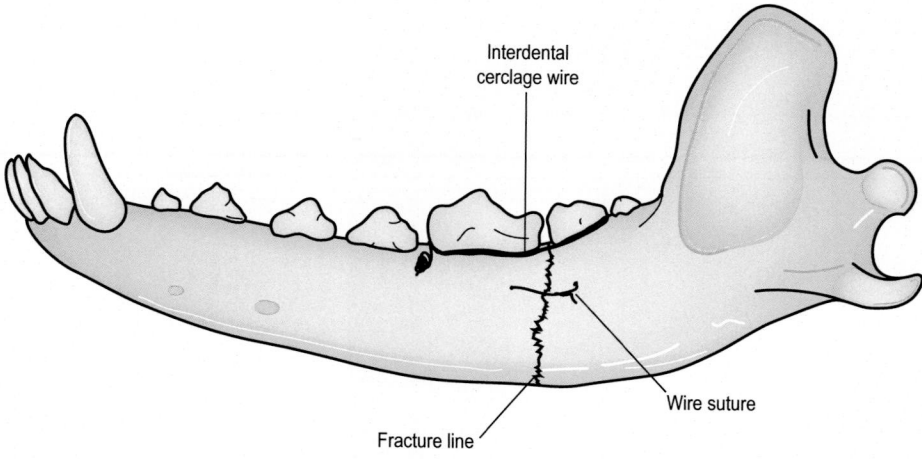

Interdental
cerclage wire

Wire suture

Fracture line

Fig. 12.31 Repair of fracture of the horizontal ramus of the mandible caudal to the 1st molar Pre- and intraoperative radiographs to avoid tooth root damage are mandatory.

The 'bumper' bar technique described above for upper jaw fractures is also applicable to the mandible. Transverse pins are placed through the mandible. Attach flexible plastic tubing to the pins to act as a mould for the acrylic bar. Ensure that normal occlusion is obtained. While maintaining normal occlusion, acrylic is poured into the plastic tubing to form the bar that will hold the pins in the correct position. Tooth roots and periapical areas should not be damaged by the placement of the pins.

Tooth-borne appliances

These techniques can be used for fracture treatment in either the upper or lower jaw. The techniques are inexpensive and easy to learn. They achieve both normal occlusion and fracture fixation. Most importantly, they avoid iatrogenic complications of other techniques. Suggested treatment options for fracture in either jaw using tooth-borne appliances are outlined below.

Upper jaw fracture

The upper jaw consists of thin bones that do not require rigid fixation.

- Intraoral splint (on the buccal surface of maxillary teeth)
- Bonding upper and lower canine teeth (as long as lower canines are in normal occlusion).

Mandibular fracture

- Favorable biomechanics – intraoral acrylic splint.
- Unfavorable biomechanics – interdental wire and intraoral acrylic splint.

Intermaxillary fixation

Intermaxillary fixation relies on maintaining occlusion by aligning and locking the upper and lower jaw together. This term is misleading as it is actually bonding the upper and lower jaw. The techniques can be used for treatment of fracture in either jaw. The fixation can be rigid and fixed, i.e. bonding the upper and lower canines together, or it can be semi-rigid and removable, e.g. tape muzzle.

Tape muzzle. In many situations, a tape muzzle for 3–4 weeks may provide sufficient stability for the fracture to heal. It can also be used as temporary support or as an adjunct to other methods of fixation. A tape muzzle is particularly useful in dolichocephalic breeds. The interdigitation of the canine teeth prevents lateral movement of the jaw so the muzzle must be tight enough to ensure that these teeth do interdigitate. A 0.5–1.0 cm gap is left to allow eating and drinking.

Commercially available soft muzzles, e.g. a Mickey muzzle, may fit on some dogs and it is worth trying to find one that fits. Otherwise, a tape muzzle (Fig. 12.32) can readily be made as follows:

1. Clip the hair.
2. Wrap wide tape around the muzzle with the sticky side out (tape A).
3. Measure the distance from the left upper canine, behind the ears and back to the right upper canine.
4. Cut a piece of wide tape twice this length (tape B).
5. Lay tape B with sticky side out by placing the middle of the tape behind the ears and bringing the ends forward to attach to tape A on either side of the muzzle.

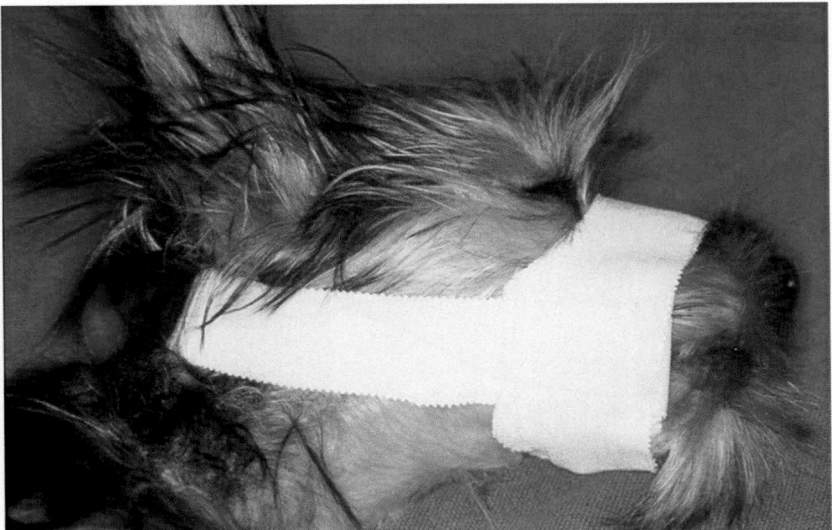

Fig. 12.32 A tape muzzle

6. Wrap another tape around the muzzle over tape A, this time with the sticky side in. This will secure tape B.
7. Fold tape B backwards, sticking it to itself.
8. Measure the distance from tape A to tape B over the forehead.
9. Cut a piece of wide tape twice this length (tape C).
10. Thread tape C, sticky side out, under tape A over the forehead and under tape B and then back over itself so it sticks to itself.

Bonding upper and lower canine teeth

The rationale for the technique is that if bonding upper and lower canines together restores normal occlusion and reduces the fracture then it provides sufficient stabilization during bone healing. It can be used for fracture in either jaw. It is remarkably well tolerated, but some animals will not settle and it may then need to be removed. Soft food, which can be lapped, is recommended for the 3–4 weeks that the appliance is left in place.

The procedure is as follows:

1. Acid etch the upper and lower canines bilaterally (Fig. 12.33A).
2. Close the mouth until there is 2 mm overlap of the tips of the canine teeth.
3. Apply acrylic to cover and lock the teeth together (Fig. 12.33B).
4. Add additional layers of acrylic to secure the lock (Fig. 12.33C).

To remove the appliance – gently close forceps around the acrylic to crack it and then bur away the excess being careful not to damage the teeth. Use acrylic of a different color from the tooth.

Interdental fixation

Interdental ligature and interdental splints

Depending on the biomechanics of a particular fracture, it can be reduced and fixed with interdental ligature alone, or with an acrylic splint alone or more often a combination of wire and acrylic. These techniques require the tongue to be folded caudally into the oropharynx to allow closure of the mouth during the manufacture of the appliances. This requires pharyngotomy intubation (see Ch. 2) or an intravenous general anesthetic technique.

Intraoral acrylic splints. Any soft-tissue injuries should be sutured or covered prior to making the splint to prevent wound contamination with acrylic. The technique (Fig. 12.34) utilizes the teeth to splint the fracture. The advantages of this technique are:

- It is not invasive
- Perfect occlusion is maintained
- It is technically easy to do
- It is a quick procedure, therefore requiring only a short anesthetic time.

The results are excellent and the technique is highly recommended.

Suitable acrylics are cold curing, i.e. the setting reaction is not exothermic. Cold cure acrylics are commonly used to rebase dentures. Light cure acrylic, e.g. Triad, is the simplest material to use.

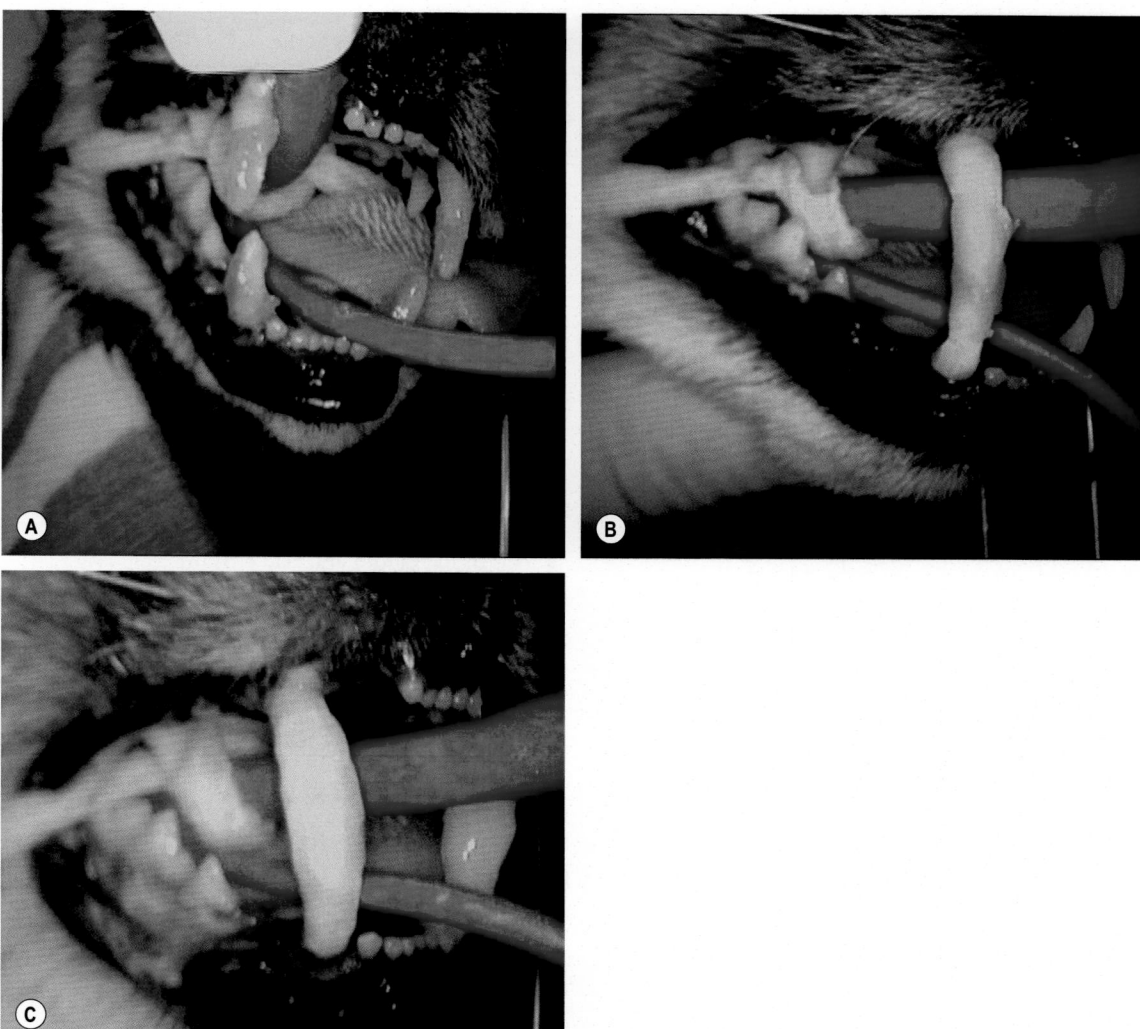

Fig. 12.33 Bonding upper and lower canines (A) Acid etch the upper and lower canines bilaterally. (B) Close the mouth until there is 2 mm overlap of the tips of the canine teeth and apply acrylic to lock the teeth together. (C) Apply additional acrylic to secure the lock.

With rebase materials, there are two techniques described, namely the 'salt and pepper' and the 'dough' technique.

The procedure to manufacture an intraoral acrylic splint using the 'salt and pepper' technique in the upper jaw is outlined below. The technique is identical for the lower jaw except the orthopedic wire is placed lingually. The wire is used for stabilization purposes and is not required if the fracture is easily reduced and stable.

1. The teeth are scaled and polished.
2. Orthopedic wire is bent to follow the buccal aspect of the dental arcade.
3. Acid etchant is applied to the teeth for 30–60 s.
4. The etchant is removed using the air/water syringe for 30 s.
5. The teeth are dried using the air syringe.
6. The mandibular teeth are covered with a thin layer of Vaseline (to prevent acrylic binding to the teeth when the mouth is closed).
7. Boxing wax is placed on the buccal and lingual aspects against the necks of the teeth to prevent acrylic from running onto the gingiva.
8. The wire is then placed against the buccal tooth surfaces coronal to the gingiva.

9. Acrylic powder is poured over the teeth and wire enclosed by the boxing wax. Liquid is added to the powder and the mouth is closed to ensure correct occlusion.

10. Once the acrylic has set, the wax is removed.

11. Any excess acrylic should be removed and rough surfaces should be smoothed. This can be done before the acrylic has set.

If using the 'dough' technique, the first six steps are identical to those above. Then, the wire is placed and a dough of mixed acrylic is placed over the maxillary teeth and the mouth is closed to ensure correct occlusion. For

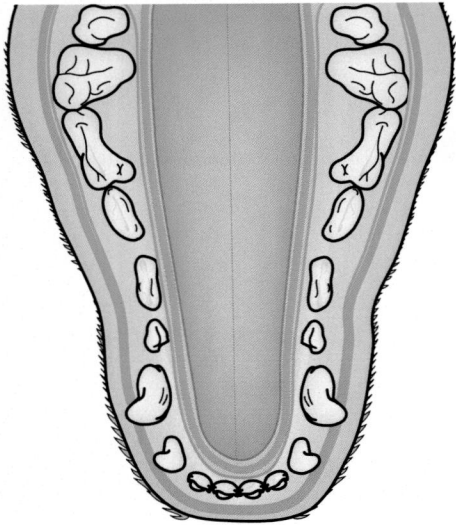

Fig. 12.34 Intraoral acrylic splint in place to repair a maxillary fracture

Triad, the technique is the same as for 'dough' and then the acrylic is light cured as the mouth is kept closed.

The appliance can usually be removed after 4–6 weeks. The easiest way to remove the splint is to drill through the wire and acrylic at several points and then gently rotate the pieces.

The procedure for interdental wire and acrylic splint fixation in the lower jaw is as follows:

1. Scale and polish the teeth
2. Assess the fracture radiographically
3. Extract diseased teeth
4. Teeth in the fracture line are managed (extract, endodontic treatment, left *in situ*)
5. Soft-tissue wounds are debrided and sutured
6. Reduce the fracture
7. Stabilize the fracture with wire (as shown in Figure 12.35A)
8. Close the mouth to check occlusion – adjust the wire if necessary, occlusion is more important than tight fixation of the fracture
9. Open the mouth and acid etch the teeth (Fig. 12.35B); rinse and dry
10. Apply Vaseline to the teeth in the upper jaw
11. Acrylic is applied (dough or Triad) predominantly to the lingual surface (Fig. 12.35C)
12. Mouth is closed and the material allowed to set with good occlusion maintained (Fig. 12.35D)
13. Appliance is smoothened with acrylic bur if required.

Postoperative care following jaw fracture repair

- Daily flushing the oral cavity clean using a chlorhexidine solution is advantageous if the animal allows it.

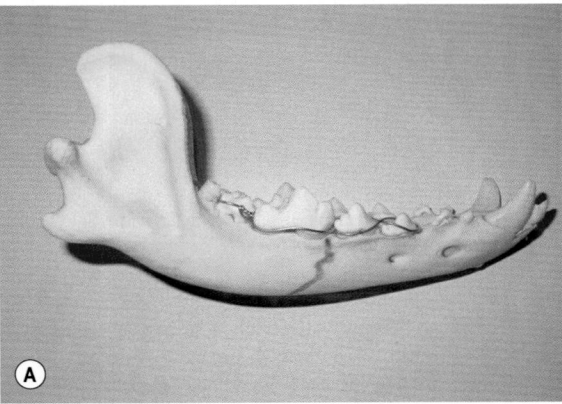

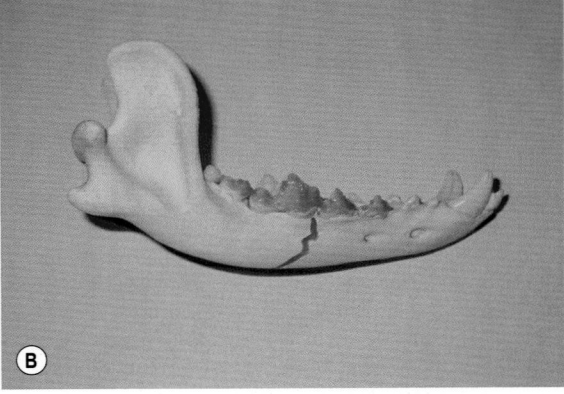

Fig. 12.35 Procedure for interdental wire and acrylic splint fixation in the lower jaw (A) The fracture has been reduced and stabilized with wire. Remember to close the mouth and check that the wire does not interfere with occlusion. (B) Acid etch is applied to the teeth. Rinse the etch away thoroughly and air-dry the teeth.

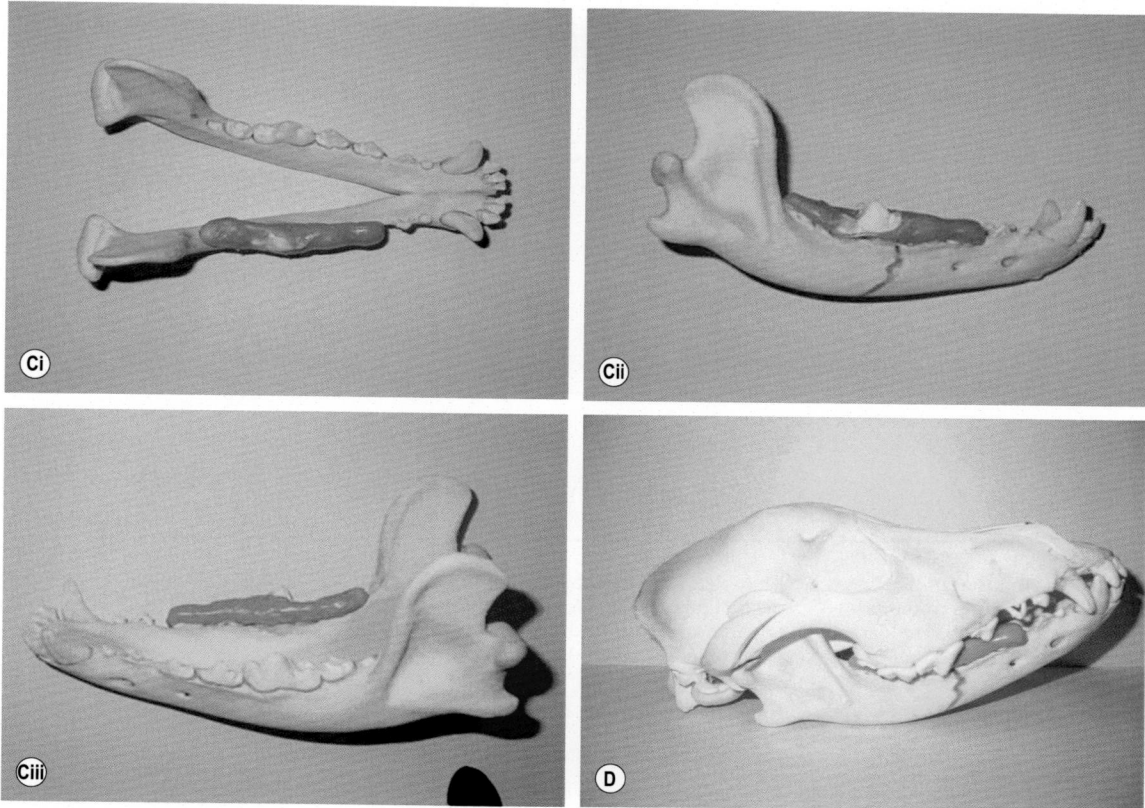

Fig. 12.35, cont'd (C) Acrylic is applied (dough or Triad) predominantly on the lingual aspects to avoid interference with occlusion, which would occur if placed predominantly buccally. (D) The mouth is closed and the material allowed to set with good occlusion maintained. Remember to put Vaseline on the upper teeth so that they do not bind to the acrylic.

- Liquid or soft food should be given for the first 3 weeks. Most animals will not need nasogastric or pharyngostomy feeding.
- Systemic antibiotics are indicated in all cases where the fracture is compound. (See Ch. 3 for more detail on the use of antibiotics.)
- Opiates and non-steroidal anti-inflammatory drugs should be administered during the early recovery phase. (See Ch. 2 for more detail on the use of analgesics.)

Complications

Many of the possible complications of jaw fractures are similar to those seen with fractures elsewhere in the body, and are dealt with in the same way. These are:

- Soft-tissue trauma
- Non-union
- Malunion
- Infection.

The two complications unique to the jaw are:

- Malocclusion
- Endodontic problems.

The use of tooth-borne appliances and managing teeth in the fracture line appropriately reduces the risk of malocclusion and endodontic problems.

Malocclusion is dealt with in Chapter 5 of this book. Teeth that have become affected by pulp and periapical disease will need endodontic therapy and should be referred to a person specializing in veterinary dentistry.

SUMMARY

- Most dental emergencies follow facial or general trauma.
- Treatment should be prioritized and initial attention given to life-threatening problems or complications.
- Good surgical principles of lavage, debridement, gentle technique and tension-free closure (if appropriate) should be followed for all oral soft-tissue injuries.
- Complicated crown fractures (pulp exposure) always need treatment by referral for endodontic therapy or else extraction.
- Root fractures can be treated by fixation (usually via referral) or extraction.
- Luxated and avulsed teeth usually require prompt referral to a specialist if the tooth is to be saved.
- Special considerations apply to jaw fractures. The emphasis should be on maintaining occlusion and minimizing iatrogenic trauma during repair.
- Intraoral acrylic splints are especially useful for mandibular fractures.

REFERENCES

Umphlet, R.C., Johnson, A.L., 1988. Mandibular fractures in the cat. A retrospective study. Veterinary Surgery 17, 333–337.

Umphlet, R.C., Johnson, A.L., 1990. Mandibular fractures in the dog. A retrospective study of 157 cases. Veterinary Surgery 19, 272–275.

FURTHER READING

Gorrel, C., 2008. Malocclusion. In: Saunders Solutions in Veterinary Practice – Small Animal Dentistry. Saunders/Elsevier, Philadelphia, pp. 129–170.

Gorrel, C., 2008. Pulp and periapical disease. In: Saunders Solutions in Veterinary Practice – Small Animal Dentistry. Saunders/Elsevier, Philadelphia, pp. 171–192.

Chapter |13|

Tooth extraction

INTRODUCTION

Tooth extraction is commonly indicated in small animal practice. The procedure is often time consuming and fraught with difficulties. The problems experienced are usually attributable to poor equipment and instrumentation, as well as lack of familiarity with extraction techniques. The purpose of this chapter is to aid the general practitioner in making optimal choices for equipment and instrumentation (see also Ch. 1) and selecting the correct techniques to extract teeth with minimal trauma.

INDICATIONS

While there are some absolute indications (i.e. no other treatment option exists) for extraction, there are often alternative treatments available (e.g. endodontic therapy and restoration of a complicated crown fracture), which would allow a tooth to be maintained. Alternative treatment is recommended for strategic teeth, i.e. the permanent canines and large posterior teeth, but only if they are periodontally sound. *However, treatment by extraction is always preferable to leaving pathology untreated.*

Common conditions that generally require extraction include the following.

Advanced periodontitis

Periodontal therapy, in combination with rigorous, life-long homecare, may allow some teeth with advanced loss of periodontal attachment to be maintained. In many instances, when the periodontal destruction is excessive and/or the owners cannot perform homecare, extraction is required.

Extensive destruction of dental hard tissue

Extensive destruction of dental hard tissue occurs with dental caries and odontoclastic resorptive lesions. Teeth with caries can be treated either with restoration alone or in combination with endodontic therapy if the pulp is also affected. In advanced caries, however, most of the crown has been destroyed and only the root(s) with inflamed or necrotic pulp tissue remain in the alveolar bone. These root(s) must be extracted to avoid periapical pathology.

Resorptive lesions are detailed in Chapter 11. The current treatment recommendation for most teeth affected by resorptive lesions is extraction. However, if there is no radiographic evidence of endodontic involvement and the roots are seen to be undergoing replacement resorption, crown amputation and flap closure is justified, but this procedure requires long-term postoperative radiographic monitoring.

Persistent primary teeth

Persistent primary teeth, i.e. primary teeth that are still in place when their permanent counterparts start erupting, may interfere with the normal eruption pathway of the permanent counterparts, resulting in the development of malocclusion. The primary incisors and canines are the most common teeth that persist. Apart from the risk of a malocclusion developing, periodontal complications are likely. Hair and other debris become trapped between the primary and permanent homologous pair and accelerate plaque-induced periodontal breakdown. Persistent primary teeth should generally be extracted early in the animal's life (ideally at around the time that the homologous permanent tooth is erupting), to reduce the likelihood of a malocclusion developing and prevent periodontal complications.

Malocclusion

Orthodontic techniques are available to correct/modify malocclusion of the permanent dentition, such that pain-free function is achieved. However, there will be owners who will not be able to afford these, usually multistage, procedures. Alternatively, the patient may not be suitable for more than a single elective anesthetic. Ethical considerations also play a role in deciding how best to treat a malocclusion. In many circumstances, extraction of maloccluding teeth, and/or their antagonist tooth, will enable adequate function.

Primary teeth involved in malocclusion should be extracted before the eruption of their permanent counterparts (i.e. at 6–8 weeks of age). This is called 'interceptive orthodontics'. It will allow the upper jaw and mandible to develop to their full genetic potential independently before the permanent dental interlock forms. Interceptive orthodontics will prevent dental interlock-induced malocclusion from developing. However, if the developing malocclusion is of skeletal origin, the value of interceptive orthodontics is negligible since the permanent teeth will form the same incorrect interlock.

Traumatic tooth injuries

Traumatic tooth injuries are common and may involve fracture of the tooth or damage to the periodontium. The management of these injuries to the permanent dentition is detailed in Chapter 12. While many tooth crown fractures can be managed by endodontic therapy and restoration, oblique crown root fractures are an absolute indication for extraction.

Pulpal and periapical disease of a primary tooth (due to a traumatic injury) may cause damage to the underlying developing permanent tooth. Consequently, a primary tooth affected by traumatic injury is also an absolute indication for extraction.

Overcrowding/supernumerary teeth

Overcrowding of teeth, often the result of a skeletal malocclusion, e.g. an upper jaw or mandible that is too short for the full complement of teeth to have sufficient space for normal occlusion, will predispose to periodontitis. In such situations, early extractions of a selected few teeth can help maintain the periodontal health of the other teeth. Supernumerary teeth should be extracted if their presence results in overcrowding and periodontal complications.

Teeth involved in a fracture line

Teeth are often involved in a fracture line. Such teeth may need removal, depending on the jaw fracture repair method employed.

CONTRAINDICATIONS

There are probably no absolute contraindications for extraction, but bleeding disorders or clotting defects should be identified, since a life-threatening hemorrhage can follow extraction in these patients.

TYPES OF EXTRACTION

There are two basic extraction techniques, namely:

1. Closed (non-surgical)
   This can be defined as extraction using simple luxation and/or elevation, without the need to remove alveolar bone. The extraction socket is either left open to heal by granulation or it may be closed by suturing the gingiva over the defect to achieve primary healing.
2. Open (surgical)
   This technique is where a mucoperiosteal flap is raised in order to access the alveolar bone. The alveolar bone overlying the buccal surface of the tooth root is usually removed in order to facilitate tooth removal. The mucoperiosteal flap is replaced to close the extraction socket, thus allowing primary healing.

CHOICE OF EXTRACTION TECHNIQUE

The choice of either a closed or an open technique will depend on several factors. The most important are:

1. Tooth morphology
2. Existing pathology
3. Operator preference.

Preoperative radiographs are mandatory to evaluate the tooth morphology and extent of pathology necessitating the extraction.

Situations where an open extraction technique is absolutely indicated (i.e. the tooth cannot technically be removed using a closed technique, since alveolar bone must be removed to free the root) include:

- Bizarre root morphology, with bends or spirals
- Extensive root resorption ± ankylosis
- Periodontally sound upper and lower canines (the roots are curved and are wider below the cemento-enamel junction than above it).

Situations where an open technique may facilitate extraction include:

- Retained root remnants
- Any multirooted tooth which is periodontally sound, i.e. there is no loss of alveolar bone (an open technique will make access to the furcation and individual roots possible)
- Feline teeth.

With the exception of teeth affected by advanced periodontitis, I generally use an open extraction technique. It enables visualization of the periodontal ligament space (instrument placement can thus be more precise and the extraction is less traumatic to adjacent tissues) and healing is more predictable. Human patients report less postoperative discomfort following an open technique than a closed technique. The same is probably true for our patients.

EXTRACTION TECHNIQUES

General considerations

Extraction of teeth is a surgical procedure. While it is not possible to achieve a sterile environment in the oral cavity, the mouth should be clean before extraction is performed. All teeth should be scaled and polished and the mouth rinsed with a chlorhexidine solution.

It is essential to know the normal anatomy of the oral cavity to prevent iatrogenic damage, e.g. severing neurovascular structures, which would result in sensory deficits and hemorrhage. Good visibility simplifies the procedure greatly. A good light source is essential. In addition, use the three-way syringe to clean the mouth out frequently during the procedure. Use water only or water and air to clean away debris, followed by air only to dry the tissues. The air spray should be used sparingly (brief bursts) to avoid soft-tissue emphysema. Suction is extremely useful and strongly recommended. Extraction is easy if the periodontal ligament space can be visualized and consequently instruments applied at the correct location. Contrary to common belief, tooth extraction requires no force. It is best achieved by planned placement of instruments and carefully working around the whole circumference of the tooth cutting the periodontal ligament, thus releasing the tooth.

As already mentioned, preoperative radiographs are mandatory to assess the extent of the pathology and identify morphologic abnormalities. The clinical findings in combination with preoperative radiographs allow selection of the best extraction technique for each tooth. Intraoperative radiographs are recommended if the procedure is not proceeding as planned. Finally, adequacy of the extraction should be verified with postoperative radiographs.

Equipment and instrumentation requirements for extraction are detailed in Chapter 1. A new extraction

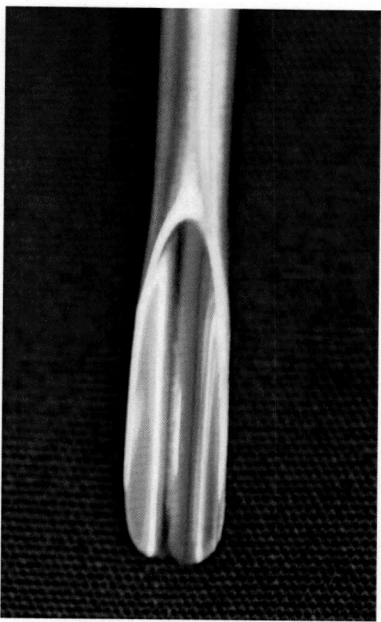

Fig. 13.1 The Extraktor This instrument has been specifically developed (by a Swedish company called Accesia) for extraction of feline and canine teeth. Its use requires modification of standard techniques. If performed correctly, the use of the Extraktor results in minimally traumatic extraction in a reasonable period of time.

instrument, called the 'Extraktor' has recently been developed (Fig. 13.1). The Extraktor has been specifically designed to fit the shape of canine and feline tooth roots, thus optimizing the forces used. It can be used to exert apical pressure and cut the periodontal ligament. It can also be used for leverage. The Extraktor can be used both as a luxator (cutting in an apical direction) and as an elevator (exerting horizontal leverage). In addition to these modes of action, the Extraktor, because of its sharp lateral edges, can be used to cut laterally, sliding around the tooth to cut the periodontal ligament. This mode of use is unique to the Extraktor. The correct use of the Extraktor is critical for success. The technique is a modification of traditional techniques using luxators and elevators and will be detailed in this chapter. Correct use always entails amputating the tooth crown to allow the Extraktors to fit snugly to the root surface. If performed correctly, the Extraktor technique results in minimally traumatic extraction in a reasonable time period.

Some guidelines for the use of dental luxators, elevators and Extraktors:

- Select the appropriate size of instrument for the size of the root
- The size of instrument required may change as the tooth loosens, i.e. smaller diameter instruments may

be required to cut periodontal ligament apically than required at the start of the extraction

- Luxators should not be used for leverage as this will damage the fine working end
- Elevators and Extraktors are used with a combination of apical pressure and leverage
- Amputating the tooth crown prior to extraction is useful when using luxators and elevators
- Amputating the tooth crown prior to extraction is mandatory when using Extraktors
- Extraktors are also used in a lateral sliding motion to cut the periodontal ligament.

Closed extraction

Single-rooted teeth

Teeth suitable for this technique are any single-rooted teeth e.g. incisors in the dog and cat, 1st premolars in the dog, upper 2nd premolars in the cat, and mandibular 3rd molars in the dog. It can also be used for canine teeth with extensive bone loss due to severe periodontitis.

Procedure – using luxators and elevators

1. Cut the gingival attachment around the whole circumference of the tooth using either a No. 11 or 15 scalpel blade in a handle or a *sharp* luxator (Fig. 13.2).
2. Select a luxator of the appropriate size. Its concave surface should equal the curvature of the root being extracted. This is often a larger size than initially estimated. The instrument is held with the handle along the palm of the hand and the index finger resting on the shaft, with the tip of the finger close to the cutting end (Fig. 13.3). The fingertip functions as an emergency stop should you slip, thereby avoiding iatrogenic damage to surrounding

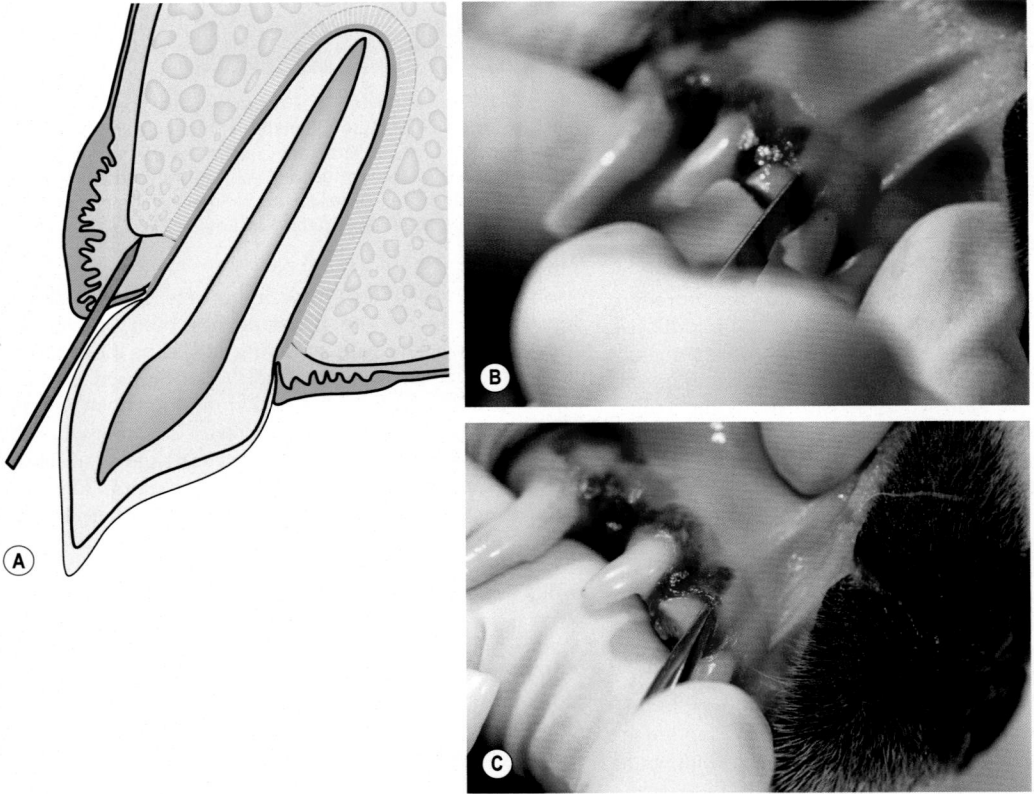

Fig. 13.2 Cutting the gingival attachment to the tooth The first step of any extraction, irrespective of whether a closed or open technique is planned, is to cut the gingival attachment around the whole circumference of a tooth. There is no attempt to enter the periodontal ligament space at this stage. The purpose of this cut is just to free the gingival attachment (A). A scalpel blade (B) or a sharp luxator or Extraktor (C) can be used to cut the gingival attachment. The sharp instrument is inserted into the gingival sulcus until the instrument contacts the margin of the alveolar bone. The gingival attachment to the tooth surface is released in this way around the whole circumference of the tooth.

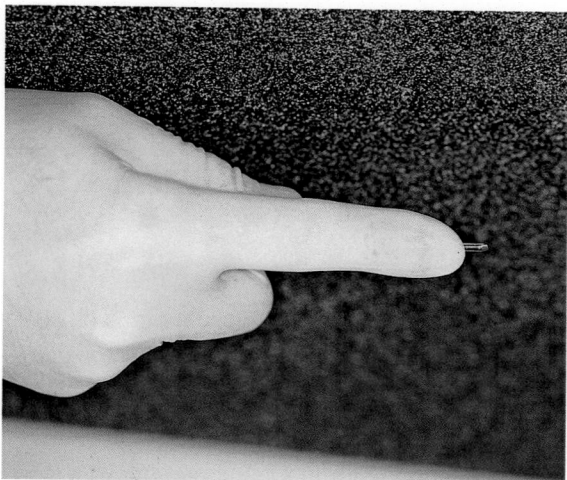

Fig. 13.3 The correct grip for a dental luxator, elevator or Extraktor The instrument is held with the handle along the palm of the hand and the index finger resting on the shaft, with the tip of the finger close to the cutting end. The fingertip functions as an emergency stop should you slip, thereby avoiding iatrogenic damage to surrounding structures.

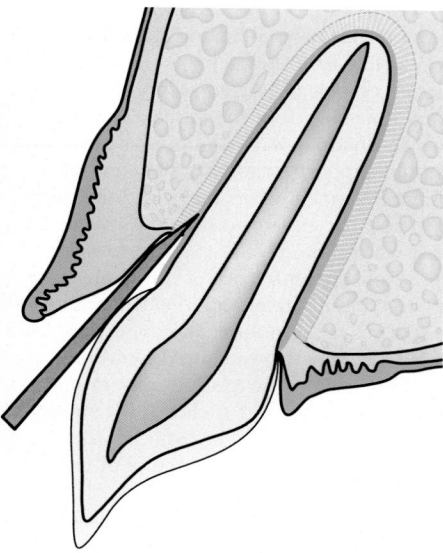

Fig. 13.4 Inserting a luxator, elevator or Extraktor into the periodontal ligament The luxator, elevator or Extraktor is advanced into the gingival sulcus at a slight angle to the tooth, i.e. following the surface of the tooth, and pressed into the periodontal ligament space.

structures. With an average-sized hand, this will leave the end of the handle resting against the wrist, where it can be gripped with the other fingers. This grip prevents the excessive force which can be applied if the handle end rests in the center of the palm, forming a straight line of force from the elbow!

3. The luxator is advanced into the gingival sulcus at a slight angle to the tooth, i.e. following the surface of the tooth, and pressed into the periodontal ligament space (Fig. 13.4). If the luxator is not inserted into the gingival sulcus in the described fashion, it is likely to slide over the margin of the alveolar bone and raise the gingiva off the bone. This will lacerate the gingiva rather than break periodontal ligament fibers!

4. The luxator is worked, applying gentle apical pressure, into the periodontal ligament space around the whole circumference of the tooth (Fig. 13.5). The sharp luxator will cut the periodontal ligament fibers. Once sufficient space has been created between the tooth and the alveolar bone, an elevator can be used. Some clinicians prefer to perform the whole extraction using luxators of increasing size, i.e. do not switch to elevators. This is acceptable procedure as long as the luxators are used in the correct fashion, i.e. in an apical direction, without rotation, to cut the periodontal ligament fibers. Luxators should not be rotated, as this will damage the fine end of the instrument.

5. The elevator (gripped in the hand in the same way as a luxator) is also worked circumferentially around

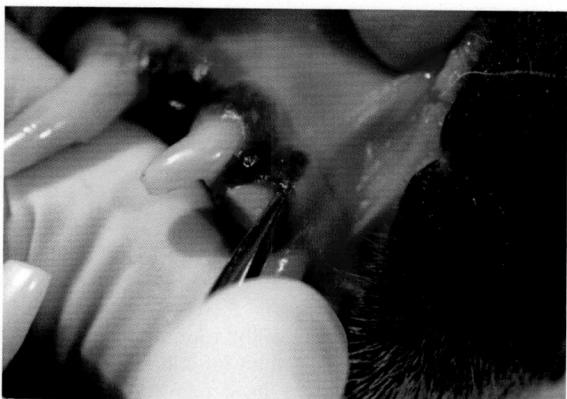

Fig. 13.5 Using a dental luxator, elevator and Extraktor These instruments are used circumferentially around the tooth. The luxator is limited to gentle apical pressure while the elevator and Extraktor can also be used with a steady gentle rotational pressure held at each point for 10–15 s to fatigue the deeper periodontal fibers. In addition, lateral pressure can be used with the Extraktor to engage the side cutting edges and slide around the tooth circumference.

the tooth, with a steady gentle rotational pressure held at each point for 10–15 s to fatigue the deeper periodontal fibers. Hemorrhage will be created at the same time, which adds hydraulic pressure to the process of breaking down the fibers. The other hand should be used to support the jaw and prevent any undue stress on the jawbone. In addition, the thumb and index finger of the other hand should be placed on the buccal and palatal/lingual aspect of the tooth root (around the alveolus of the tooth). This will allow tactile feedback as well as minimize iatrogenic damage should slippage occur with the elevator. As the periodontal ligament fibers break and the tooth begins to loosen, the elevator can be pushed further apically, and rotated more. It is essential to work around the whole circumference of the tooth. It is tempting to concentrate elevation at the points where the tooth is most mobile. The opposite should be performed, i.e. the elevator should be worked more in positions where the tooth is least mobile. When the tooth is loose in its socket, it is tempting to use extra force to speed up the extraction. Try to avoid this, as it usually results in fracture of the root, which then needs to be retrieved.

6. When the tooth is loose, it can be drawn out of the socket with fingers or forceps. In my experience, the use of dental forceps usually results in fracture of the apical portion of the root. I do not use them or recommend their use. However, if they are used, make sure that the forceps are applied as far apically as possible on the root and use gentle rotational force applied in a back and forth manner along the long axis of the tooth.

Procedure – using Extraktors

1. Cut the gingival attachment around the whole circumference of the tooth using either a No. 11 or 15 scalpel blade in a handle (Fig. 13.2B) or a *sharp* Extraktor (Fig. 13.2C).
2. Amputate the tooth crown at the cemento-enamel junction.
3. Select an Extraktor of the appropriate size. Its concave surface should equal the curvature of the mesial and distal surface of the root being extracted. This is often a larger size than initially estimated. The instrument is held in the same way as a luxator or elevator (Fig. 13.3).
4. The Extraktor is advanced into the gingival sulcus at a slight angle to the tooth, i.e. following the surface of the tooth, and pressed into the periodontal ligament space (Fig. 13.4).
5. The Extraktor is worked, applying gentle apical pressure, into the periodontal ligament space at the mesial and distal surfaces of the tooth root (Fig. 13.5). The instrument is also encouraged to slide buccally and palatally/lingually (Fig. 13.6) to cut periodontal ligament fibers around the whole circumference of the tooth. The spoon-shaped Extraktor is sharp at its apical termination but also on part of its lateral wings and will thus readily slide

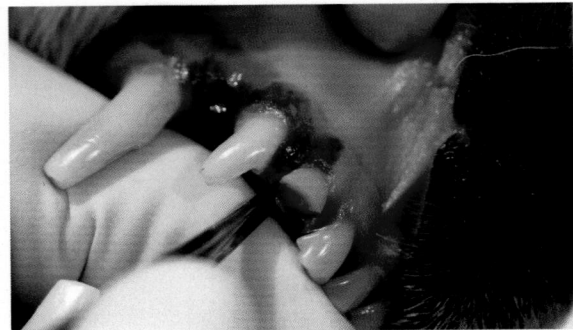

Fig. 13.6 Engaging the side cutting edges with the Extraktor The instrument is encouraged to slide buccally/palatally.

bucally and palatally/lingually. Extraktors are also of sufficient metal thickness to allow some rotation (unlike luxators).

6. As the periodontal ligament fibers break and the tooth begins to loosen, the Extraktor can be pushed further apically, and rotated more. It is essential to work around the whole circumference of the tooth.
7. When the tooth is loose, it can be drawn out of the socket with fingers or careful use of forceps.

Multirooted teeth

The tooth is sectioned into single-rooted units, such that each unit can be removed as a single-rooted tooth. The reason for sectioning is that the roots of multirooted teeth diverge away from each other, which gives the tooth greater stability in the mouth, but also makes it impossible to extract the tooth as a single unit. For a visual analogy, imagine the periodontally sound maxillary 4th premolar as a tripod embedded in concrete. Each root, therefore, needs to be drawn out at a different angle to its neighbor during the extraction process. The obvious exception is the tooth with such advanced periodontitis that has so little bone support left that it is already mobile and will, after careful breaking down of the remaining periodontal fibers, come out as a unit. I would still recommend sectioning to avoid iatrogenic root fracture.

The three-rooted teeth are the maxillary 4th premolars in cats and the maxillary 4th premolars and the maxillary 1st and 2nd molars in dogs. All other multirooted teeth have two roots. Note, however, that supernumerary roots are quite common. Preoperative radiographs will allow detection of extra roots and allow optimal sectioning into single-rooted units. Different methods of sectioning the multirooted teeth have been described. My preferred methods for sectioning of the maxillary 4th premolar and 1st molar in dogs and the mandibular 1st molar in dogs and cats are shown in diagrammatic form in Figures 13.7–13.9.

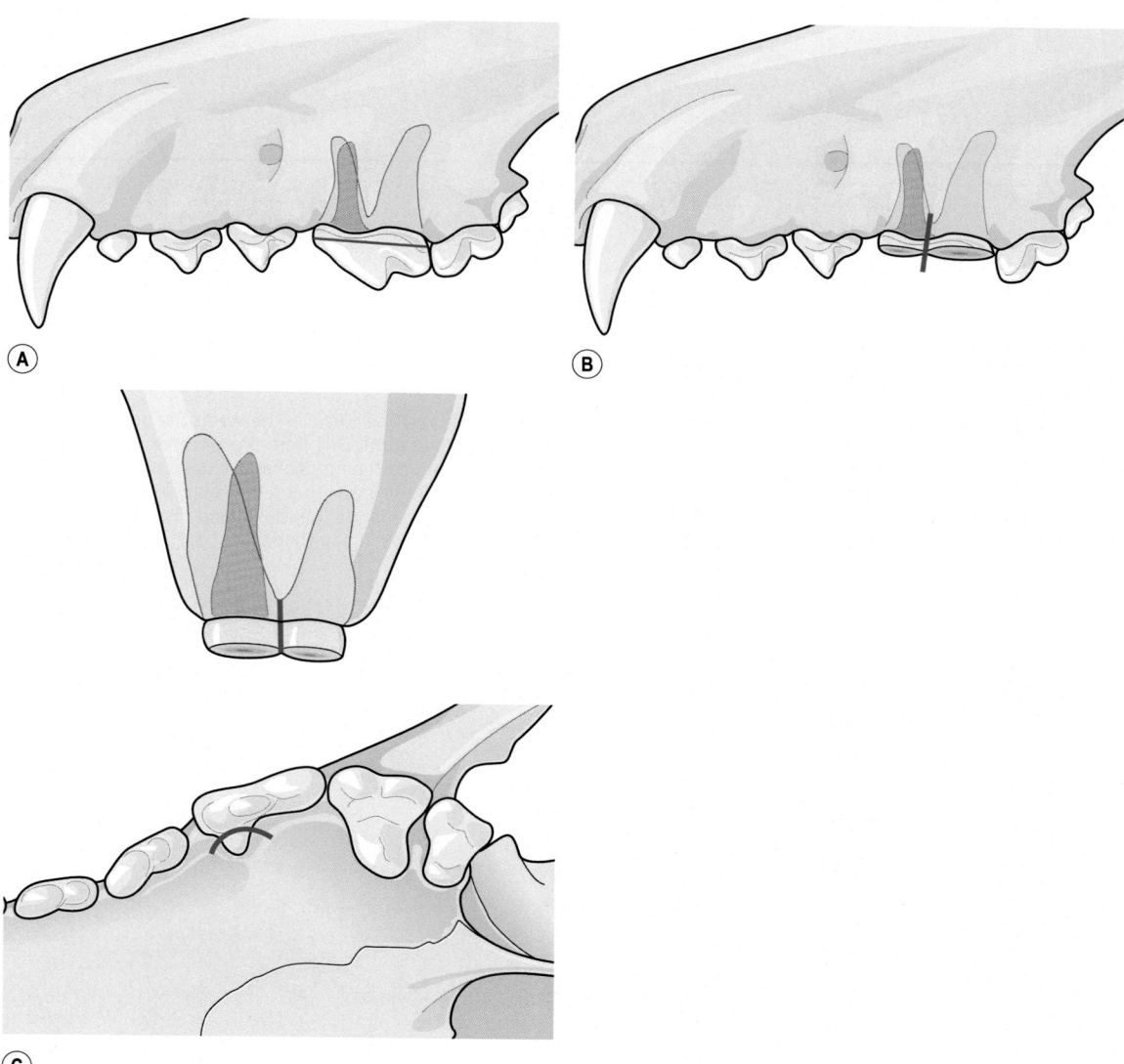

Fig. 13.7 Tooth sectioning – maxillary 4th premolar (A) Shorten the crown (horizontal cut through tooth) using either a fissure bur or a round bur to improve access to the furcation. (B) Identify the furcation between the mesiobuccal and distal roots. Insert a round bur into the furcation and drill through the furcation creating a tunnel in the alveolar bone under the furcation before cutting up into the crown. This separates the tooth into two units. (C) In the periodontally sound tooth, it can be difficult to clearly identify the furcation between the mesiobuccal and mesiopalatal root and sectioning may need to be performed by drilling from the occlusal surface towards the furcation area. It is relatively easy to miss the furcation. Another option is to extract the distal crown/root unit before sectioning the mesial tooth structure into its two crown/root units. Visualization is greatly improved when the distal portion has been removed. A tunnel can be drilled under the furcation of the two mesial roots and the cut then extended up through the crown.

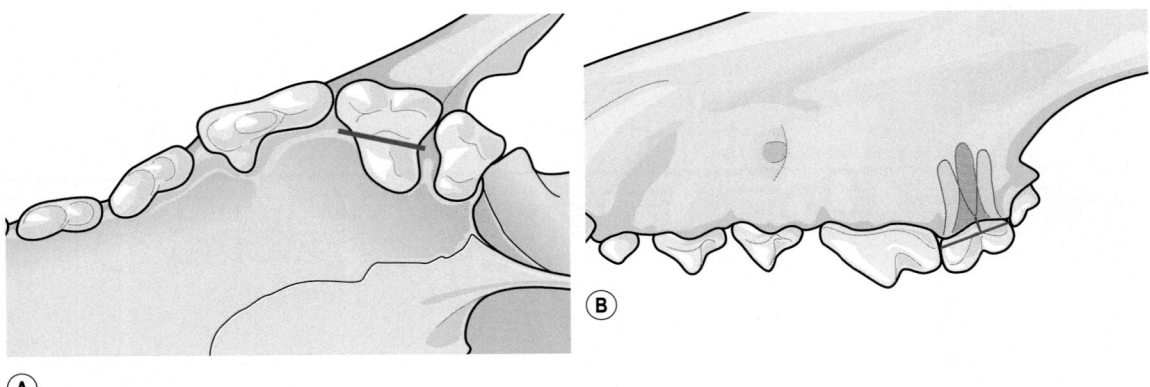

Fig. 13.8 Tooth sectioning – maxillary 1st molar (A) Shorten the crown. Identify the furcation between the buccal tooth unit (contains the mesial and distal roots) and the palatal unit (contains the palatal root). Drill from the furcation in a coronal direction to separate the tooth into these two units. (B) Identify the furcation between the mesial and distal roots and drill from the furcation up through the crown to separate the mesial and distal tooth/root units. There is no absolute rule that the above needs to be the sequence of events. In many situations, it may be easier to separate the mesial and distal tooth/root units first. Use the technique that is most reproducible and creates least tissue trauma in your hands.

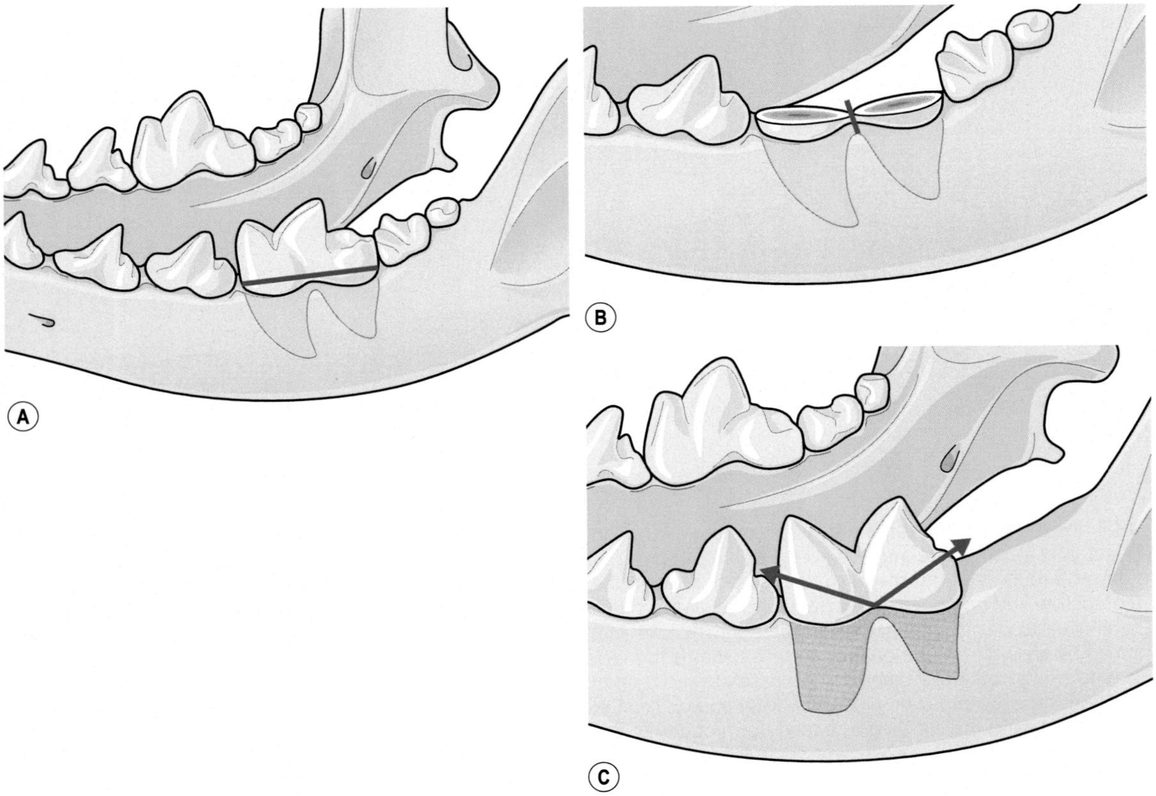

Fig. 13.9 Tooth sectioning – mandibular 1st molar The two-rooted teeth can be sectioned in one of two ways. The first is described in (A) and (B) and the second, which is often my preference, in (C). (A) Shorten the crown. (B) Identify the furcation between the mesial and distal roots and drill from the furcation up through the crown to separate the mesial and distal tooth/root units. (C) Identify the furcation and make one cut mesial and one distal towards the gingival margin. These cuts will separate the tooth into two single-rooted units and remove the bulk of the crown.

Procedure

1. Cut the gingival attachment as described earlier.
2. Unless the furcation of the roots is exposed by gingival recession, the gingiva will need to be elevated to visualize these sites. This is best achieved with a round-ended periosteal elevator of the 'wax spatula' type. A periosteal elevator can be held in the classic modified pen grip traditionally used for dental instruments. It can also be gripped in the same fashion as described for a dental luxator or elevator. My preference is the latter, as it minimizes the potential trauma induced by accidental slippage. The periosteal elevator is inserted into the space between the gingiva and the tooth pointing apically until contact is made with the margin of the alveolar bone. The periosteal elevator is advanced and gently rotated, peeling the attached gingiva off the underlying bone, to raise a full thickness gingival flap. Keep the elevator close to the bone to ensure that the flap is full thickness. Holding around the alveolus with the thumb and index finger of the other hand is useful; it facilitates keeping the elevator close to the bone and minimizes potential trauma if slippage occurs.
3. The tooth is sectioned into single-rooted units (Fig. 13.10) using a bur in either a slow- or high-speed hand piece. Traditionally, a 701 taper fissure cut bur has been recommended for sectioning teeth. It is inserted into the furcation and the cut is then extended coronally (i.e. towards the occlusal surface). I find fissure burs difficult to use for this purpose, unless the furcation is open, as they do not cut efficiently when the end is used (the cutting surfaces of a fissure bur are its sides). In my hands, a better method is to use a round bur (size 4–6 for cats and 6–8 for dogs), since this can be used to cut a tunnel in the alveolar bone under the furcation before cutting up into the crown. Using a round bur will usually create a larger slot in the crown than if a fissure bur is used. This aids insertion of the luxator or elevator between the two crown/root units created. At all times, water cooling is essential to prevent thermal damage to surrounding tissues. An alternative to the round bur is a pear-shaped bur, e.g. 331L type, which cuts both on the end and on the shank.
4. Luxate and elevate the single-root units as already described for a single-rooted tooth (Fig. 13.11). In addition to using the elevator in an apical direction, it can be inserted in a horizontal fashion between the tooth root and bone, and rotated to lift the tooth roots out of their alveoli (Fig. 13.12). If using Extraktors, then ensure that the crown has been amputated at the cemento-enamel junction to ensure good adaptation of the correct size of Extraktor to

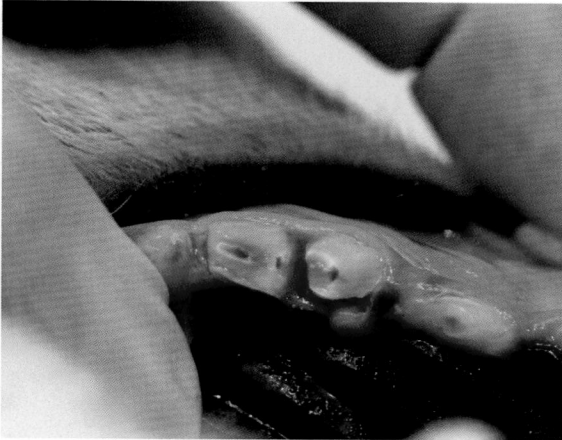

Fig. 13.10 Sectioned upper 4th premolar The right upper 4th premolar has been sectioned into its three component roots.

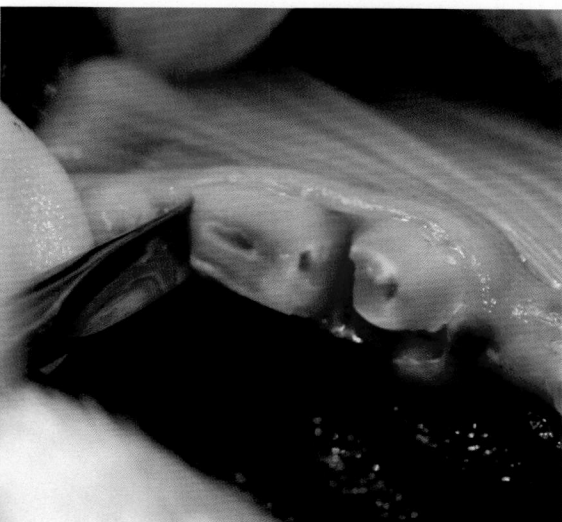

Fig. 13.11 Extracting the distal root An Extraktor of appropriate size has been inserted into the distal periodontal ligament space. The instrument will be used around the whole circumference of the distal root to break the periodontal ligament fibers and enable extraction of the tooth. It is recommended to always extract the distal root first. Once the distal root has been removed, it is easier to section the two mesial roots correctly and remove any bone in the furcation to facilitate extraction.

the tooth root. In addition to using the Extraktor in an apical direction (initial points of entry into the periodontal ligament space on the mesial and distal surfaces and then sliding buccally and palatally/lingually), the Extraktor can be inserted in a

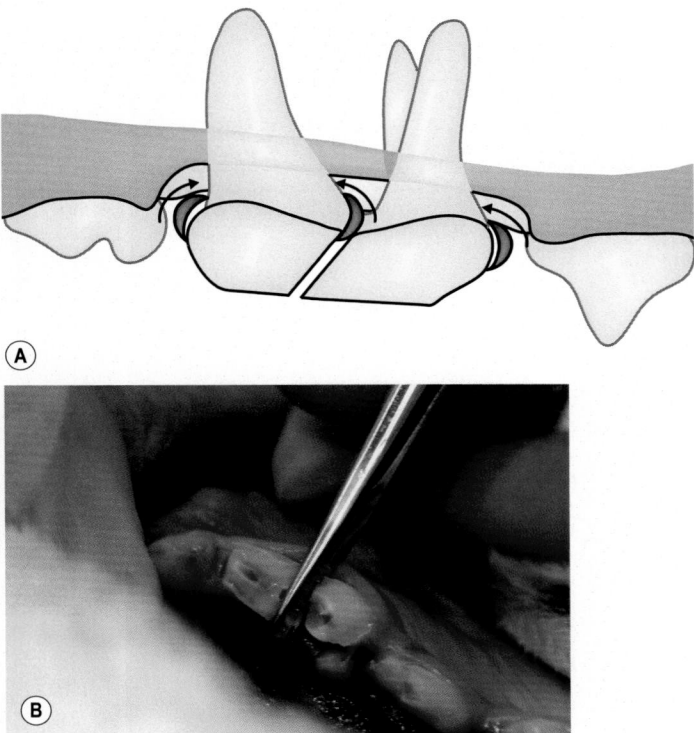

Ⓐ

Ⓑ

Fig. 13.12 Using a dental elevator or Extraktor in a horizontal fashion (A) In addition to using the elevator or Extraktor in an apical direction, it can be inserted in a horizontal fashion between the tooth sections (shown in cross-section here) and rotated on its long axis to help tear periodontal fibers, so loosening the root. It can also be used mesially and distally; in which case, ensure that the alveolar margin is used as the fulcrum, not the adjacent tooth. (B) The Extraktor is shown inserted between the tooth sections and gently rotated. Note that it is the thicker section of metal, i.e. not the fine tip, which is used for horizontal leverage.

horizontal fashion between the tooth root and bone and rotated to lift the roots out of their alveoli. Ensure that the Extraktor is inserted sufficiently far between the root and bone (Fig 13.12B) for the thicker section of metal to become engaged, i.e. do not use the fine tip for horizontal leverage.

5. Any sharp bony edges should be removed with a round bur or bone cutters. The loose gingiva should be protected, e.g. with a plastic spatula.

6. Unless the gingiva lies flat against the alveolar bone after extraction, suturing the extraction socket closed should be considered to speed healing, prevent infection, and reduce postoperative pain. Suturing is mandatory following multiple mandibular premolar and molar extractions since the gingiva tends to fall away from the extraction site, leaving exposed bone. Always elevate sufficient gingiva to allow suturing without tension, or wound breakdown will inevitably occur.

Open extraction

An open extraction technique can be used for all teeth. In open extractions, a mucoperiosteal flap is raised (usually on the buccal aspect of the tooth) to expose the alveolar bone. Releasing incisions (from the gingival margin to beyond the mucogingival line) are usually placed at one or both ends of the initial incision to allow the flap to be raised past the mucogingival junction, thus exposing most of the buccal bone plate. The incisions should be placed over bone. The number, length and position of the releasing incisions depend on the exposure required to perform the extraction. The flap needs to be large enough for good visualization. It also needs to allow enough space to remove alveolar bone without damaging the flap. A large flap will heal at the same speed as a small flap. My recommendation is to start large; with increasing experience and skill, smaller flaps will be required. It is essential to protect the flap during the procedure, as this is the tissue that will be used to suture over the extraction socket. Plastic spatulas or gingival retractors can be used to keep the flap intact. Asking an assistant to work the spatula or retractors will make the extraction easier and quicker, as well as prevent iatrogenic damage to the flap.

Once the tooth has been removed, the flap is replaced and sutured to the palatal/lingual mucosa to close the extraction socket. *There must be no tension on the suture line.* If there is tension, wound healing is compromised and the flap is likely to dehisce. If necessary, bluntly dissect the flap submucosally towards the lip margin in order to gain more tissue. In addition, ensure that the edge of the palatal/lingual mucosa is free by gently inserting the periosteal elevator between the bone and soft tissue. Lowering the margin of remaining alveolar bone will also help reduce tension. If it is not possible to fully close the flap without tension, then leave an opening. *Leaving an opening is preferable to tension!* The opening will heal by granulation.

In the following, the maxillary canine tooth will be used to exemplify the details of the open extraction technique. Differences for other teeth will be highlighted as required.

Maxillary canine

Procedure

1. The gingival attachment around the whole circumference of the canine is cut (Fig. 13.13A). This incision is then extended distally to the mesial or distal aspect of the 2nd premolar using a No. 11 or 15 blade in a handle. This involves cutting the buccal gingival attachment of the 1st and 2nd premolars.
2. A vertical releasing incision (extending from the gingival margin to just beyond the mucogingival line) is placed at the rostral end of the initial incision, i.e. mesial to the canine tooth (Figs 13.13A, 13.14A). Make the releasing incision parallel or slightly divergent to ensure that the base of the flap is broader than the edge and the blood supply to the flap is thus not compromised.
3. Periosteal elevators are used to lift the gingiva and mucosa from the bone overlying the buccal aspect of the canine root (Figs 13.13B,C, 13.14B). Extend the rostral releasing incisions if greater access is required. I usually work the periosteal elevators from the gingival incision in an apical direction. Use a gentle technique, especially at the mucogingival junction, to prevent tearing of the flap with the periosteal elevators. Remember that this tissue will be required to close the extraction socket.
4. The buccal bone plate overlying the root is drilled away (Fig. 13.13D). It is usually not necessary to remove bone to the apex, only to two-thirds of the root length. A size 2 or 4 bur is best for cats; a size 6 for dogs; and size 8 for giant breeds. A shallow

trough or gutter is then created between the root and the buccal bone using a small round bur (Fig. 13.13E). Water cooling of the bur is mandatory to avoid thermal damage to the bone. I prefer to use slow speed for bone removal to minimize the risks of thermal damage and emphysema. A feather-light, stroking motion with the bur enables removal of the bone without digging into the tooth substance. Bone can readily be differentiated from tooth: bone has a grayish color and bleeds, cementum/dentine is white and avascular.

5. Amputate the tooth crown at the cemento-enamel junction (Fig. 13.14C). This is useful for correct placement of the instrument (luxator, elevator or Extraktor) as the cervical bulge of the crown forces the instruments in the wrong direction. Remember, luxators, elevators and Extraktors are designed to fit the shape of the root.

If using Extraktors:

6. Use a size of Extraktor that fits the contour of the mesial and distal tooth root surfaces. Insert the Extraktor into the periodontal ligament space on the mesial root surface and exert pressure in an apical direction (Fig. 13.13F). Also gently slide palatally to cut the attachment on this surface (Fig. 13.14D). Repeat on the distal aspect of the tooth (Fig. 13.13G). Alternate between mesial and distal, sliding palatally and progressing in an apical direction until the tooth is so loose it can be lifted out with fingers.

If using luxators and elevators:

7. Place an elevator in one of the troughs and rotate the elevator along its long axis. This action will rotate the tooth along its long axis. The aim is to break down the palatal periodontal fibers and those of the root tip, but avoid levering the root tip into the nasal cavity. The elevator is rotated to stretch the fibers, and held for 10–30 s at a time, repeating each side until the tooth becomes loose, and can be easily removed. It is useful to also use a luxator to cut the buccal apical periodontal fibers.

For all techniques, the next steps are:

8. The bur is used to smooth the edges of the alveolus. If the socket is filled with debris, this should gently be flushed out prior to closure. Ensure that a clean clot forms in the socket (Fig. 13.14E).
9. The flap is replaced and sutured to the palatal mucosa to close the extraction socket. There must be no tension on any of the sutures. Ensure that the edge of the palatal mucosa is free (Fig. 13.13H). If necessary, bluntly dissect the flap submucosally towards the lip margin in order to gain more tissue. Use simple interrupted sutures (Fig. 13.13I, 13.14F) and an absorbable suture material with a swaged on needle. Proper placement of releasing incisions should ensure that all edges at the time of repair are

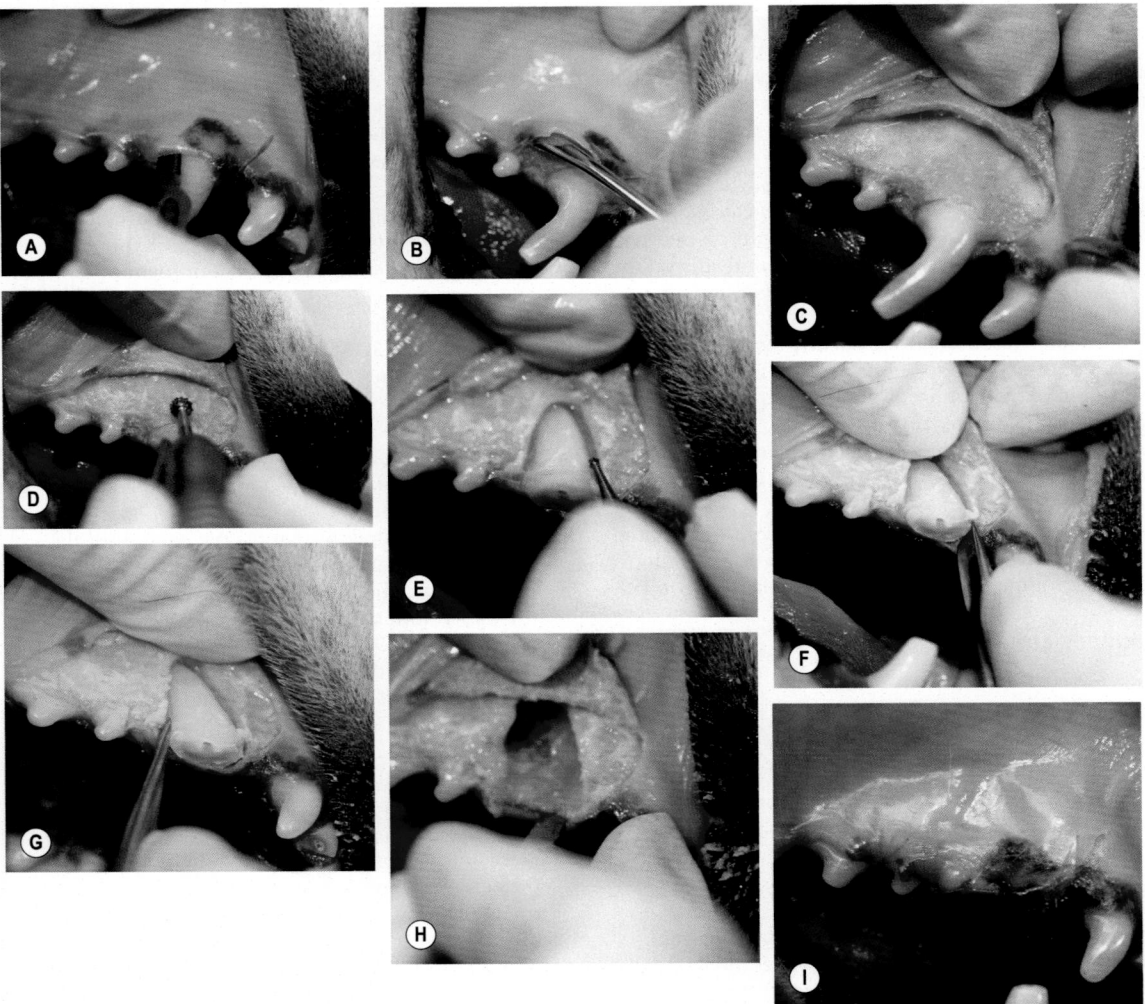

Fig. 13.13 Open extraction – maxillary canine (clinical slides) (A) Cutting the epithelial attachment. A rostral vertical releasing incision has been placed. (B) A full thickness flap extending from the gingival margin past the mucogingival junction has been started working from the gingival incision in an apical direction. (C) The full thickness flap has been elevated to expose most of the buccal alveolar bone plate. (D) The buccal bone plate will be removed using a slow-speed hand piece. (E) Approximately two-thirds of the buccal bone plate overlying the root has been drilled away. The bone overlying the apical third of the root has not been removed. In addition, a gutter between the bone and tooth has been created on the mesial and distal aspects of the tooth. (F) An appropriately sized Extraktor has been placed into the periodontal ligament space on the mesial root surface and pressure is exerted in an apical direction. (G) An appropriately sized Extraktor has been placed into the periodontal ligament space on the distal root surface and pressure is exerted in an apical direction. Alternate between working mesially and distally, sliding palatally and progressing in an apical direction until the tooth is so loose it can be lifted out with fingers. (H) Ensure that the edge of the palatal mucosa is free. Here a scalpel blade is being used to do so. Another option to free the palatal mucosa would be to insert a periosteal elevator between the bone and soft tissue. (I) The flap has been replaced and sutured to the palatal mucosa to close the extraction socket. There must be no tension on the suture line.

supported by bone. If it is not possible to fully close the flap without tension, then leave an opening. Leaving an opening is preferable to tension! The opening will heal by granulation.

Mandibular canine

Extraction of a periodontally sound mandibular canine is difficult. Patience and gentle technique are encouraged.

This tooth can be extracted using either a buccal or a lingual approach. If using a buccal approach, be careful to avoid damage to the neurovascular bundle exiting the mental foramina while raising the flap. A lingual approach is possible, but gives poor visualization.

My preferred method is a combined buccal and lingual approach as follows:

1. The buccal flap is raised in a similar fashion to that described for the maxillary canine. The large

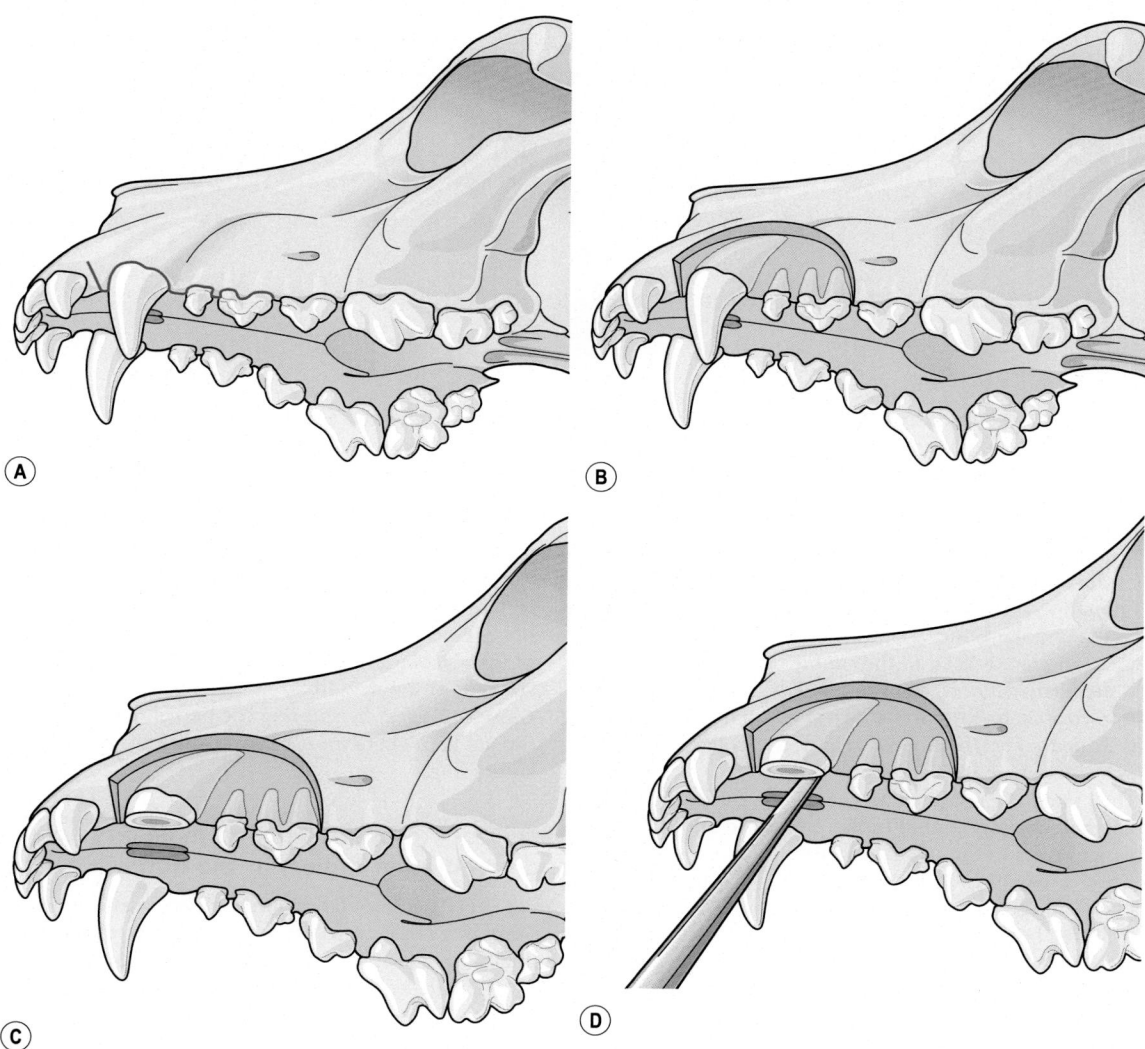

Fig. 13.14 Open extraction – maxillary canine (diagrammatic representation) (A) The primary incision and the rostal vertical releasing incision have been placed. (B) The flap has been raised and reflected. (C) The crown has been amputated at or below the cemento-enamel junction. (D) Buccal bone plate has been removed and the mesial and distal gutters between bone and tooth have been created. The Extraktor is worked mesially and distally while sliding palatally, while exerting force in an apical direction. If working with elevators they are inserted into the mesial and distal gutters and force is applied to rotate the tooth along its long axis to break the periodontal ligament fibers.

Continued

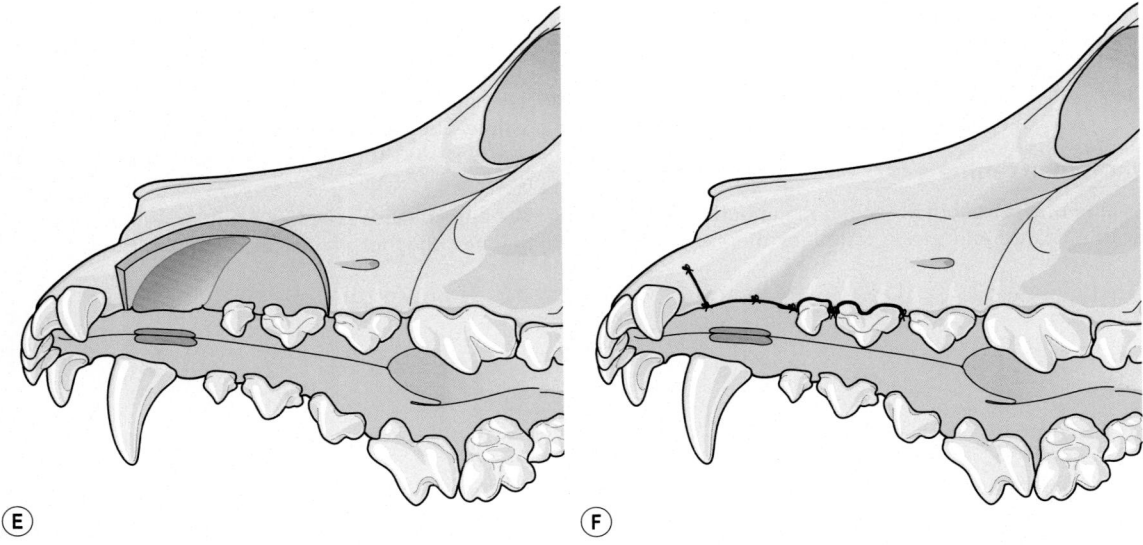

(E)   (F)

Fig. 13.14, cont'd (E) Ensure that a clean clot forms in the extraction socket. (F) The flap has been sutured in place with no tension.

neurovascular bundle exiting at one of the mental foramina (usually the middle foramen) must not be transected. It is visualized and carefully dissected free so that it can be reflected together with the flap (Fig. 13.15).

2. A gingival flap is also raised on the lingual aspect of the tooth (Fig. 13.16). It needs to be just large enough to provide access to the lingual margin of the alveolar bone. A short lingual releasing incision placed distal to the canine tooth is used if necessary.

3. Approximately 30% of the buccal alveolar bone plate is drilled away. The bone is removed to a level just apical to where the root is at its widest.

4. The crown is amputated just above the cemento-enamel junction (round or fissure bur) to allow easier access to the lingual surface.

5. Approximately 20% of the lingual alveolar bone plate is drilled away. Ensure that the flap is protected from the bur.

6. Mesial and distal gutters between the tooth root and bone are created bucally as described for the maxillary canine.

7. To loosen the tooth, elevators or extraktors are used in the buccal mesial and distal gutters as described for extraction of the maxillary canine. Extraktors are particularly useful as they have a cutting edge laterally and can thus be used in a sliding motion from mesial or distal to lingual. Also, extraktors can be used to cut the buccal apical periodontal fibers. If Extraktors are not available, then luxators should be

used to cut the buccal apical periodontal fibers and to cut the fibers on the lingual aspect and create enough space for elevators of increasing size to be used. Working in this fashion, the periodontal ligament is progressively destroyed around the whole circumference of the root until the tooth is loose and can be lifted out with your fingers.

8. It may be necessary to remove additional alveolar bone, especially lingually. Try to maintain as much of the alveolar bone as possible to preserve the strength of the mandible.

9. Close the defect by suturing the buccal flap to the lingual flap. There must be no tension on the suture line.

Maxillary 4th premolars and maxillary and mandibular molars in the dog

These teeth, if periodontally compromised, can be removed by sectioning, and closed extraction. If the teeth are periodontally sound, open extraction is recommended.

The flap for the maxillary 4th premolar extends from the mesial aspect of the 3rd premolar to the distal edge of the 1st molar. After cutting the gingival attachment around the whole circumference of the upper 4th premolar, the incision is extended rostrally to the mesial aspect of the maxillary 3rd premolar and caudally to the distal edge of the 1st molar. One divergent releasing incision extending just past the mucogingival line is made at the distal aspect of the 1st molar (Fig. 13.17). Placing only the one releasing incision distally avoids damage to the

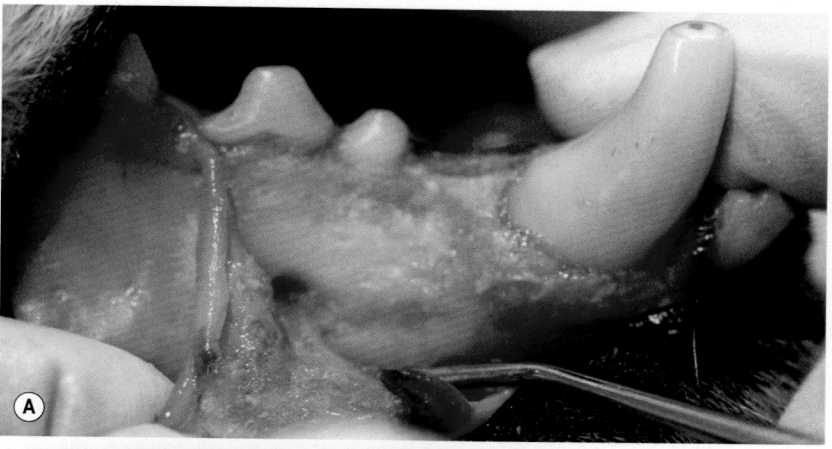

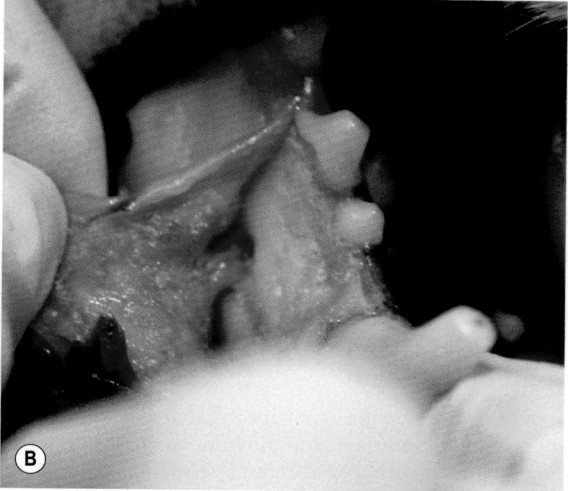

Fig. 13.15 Open extraction – mandibular canine The inferior alveolar nerve, artery and vein exit at one of the mental foramina. It is visualized (A) and carefully dissected free (B) so that it can be reflected together with the buccal access flap.

neurovascular bundle exiting at the infraorbital foramen, dorsal to the 3rd premolar.

The flap for the maxillary 1st molar needs to extend from the mesial or mid-buccal aspect of the 4th premolar to the distal aspect of the 2nd molar. Vertical releasing incisions are generally not required, but I would use the distal aspect of the 2nd molar if further access is needed.

The flap for the maxillary 2nd molar extends from the mesial or mid-buccal aspect of the 1st molar to the distal aspect of the 2nd molar. No releasing incisions are usually required.

The flap for the lower molars usually only needs to extend to the adjacent teeth, with the releasing incisions at each end diverging as they pass through the muco-gingival line.

In all teeth, buccal bone is removed to expose the furcation and the tooth is sectioned into its constituent root/crown units. Further removal of alveolar bone (start with approximately 30% of the alveolar bone plate) will facilitate extraction. If necessary, e.g. ankylosis, the whole buccal bone plate can be removed. However, use caution when removing large amounts of buccal bone. It is essential to know the anatomy of your patient, e.g. the mesiobuccal root of the maxillary 4th premolar is close to the infraorbital canal and the mandibular 1st molar root tips are adjacent to the mandibular canal.

It is always useful to amputate the crown to allow correct placement of luxators, elevators or Extraktors without interference from the enamel bulge. When using Extraktors, crown amputation is mandatory.

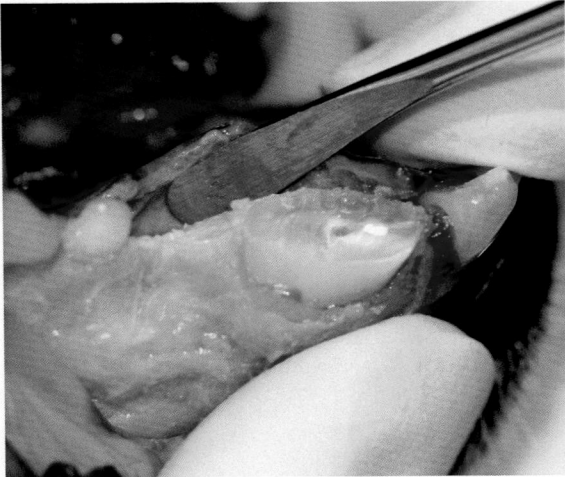

Fig. 13.16 Open extraction – mandibular canine
A lingual access flap has been raised.

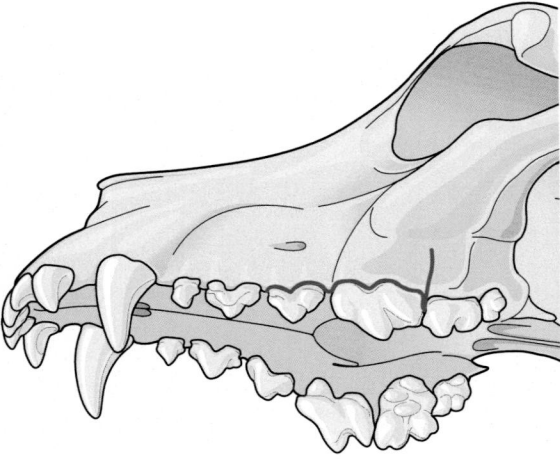

Fig. 13.17 Open extraction – upper 4th premolar The proposed flap design for open extraction of an upper 4th premolar is depicted. Placing only one releasing incision distally avoids damage to the neurovascular bundle exiting at the infraorbital foramen, dorsal to the 3rd premolar.

To reduce tension on the suture line, remember to free the palatal/lingual mucosa from the underlying bone.

Primary teeth

Primary teeth can be extracted using either a closed or an open technique. Preoperative radiographs are mandatory to give information as to the position and extent of primary tooth root resorption and the location and stage of development of the adjacent permanent tooth.

Closed extraction is indicated when the root is virtually resorbed. In most other situations, visualization will aid the procedure and open extraction is my technique of choice. The details of the extraction procedure are the same as for permanent teeth but use care to avoid damage to adjacent developing permanent dentition.

Special considerations with feline teeth

The most common diseases necessitating tooth extraction in cats are resorptive lesions, periodontitis and traumatic dental injuries resulting in pulpal exposure.

Small single-rooted teeth

In the cat, the incisors, the maxillary 2nd premolar and the maxillary molar are small single-rooted teeth. They can generally be removed using a closed technique. The technique is the same as already described for the dog, but use a gentle approach and make sure that the luxators, elevators or Extraktors used are of an appropriate size for the tooth.

Canine teeth

The canine teeth, unless affected by severe periodontitis, require an open extraction technique as described for the dog.

Multirooted teeth

In the cat, these are the maxillary and mandibular 3rd and 4th premolars and the mandibular molar. These teeth are every veterinary surgeon's nightmare owing to the ease with which they fracture during extraction. This leaves roots, with or without pieces of crown attached, which must be removed. Although it might be tempting to leave these roots and hope they will resorb, or the gingiva will grow over them, this is negligent. Every attempt should be made to retrieve such root remnants. If this is not technically possible, the owner must be informed that extraction was incomplete. Postoperative clinical and radiographic monitoring is mandatory. While some root remnants may resorb, others may result in inflammatory disease. In the latter case, a second attempt to retrieve them should be performed.

Multirooted teeth in the cat can be removed using either a closed or an open technique. The closed technique is identical to that described for the dog. Gentle technique is essential. In addition, ensure selection of appropriately sized instruments to avoid iatrogenic root fracture. Open extraction is similar to that described for the dog. Suggested modifications in the cat will be covered in the next paragraph. Irrespective of extraction technique, multirooted teeth always need to be sectioned into single-rooted

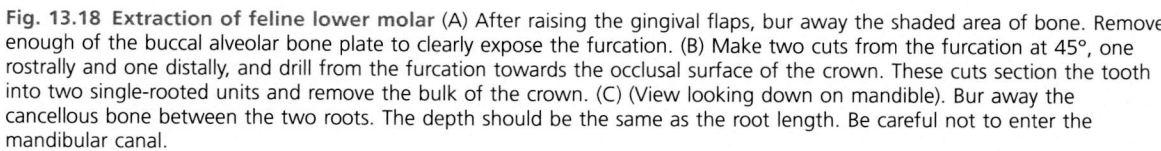

Fig. 13.18 Extraction of feline lower molar (A) After raising the gingival flaps, bur away the shaded area of bone. Remove enough of the buccal alveolar bone plate to clearly expose the furcation. (B) Make two cuts from the furcation at 45°, one rostrally and one distally, and drill from the furcation towards the occlusal surface of the crown. These cuts section the tooth into two single-rooted units and remove the bulk of the crown. (C) (View looking down on mandible). Bur away the cancellous bone between the two roots. The depth should be the same as the root length. Be careful not to enter the mandibular canal.

segments. My preference in the cat is open extraction unless there is severe periodontitis and the tooth is very mobile.

A modified technique for extracting multirooted teeth in the cat is proposed. The aim of the modification is to simplify removal and preserve alveolar bone. In the following, it is described for the mandibular teeth. The method can be adapted for removal of the maxillary multirooted teeth.

1. Raise a gingival flap both buccally and lingually.
2. Remove enough alveolar bone to expose the furcation (Fig. 13.18A).
3. A small round bur, size 2 usually, is used to make two cuts from the furcation at 45°, one distally and one rostrally (Fig. 13.18B). These cuts will remove the bulk of the crown, leaving only a small point of crown on each individual root.
4. Use either a size 2 or a size 4 round bur to remove the cancellous bone between the two roots. The depth should be the same as the root length, but not long enough to enter the mandibular canal (Fig. 13.18C). If in doubt, measure the distance on your radiographs.

5. Each root is then only supported by bone on three sides. A small luxator, elevator or Extraktor can be eased into the space created by the bur and the roots can be loosened and removed.
6. If necessary, remove additional buccal bone.
7. Remove any sharp bony edges.
8. Suture the buccal flap to the lingual flap.

COMPLICATIONS OF EXTRACTION

Thermal bone injury

Adequate water cooling of the bur (whether used in a high- or slow-speed hand piece) is mandatory. Overheating will result in damage to both the soft tissue and bone. Thermal necrosis of bone usually results in the development of a bone sequestrum that needs to be surgically retrieved as a second procedure.

I prefer to use a slow-speed hand piece to remove bone. It is more accurate and probably safer as it reduces the risk of thermal injury. It is equally quick to using a high-speed hand piece.

187

Tooth fracture

Extraction may result in fracture of the tooth, either the crown or the root. Fracture of the crown is usually due to excessive force with elevators or using dental forceps. If the root is in one piece and can be visualized, it is removed using small luxators, elevators or Extraktors to cut the remaining periodontal ligament fibers. This is where a small (2 mm) luxator or Extraktor come in handy. Visibility is essential to be able to place instruments in the periodontal ligament space. Use the water spray to remove blood.

If the root fractures, a radiograph is required to assess how much root is still in place and its position. Based on the radiographic findings, the extraction can be planned. An open extraction may be required to access the root remnant. If the root tip cannot be removed, the client must be informed and the affected jaw monitored clinically and radiographically for evidence of pathology.

Oronasal communication

A communication between a maxillary tooth alveolus and the nasal chamber may occur. Established fistulae are lined by epithelium and will, therefore, not heal spontaneously. The three most common causes of oronasal fistula formation involving the maxillary alveolus area are:

- Advanced periodontal disease
- Periapical lesions
- Iatrogenic.

An oronasal fistula in the region of the canine tooth is usually the result of advanced periodontal disease where the process caused destruction of the medial bony wall of the alveolus. Periapical pathology of the maxillary canine teeth and premolars can also cause perforation of the medial bony wall of the alveolus. Extraction of a maxillary canine tooth may also cause perforation of the medial bony wall when an incorrect technique is used. A small iatrogenic perforation will probably heal if the gingival flap is replaced and sutured. Large fresh defects or long-standing defects causing clinical signs, such as nasal discharge, food impaction and chronic infection, should be surgically repaired. The repair of persistent symptomatic oronasal communication is covered in Chapter 12.

Emphysema

Emphysema can occur if the high-speed hand piece is angled in such a way that air is blown into the bone and soft tissues. The risk of emphysema is one of the reasons why high speed is best avoided for bone removal during extraction. Continuous air-drying, especially if the air is directed into the alveolus, can also lead to emphysema. Cats seem particularly prone and, on recovery, have swelling across the base of the nose and forehead. There is obvious crepitus on palpation of the swelling. Alternatively, the floor of the mouth is swollen. The condition usually resolves over a few hours/days. The owners are often concerned and it is best avoided.

Sublingual oedema

Traumatizing the lingual mucosa may result in sublingual oedema. If severe, it may require medical management with anti-inflammatory drugs and sometimes diuretics. It is easily avoided by using a gentle technique.

Jaw fracture

Advanced periodontal disease around mandibular teeth will weaken the mandible itself, and jaw fractures can and do happen. Extreme caution should be used in elderly toy and small breeds who seem most prone to this. The principles of and techniques for jaw fracture repair are covered in Chapter 12.

Hemorrhage

Clotting defects may not be apparent until after you have extracted a tooth, when the associated hemorrhage does not stop after a few minutes, but continues copiously and can become life-threatening. Suturing the gingiva with a hemostatic gauze or plug in the alveolus can help.

SUMMARY

- ◆ Tooth extraction demands suitable equipment, instrumentation and surgical technical skills if patient morbidity is to be minimized.
- ◆ Sufficient time should be allocated for the procedure.
- ◆ Extraction is performed under radiographic control including, in problem cases, intraoperative radiographs.
- ◆ Closed (non-surgical) and open (surgical) techniques are possible, but the latter generally cause fewer problems and result in greater patient comfort when executed well.
- ◆ Each tooth should be approached using one of the prescribed techniques for that location.
- ◆ When mucoperiosteal flaps are used, care should be taken to ensure that their replacement is tension free, using appropriate suture materials and technique.

FURTHER READING

Gorrel, C., Robinson, J., 1995. Periodontal therapy and extraction technique. In: Crossley, D., Penman, S. (Eds.), BSAVA Manual of Small Animal Dentistry. BSAVA, Cheltenham, pp. 139–149.

Holmstrom, S., Frost, P., Eisner, E., 2004. Exodontics. Veterinary Dental Techniques. WB Saunders, Philadelphia, pp. 291–338.

Mulligan, T., Aller, M., Williams, C., 1998. Atlas of Canine and Feline Dental Radiography. Veterinary Learning Systems, Trenton.

Chapter 14

Dental diseases in lagomorphs and rodents

with Leen Verhaert

INTRODUCTION

Lagomorphs and rodents are increasingly popular pets. These 'pocket pets' have a high incidence of oral/dental problems that the general practitioner needs to be able to identify and manage. Most of the problems are related to the anatomic peculiarities of their dentition in combination with poor husbandry, i.e. feeding a non-abrasive diet resulting in abnormal wear and malocclusion.

While there are many similarities between lagomorphs and rodents with regards to type of dentition, oral/dental conditions and treatment options, there are also significant differences. In addition, there are differences within the rodent group.

This chapter will describe the normal anatomy of the dentition and the common oral/dental conditions of lagomorphs and rodents. As with other species, it is essential to know what is normal in order to identify disease. Dental procedures, i.e. tooth trimming and extraction techniques, are detailed separately at the end of the chapter.

Types of teeth

There are two basic types of teeth:

- Brachyodont
- Hypsodont.

The *brachyodont* tooth has a short crown : root ratio, with a true root. Once the tooth has matured, the root apex closes and the potential for further tooth growth ceases. Humans, dogs, cats and ferrets have a brachyodont dentition.

The *hypsodont* tooth is a tooth with a long anatomic crown, and a comparatively short root. The subgingival part of the crown is called the reserve crown. Hypsodont teeth are either radicular or aradicular. The radicular hypsodont tooth eventually forms a true root. The tooth grows for most of the life of the animal, but late in life, the root apex closes and tooth growth ceases. Horses and cows have radicular hypsodont teeth. The aradicular hypsodont tooth never forms a true root with an apex and the tooth grows continuously throughout the animal's life. Rabbits, guinea pigs, chinchillas and degus have aradicular hypsodont teeth. The incisors of all rodents are aradicular hypsodont, while the cheek teeth are either aradicular hypsodont or brachyodont depending on the species.

If eruption of continuously growing teeth is hindered, e.g. mechanical obstruction due to a malocclusion resulting in abnormal occlusal forces, the continued growth of the tooth will result in destruction of the alveolar bone and apparent 'apical growth' of the tooth. This may result in perforation of the cortical bone of the jawbones. In advanced stages, the tooth itself may show severe deformation in the more apical portion.

DENTAL ANATOMY

Lagomorphs

The Order of Lagomorphs includes rabbits, hares, cottontails and pikas. All teeth in lagomorphs are aradicular hypsodont. They have four incisor teeth in the upper jaw. This clearly differentiates them from rodents who only have two incisors in the upper jaw. The lagomorphs do not have canine teeth (Box 14.1).

The four incisor teeth in the upper jaw are placed in two rows with the two large incisors located labially and the

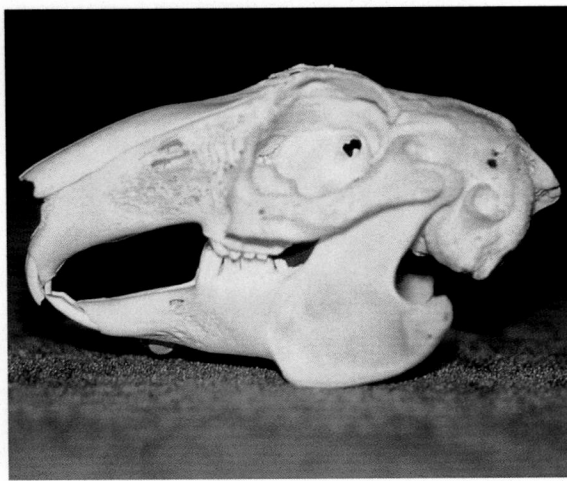

Fig. 14.1 Normal rabbit skull At rest, the incisors are held in occlusion and the cheek teeth are out of occlusion.

two smaller rudimentary incisors (peg teeth) located palatally. In occlusion, the crown tips of the mandibular incisor teeth rest between the 1st and 2nd row of upper jaw incisors. At rest, the incisors are held in occlusion and the cheek teeth are held out of occlusion (Crossley 1995a). A relatively normal rabbit skull is depicted in Figure 14.1.

Rabbits do not gnaw like rodents, unless there is some cheek tooth problem interfering with normal mastication (Crossley 1995a). The incisors are mainly used in a lateral slicing motion, so they more or less cut their food into smaller apprehensible pieces. The large upper incisors grow at an average rate of 2.0 mm per week and the lower incisors at a rate of 2.4 mm per week (Wiggs and Lobprise 1995). A rabbit with normal incisor occlusion, eating a normally abrasive diet such as hay, grass and fresh greens, will wear down the teeth at a similar rate. The incisor teeth have thick white enamel on the labial surface and almost no enamel on the palatal/lingual surface. Normal tooth wear thus results in a chisel-shaped tooth as the softer dentine wears down faster than the thick enamel.

A large diastema separates the incisor teeth from the cheek teeth (premolar and molar teeth).

The upper jaw is wider than the mandible (anisognathic) and when there are no cheek tooth problems, and no other interference such as overgrown incisors, the rabbit chews its foods using a wide lateral (side to side) motion.

Rodents

Rodentia is the largest Mammal Order, with weights ranging from 4 g to over 50 kg. All rodents are 'gnawers', with a wide rostrocaudal movement range in the temporomandibular joint and chisel-shaped continuously growing incisor teeth designed for this dorsoventral motion. They are anisognathic, but, in contrast to the lagomorphs, the mandible is wider than the maxilla.

While the incisors are aradicular hypsodont, the cheek teeth are either aradicular hypsodont or brachyodont depending on species. The strict herbivores eating a highly abrasive diet have aradicular hypsodont cheek teeth, e.g. guinea pigs, chinchillas and degus. Species eating less abrasive diets, e.g. mice, rats, hamsters and prairie dogs have brachyodont cheek teeth.

The dental formula (Box 14.2) varies among the species, ranging from 16–22 teeth. However, all rodents have four incisors (one in each quadrant) and no canine teeth. A diastema separates the incisors from the cheek teeth.

At rest (Fig. 14.2A), the mandible is in a caudal position and the incisors are out of occlusion (Crossley 1995b). During gnawing, the incisors are held in occlusion (Fig. 14.2B).

As in lagomorphs, the enamel layer of the incisors is thickest on the labial surface, with almost none present at the palatal/lingual aspect, resulting in a chisel-shaped pattern of tooth wear. The enamel is usually orange-yellow in color. However, the guinea pig has white enamel.

HUSBANDRY

By far, the most common dental problem in rabbits is tooth overgrowth. While incisor overgrowth due to an inherited skeletal malocclusion does occur, the most common cause of tooth overgrowth is insufficient wear of the continuously growing teeth caused by feeding a non-abrasive diet, e.g. dry pellets only. The affected animal is often presented late in the process. In many cases, the patient is presented when disease is too advanced to be amenable to intervention and euthanasia is required for a condition which could have been prevented. Weekly weighing of every pocket pet is strongly recommended.

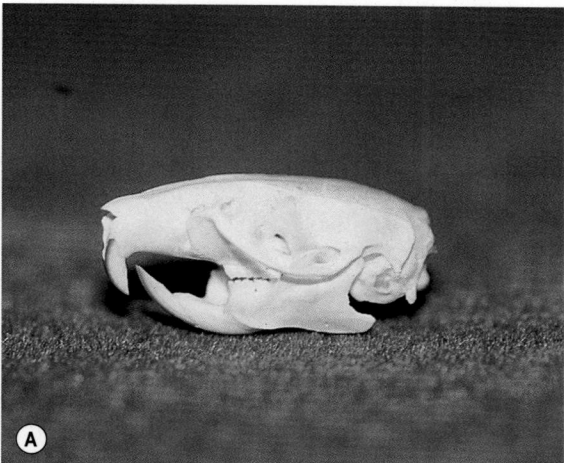

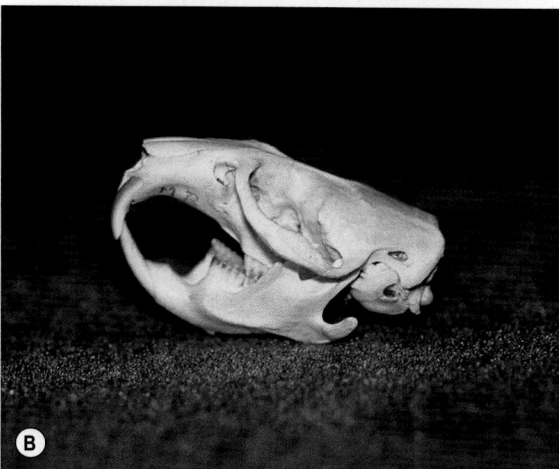

Fig. 14.2 Normal rat skull (A) At rest, the mandible is held in a caudal position. The incisors are then out of occlusion and the cheek teeth are in occlusion. (B) For gnawing, the mandible is moved rostrally so that the incisor teeth are brought into occlusion.

Weight loss requires investigation. Disease may thus be identified and treatment instituted earlier.

The ideal diet for the strictly herbivorous pocket pets consists of grass and coarse hay as the main components. This may be supplemented with fresh vegetables and dry pellets. If dry pellets are fed, they should only form a maximum of 10% of the total diet. A diet such as this will not only help in preventing dental overgrowth, but is also healthier for the gastrointestinal system. All rodents need material to gnaw on.

Guinea pigs need vitamin C supplementation (Flecknell 1991; Schaeffer and Donnelly 1997). A daily dose of 10 mg/kg is recommended for normal activity; this should be increased (up to 30 mg/kg) in situations of stress (e.g. change of environment, pregnancy, illness, new pet). There are commercially available vitamin C drops, powders and tablets that can be added to the food or the water. However, Vitamin C is unstable (easily oxidized by light and air) and therefore adding to food is preferable to putting in drinking water.

Consequences of tooth overgrowth

Tooth overgrowth commonly results in malocclusion. Complications to malocclusion include:

- Traumatization of oral soft tissues (cheeks, tongue) by the overgrown teeth
- Apical overgrowth with resultant penetration of upper teeth into the ocular sockets and/or sinuses
- Apical overgrowth of the mandibular teeth with resultant penetration of the ventral border of the alveolar bone in the mandible
- Retrobulbar and/or facial abscessation
- Inability to close the mouth
- Inability to chew (lateral slicing motion in lagomorphs; gnawing in rodents).

With advanced disease, the animal is unable to eat and weight loss occurs. The oral discomfort is often associated with excessive salivation ('slobbers'), which predisposes to moist dermatitis (wet dewlap).

EXAMINATION

General considerations

A full history should be taken. Husbandry details (housing, diet) need to be known. A full physical examination is required to assess general condition and anesthetic risk. Signs that may be due to dental disease include:

- Selective food intake
- Dropping food from mouth
- Anorexia
- Ocular discharge
- Nasal discharge
- Continuous tooth grinding
- Salivation, wet chin, dirty forelimbs
- Changes in grooming behavior
- Accumulation of cecotrops around anus (predisposing to 'fly strike').

It must be emphasized that the above signs can occur with other disease processes. Anorexia is a very common sign of advanced oral disease, but it is also a sign of almost any disease in these animals. Rabbits and rodents in pain usually stop eating. Tooth grinding is more commonly associated with abdominal discomfort than with dental disease.

Since animals with oral/dental disease are presented late in the disease process, they are often emaciated, dehydrated and obstipated. In addition, they are usually severely stressed from chronic discomfort/pain. Extreme care must be used in selection of medications (antibiotics, antiinflammatory drugs, analgesics and fluid treatment) as lagomorphs and rodents have sensitivities and toxicities to many drugs. It is outside the scope of this chapter to cover these issues. Several excellent texts on rabbit medicine, with extensive drug information, are available and the reader is encouraged to refer to these.

It may be necessary to stabilize the patient before anesthesia. While some authors recommend hospitalization to achieve this, in our experience it is not wise to hospitalize these stress-sensitive animals for long periods. A common response to stress is anorexia. If hospitalization is required, all should be done to decrease stress, i.e. the area should be quiet, as odor-free as possible, and a hiding area should be offered.

Examination of the face and oral cavity

Inspection and palpation of the face and oral cavity is the next step (Box 14.3).

Valuable information can be gained from oral examination of the conscious animal. Although the mouth cannot be opened, a reasonable view can be achieved using an otoscope or a bivalve nasal speculum. Excessive amounts of saliva, overgrowth of cheek teeth, tongue lacerations and wounds of the buccal mucosa may be identified in this way. Less severe problems will not be identified.

As in other species, thorough intraoral examination requires general anesthesia. Sedation and anesthesia in pocket pets is covered in other texts and will not be dealt with here. Aids such as mouth gags and cheek dilators are necessary to open the mouth. We do not use mouth gags in rabbits. Instead, we use cheek dilators as shown in Figure 14.3. We do use a light model mouth gag for most other species. Risks associated with using a mouth gag are damage to the teeth and damage to the temporomandibular joint (if the mouth is opened excessively).

Additional tools include spatulas to depress the tongue or push it aside. Good lighting is mandatory, and often not easy to achieve – a pen torch or headlight is useful. Endoscopy using a rigid endoscope is useful to identify subtle lesions (Capello et al. 2005a). Crown elongation, spikes, lacerations of tongue and oral mucosa, and missing teeth should be noted and recorded. The sulcus of each tooth should be examined with a periodontal probe to identify pathologic periodontal pockets. Even under general anesthesia, it is estimated that only 50% of pathology will be detected (Crossley 2000). In other words, disease is underestimated and oral examination under anesthesia needs to be complemented by imaging (radiography or CT scan, ultrasonography and MRI for abscesses).

Radiographic examination

Radiographs are mandatory to identify type and extent of pathology. Without such information, accurate diagnosis allowing appropriate treatment is not possible.

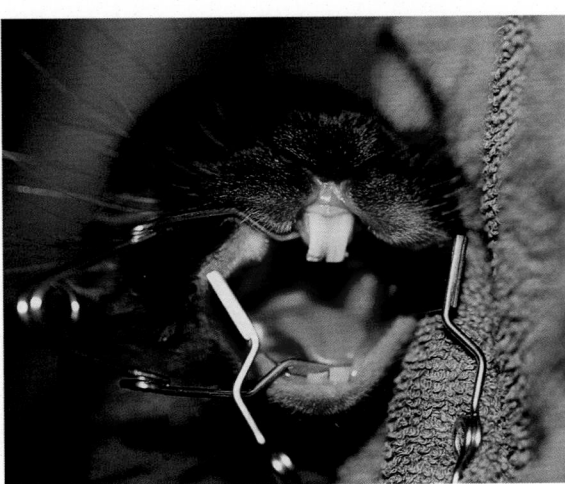

Fig. 14.3 **Access to the oral cavity** Cheek dilators can be used to open a rabbit's mouth. We rarely use mouth gags in rabbits. This method gives both good visibility and access. It can be used even when the incisor teeth have been extracted.

Box 14.3 **Checklists for inspection and palpation**

Inspection

- Salivation (wet chin, dirty forelimbs)
- Ocular discharge
- Nasal discharge
- Ocular protrusion
- Occlusion at rest (incisors should be in occlusion in rabbits, out of occlusion in rodents)
- Overgrown incisors, loss of chisel-shaped wear pattern, occlusal plane deviated from the perfectly horizontal plane
- Structure of the incisors: horizontal grooves, ribbing, discoloration.

Palpation

- Swelling, deformity of upper jaw and/or mandible
- Pain or discomfort on palpation
- Apply pressure on the eyes to identify potential retrobulbar abscessation.

Three basic skull views need to be taken, namely lateral, dorsoventral and rostrocaudal. Of these, the lateral view is usually the most informative. Additional oblique lateral views are necessary for most patients. When possible, additional intraoral views to avoid superimposition of adjacent structures are recommended. The techniques for intraoral radiography are outlined in Chapter 7. Detail is essential, so non-screen films are required.

Suggested exposure time for the rabbit, guinea pig and chinchilla is as follows:

- Standard radiography unit: 15 mA and 75 kV; 50 cm film–focus distance as a starting point.
- For rostrocaudal views, higher exposures will be needed.

Using a dental radiography unit, an exposure time comparable to that for radiography of the canine teeth in a medium to large breed dog (depending on the size of the animal) should be appropriate.

Further examination

Even with radiographic examination, a lot of the pathology will be missed. Radiographic interpretation by an experienced examiner will only reveal around 85% of the pathology present (Crossley 2000). CT-scan will give more information, especially for the detection of early cheek tooth pathology (Crossley et al. 1998; Van Caelenberg et al. 2010). Other examinations that may be indicated are ultrasonography (for retrobulbar abscesses) or MRI (for soft tissue lesions).

RABBITS

The healthy mouth

Incisor teeth

- The maxillary incisors have vertical grooves on the labial surfaces
- Held in occlusion at rest (with the crown tips of the mandibular incisors resting between the 1st and 2nd row of maxillary incisors)
- Occlusal plane is horizontal
- Have chisel-shaped wear pattern.

Cheek teeth

- The maxillary cheek teeth should be worn almost level with the gingiva
- The mandibular cheek teeth show only a few millimeters of crown (depending on the size of the rabbit)
- The occlusal plane is almost horizontal (10°)
- No spikes on any of the teeth.

Normal radiographic features

Lateral view (Fig. 14.4)

- The palatine shelf and the dorsal border of the mandible converge rostrally
- Ideally, with the incisors in occlusion, the cheek teeth should be out of occlusion. This is rarely seen in pet rabbits. As soon as both are in occlusion, there is some degree of cheek tooth overgrowth. However, as long as the maxilla and mandible converge rostrally, this is not a clinical problem
- Smooth ventral mandibular border
- Normal radiolucencies of the periapical germinal tissues
- The apices of the maxillary incisor teeth should not penetrate the palatine shelf
- The apices of the maxillary incisor teethe are located halfway along the diastema
- The apices of the mandibular incisors are located level to, or just rostral of, the first mandibular cheek teeth.

Dorsoventral view

- Smooth bony contours, with only the facial tuberosity sticking out
- Orbits clear with smooth borders

Rostrocaudal view

- Occlusal plane: almost horizontal
- No spikes visible
- No tipping of teeth.

The dorsoventral view does not usually contribute much extra information in the rabbit and we often omit it.

Incisor overgrowth

Incisor overgrowth is common in rabbits. The condition can be classified as primary or secondary, depending on its cause. Primary incisor overgrowth occurs early in life (within the first year) and is the consequence of an inherited skeletal malocclusion (maxillary brachygnathism resulting in a relative mandibular prognathism). In contrast, secondary incisor overgrowth occurs later in life (adult, usually more than 1 year old) and is the consequence of cheek tooth overgrowth. Primary incisor overgrowth is over-diagnosed. Most rabbits presented for treatment of incisor overgrowth have developed the incisor overgrowth secondary to cheek tooth overgrowth.

Primary incisor overgrowth is seen in young animals. It occurs regularly in dwarf rabbits. Due to the jaw length discrepancy (i.e. the mandible is too long with respect to the maxilla), normal incisor occlusion is not established. The mandibular incisors occlude either level with or rostral to the large labial row of maxillary incisors. The result is that normal incisor wear does not occur. The

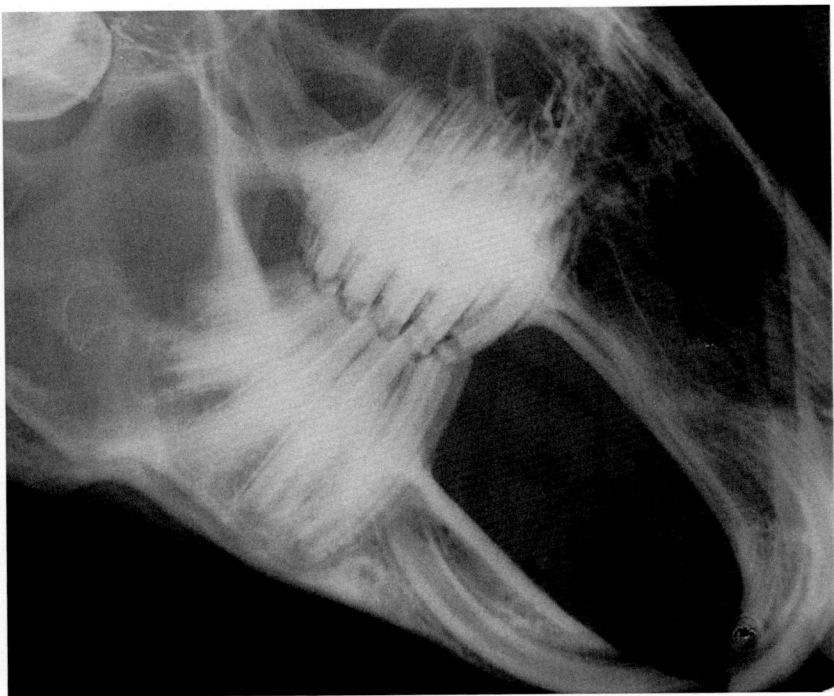

Fig. 14.4 Lateral radiograph of a normal rabbit Note that the palatine shelf and the dorsal border of the mandible converge rostrally.

upper incisors may curl inward (Fig. 14.5A) or flare out laterally (Fig. 14.5B), and the mandibular incisors protrude from the mouth. If eruption of the maxillary incisors is hindered, e.g. mechanical obstruction by abnormal occlusal forces, then tooth growth will occur in an apical direction and may result in perforation of the palatine shelf. When significant incisor malocclusion has developed, the animal cannot close its mouth normally and secondary cheek tooth overgrowth will develop over time. Radiographic features of primary incisor overgrowth are shown in Figure 14.6. If the condition is identified early, i.e. before excessive secondary cheek tooth overgrowth has occurred, the prognosis is relatively good with appropriate treatment.

The first step in treating incisor overgrowth, whether primary or secondary in origin, consists of correcting any *cheek tooth overgrowth*. Overgrown cheek teeth should be shortened to a normal level. Once that is done, two options exist for the incisor teeth. The teeth can be extracted, or they can be trimmed down every 3–5 weeks, as necessary. It is essential that feeding regimens that ensure adequate tooth wear be instituted. If the incisors are extracted, food needs to be cut into small pieces since the rabbit can no longer cut it itself.

Cheek tooth overgrowth

Cheek tooth abnormalities are very common in pet rabbits. As already mentioned, most rabbits presented for treatment of incisor tooth overgrowth have the incisor overgrowth secondarily to the cheek tooth overgrowth, i.e. the cheek tooth overgrowth is the primary cause. Although calcium and vitamin D deficiency may be involved in the etiology (Harcourt-Brown and Baker 2001), the primary cause of cheek tooth overgrowth is thought to be feeding diets that provide insufficient abrasion (Crossley 1995a; Redrobe 1997).

Early cheek tooth overgrowth is not obvious without examination under general anesthesia and radiography. The incisors may still be normally occluding and wearing. Consequently, animals with cheek tooth overgrowth are usually presented late in the disease process. In fact, it is often when the animal is unable to close its mouth and secondary incisor overgrowth and malocclusion has occurred that treatment is sought. The owners assume that the problem is isolated to the incisor teeth. Client communication and education is essential.

Late-stage disease is easy to diagnose. On conscious intraoral examination with an otoscope, the massive

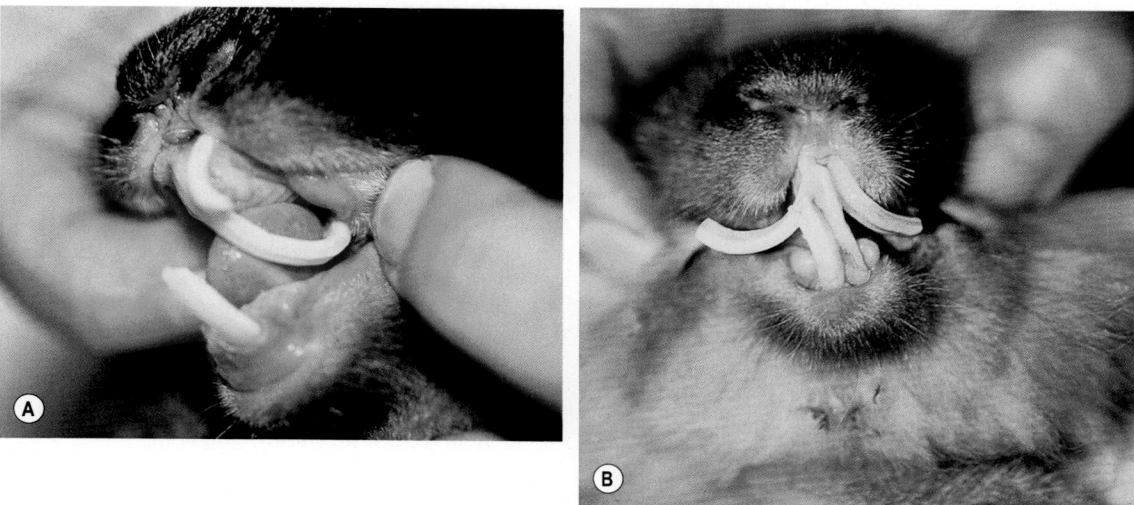

Fig. 14.5 Rabbit – incisor overgrowth (clinical presentation) (A) The upper incisors curl into the oral cavity. (B) The upper incisors flare out laterally.

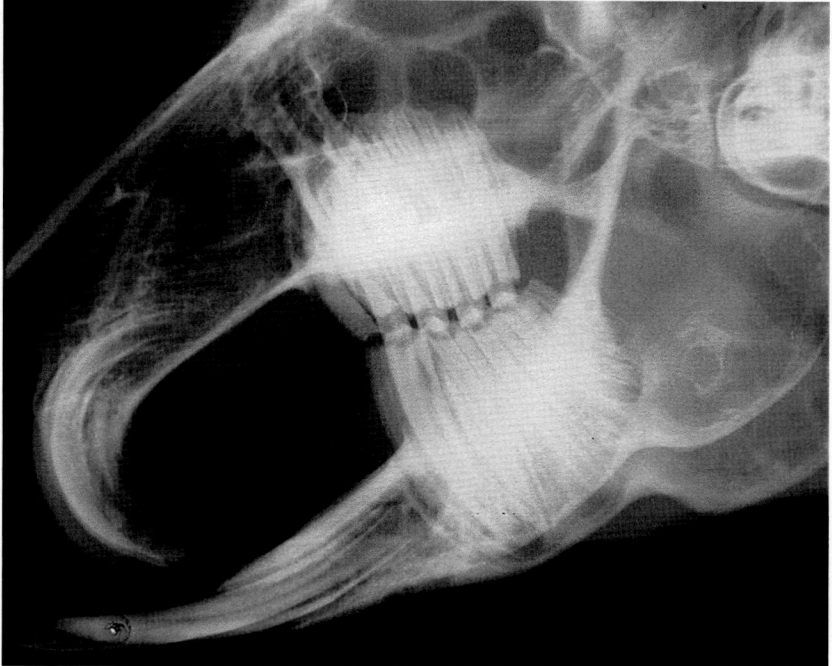

Fig. 14.6 Rabbit – primary incisor overgrowth (lateral radiograph) There is slight overgrowth of the cheek teeth, which causes the palatine shelf and dorsal border of the mandible to be parallel rather than converge rostrally.

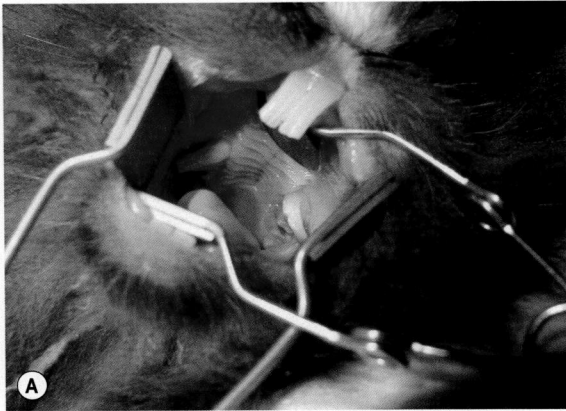

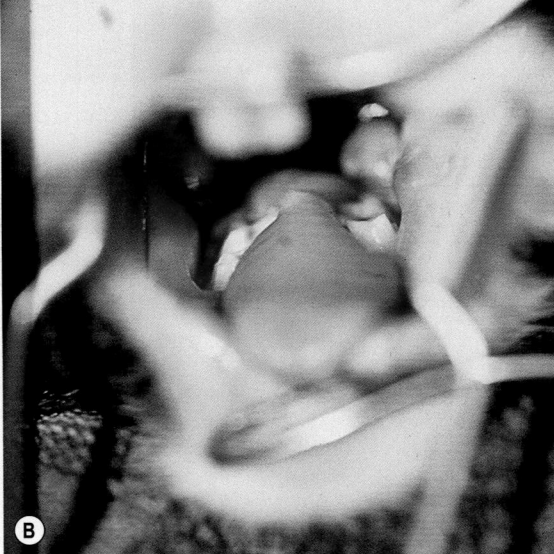

Fig. 14.7 Rabbit – cheek tooth overgrowth (clinical presentation) (A) The maxillary cheek teeth are flaring out buccally, traumatizing the soft tissues of the cheek. (B) The mandibular cheek teeth are developing lingual spikes, which may traumatize the tongue.

overgrowth of the cheek teeth is usually clearly visible. The upper cheek teeth flare out buccally (Fig. 14.7A), causing buccal ulceration and wounds. The lower cheek teeth show spikes on the lingual side (Fig. 14.7B), often associated with wounds on the tongue. The rabbit at this stage is unable to use the normal lateral chewing movements. It may be anorectic but if it is still eating, then it will only be able to consume soft fresh food or dry food, which does not need much chewing.

Figure 14.8 demonstrates many of the radiographic features of severe cheek tooth overgrowth (Box 14.4). The more abnormalities are found, the worse the prognosis.

Overgrowth of the cheek teeth may be complicated by abscess formation on one or more teeth, aggravating the disease and worsening prognosis considerably (Fig. 14.9).

Once the alveolar bone is perforated, the condition cannot be cured, but it may be controlled in some cases. Pain relief is of utmost importance when alveolar perforation is present. In many cases, the situation is really beyond treatment, and euthanasia is the only humane treatment (Figs 14.8, 14.9).

The treatment of cheek teeth overgrowth is to recreate as normal an occlusion as possible. The cheek teeth should be radically trimmed down. After treatment, the palatine shelf and the dorsal border of the mandible should again converge rostrally. The incisors should also be trimmed down, and a chisel-shaped occlusal plane should be created. Change of feeding regimen is extremely important to prevent or at least slow down further disease.

Facial abscess

The development of facial abscesses is common in rabbits. They are usually associated with diseased teeth (Fig. 14.9), but may also occur due to mucosal perforation by overgrown teeth (dental spikes), foreign bodies (e.g. straw), or due to external wounds. While abscesses caused by mucosal trauma from overgrown teeth, foreign bodies or external wounds are easy to treat, the abscesses arising due to dental pathology are more difficult to manage.

'Dental' abscesses can be of endodontic origin (pulpal disease) or periodontic origin. In the latter, foreign material (food) that is impacted into the periodontal ligament causes destruction of the periodontium, which may be so extensive that the endodontic system becomes involved secondarily. The lesions are often large at the time of diagnosis and the prognosis for complete cure is usually poor. In fact, euthanasia is often indicated.

The abscesses present clinically as enlargement of the jawbones. The cheek teeth are usually the teeth affected, but abscessation associated with incisors also occurs. In the latter case, the common practice of clipping overgrown incisors with nail cutters is often implicated. The use of nail cutters exposes the pulp and often results in longitudinal fractures that extend subgingivally. The resultant pulpal pathology may lead to the formation of a periapical abscess. Due to the position of the incisor root apices, an abscess associated with a diseased incisor tooth can be difficult to distinguish from one associated with a diseased cheek tooth. Radiographs are mandatory to identify the tooth involved and assess the precise location and extent of the destructive process.

Successful treatment relies on identifying and removing the cause, i.e. the diseased tooth, in combination with surgical removal of the actual abscess. In the case of retrobulbar abscesses eye enucleation is often also indicated. Tooth removal is difficult. Often teeth that are not actually

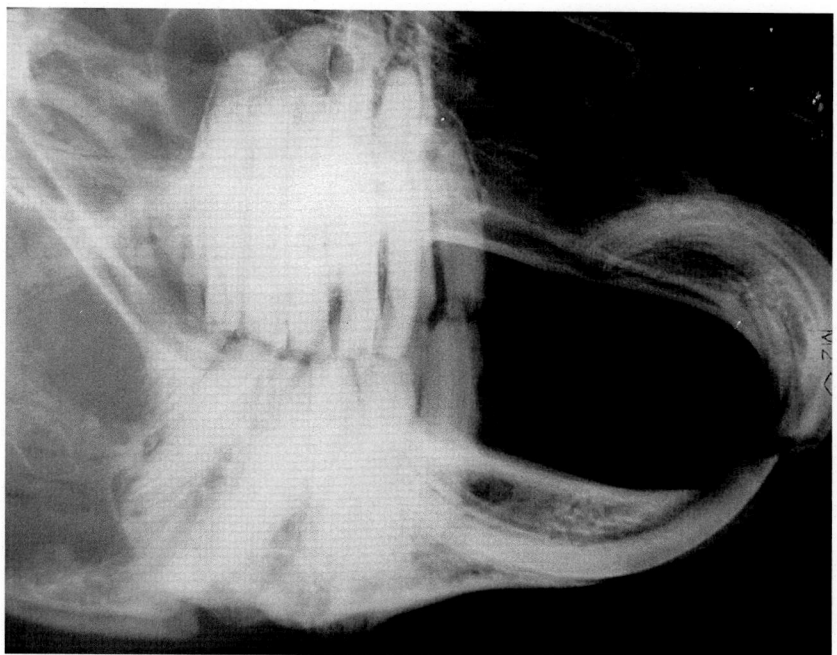

Fig. 14.8 Rabbit – severe cheek tooth overgrowth (lateral radiograph) This rabbit has severe cheek tooth overgrowth. The palatine shelf and dorsal border of the mandible are parallel. The roots of the cheek teeth are grossly deformed. The ventral border of the mandible has been perforated. There is secondary incisor overgrowth and malocclusion (level bite). The palatine shelf has almost been perforated. Once the alveolar bone is perforated, the condition cannot be cured. With appropriate management, it can be controlled in some cases. Euthanasia should be considered, and may be the most humane option, for an animal with this severity of disease.

Box 14.4 Cheek tooth overgrowth: Points to look at on lateral radiographs

- Incisor tooth position and length
- Periapical region of the incisor teeth
- The palatine shelf and dorsal border of the mandible may still converge rostrally, but are often either parallel or diverging rostrally
- Cheek tooth occlusion: straight line or extremely zigzag ('step-mouth', wave mouth)
- Cheek teeth may show resorption, curving, extensive periapical lucencies
- Thinning of the ventral border of the mandible
- Perforation of the ventral border of the mandible.

---

themselves diseased but have been secondarily involved in the destructive process also need to be removed. Moreover, complete surgical removal of the abscess may not be technically possible. The adjunctive use of systemic antibiotics may be useful and the choice of antibiotic agent should be based on culture and sensitivity results. The culture should be from the abscess wall, i.e. not from the pus; anaerobes often play a major role. The prudent use of antibiotics in lagomorphs is covered in other texts.

Many options for cure/control have been described. The options include local application of antibiotics into the abscess wall (Brown and Rosenthal 1997b), inserting a dextrose-soaked drain into the abscess cavity or packing the abscess cavity with calcium hydroxide (Remeeus and Verbeek 1995). Due to the poor success rate and in the case of calcium hydroxide excessive tissue necrosis, these options are mainly of historical interest and we do not recommend them.

Two commonly used techniques are outlined below.

1. After tooth extraction and surgical debridement of as much of the abscess as possible, the area is packed with antibiotic impregnated beads (Klaus and Bennett 1999; Bennett 2007b) and sutured closed. The beads are made of polymethylmethacrylate (Surgical Simplex P Radiopaque Bone Cement; Howmedica Inc, Rutherford, NJ). The antibiotic is mixed thoroughly with the copolymer powder prior to adding the liquid monomer, and while the mixture is still quite thin, it is placed within a syringe. The mixture is pressed out on a sterile drape

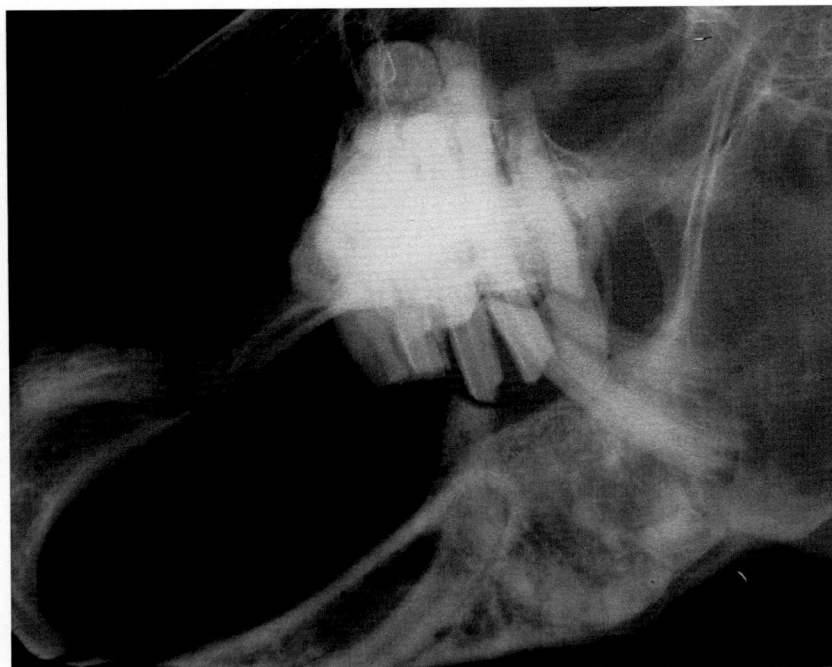

Fig. 14.9 Rabbit – severe tooth overgrowth and abscessation (lateral radiograph) This rabbit has extensive tooth overgrowth (cheek tooth and secondary incisor tooth). The palatine shelf and dorsal border of the mandible are parallel. The maxillary cheek teeth show gross root elongation with associated abscess formation. The upper incisors are almost penetrating the palatine shelf. Most of the roots of the mandibular cheek are resorbing. The lower incisors are also showing gross root elongation. Euthanasia may be the most humane option for this animal.

and cut into small pieces using a scalpel. The details of how to prepare the beads can be found in Klaus and Bennett (1999). There is no agreement as to whether the beads need to be removed or not, although in our experience they usually do need removal. Monitoring outcome of the treatment may help in deciding whether to leave or remove them.

2. After tooth extraction and aggressive surgical debridement of as much of the abscess as possible marsupialisation is used to keep the abscess cavity open as long as possible thus allowing continuous drainage (Capello et al. 2005b). An antimicrobial is applied locally (e.g. antibiotic or antiseptic ointment) and the wound is flushed daily, debridement may be needed at regular intervals.

Of these two options, the second one has the highest success rate. Systemic antibiotic treatment as an adjunct to surgical treatment may give better results especially if the abscess cannot be fully removed. A combination of benzathine penicillin and procaine penicillin used parenterally every 3–4 days is a valid option in rabbits. However, it has been reported that that this is a high risk antibiotic regimen for causing enterotoxemia (Harcourt-Brown

2002). Cultures from odontogenic abscesses have shown the bacteria to be predominantly periodontal and the more commonly used antibiotics such as enrofloxacin and potentiated sulphonamides are usually ineffective while penicillin has a much higher sensitivity (Tyrrell et al. 2002). Good intra- and postoperative analgesia is mandatory to prevent gastrointestinal stasis from stress. Animals should start eating as soon as possible and force feeding with commercial hand-feeding products (e.g. Oxbow Critical Care) may be indicated.

Other dental conditions

Periodontal disease, i.e. plaque-induced inflammation of the periodontium, is reportedly not as common in the rabbit as in the dog and cat (Wiggs and Lobprise 1995). However, periodontal disease does occur; it is probably under-diagnosed. The sulci of all teeth should be investigated with a periodontal probe. Treatment is similar to that for other species, i.e. professional cleaning and extraction of severely affected teeth. In the rabbit, loss of periodontal attachment is more often caused by food impaction triggering destruction of the periodontium rather than irritation from plaque accumulation (Redrobe

1997). Often the periodontal destruction is severe and spreads to involve the endodontic system, usually resulting in the formation of a periapical abscess. Once this complication has occurred, prognosis is poor and often warrants euthanasia of the affected animal. If treatment is attempted, it consists of tooth extraction and abscess management as detailed in the previous section.

Both caries and root resorption have been described in rabbits. When the lesions are small, they may wear away. Extensive lesions require extraction of the affected tooth or possibly restoration. The latter option requires referral to a specialist.

GUINEA PIGS

Guinea pigs are strictly herbivorous rodents, and have aradicular hypsodont cheek teeth.

The healthy mouth

- Incisor enamel is white in color (in contrast to most other rodents)
- Incisors are worn down in a chisel-shaped pattern
- The occlusal plane of the incisors is horizontal
- At rest, the mandible is held in a caudal position and the incisor teeth are out of occlusion
- The mandible is wider than the maxilla
- The cheek teeth tip (the maxillary teeth buccally and the mandibular teeth lingually)
- The occlusal plane of the cheek teeth has a 30° angle (Fig. 14.10)

- The palatine shelf and dorsal border of the mandible converge rostrally
- The crowns of the cheek teeth are almost level with the gingiva.

Incisor overgrowth

Primary incisor overgrowth is considered rare. When incisor overgrowth occurs, it is usually secondary to cheek tooth overgrowth. It may also be secondary to facial trauma.

Cheek tooth overgrowth

Most pet guinea pigs have some degree of cheek tooth overgrowth, and in many, it will cause severe problems at some stage in life. The problems include:

- Tongue entrapment by the mandibular cheek teeth (Fig. 14.11)
- Lacerations of the buccal mucosa by dental spikes on the overgrown maxillary teeth
- Overgrowth, abnormal wear patterns and malocclusion of the incisor teeth (Fig. 14.12)
- Apical overgrowth of the cheek teeth with resultant perforation of the alveolar bone.

The radiographic features of cheek tooth overgrowth in guinea pigs are shown in Figure 14.13. In guinea pigs, the rostrocaudal view provides valuable information.

There is an association between cheek tooth overgrowth and hypovitaminosis C (Klaus and Bennett 1999; Brown and Rosenthal 1997a). The condition is often exacerbated by a vitamin C deficiency, which leads to collagen defects and resultant tipping of the teeth and/or eruption

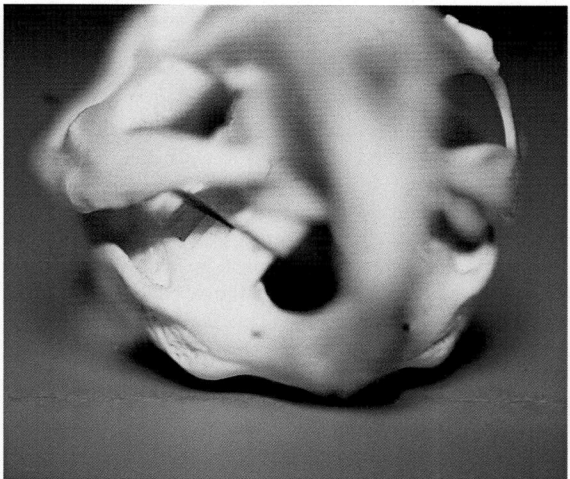

Fig. 14.10 Normal guinea pig skull The occlusal plane of the cheek teeth has a 30° angle.

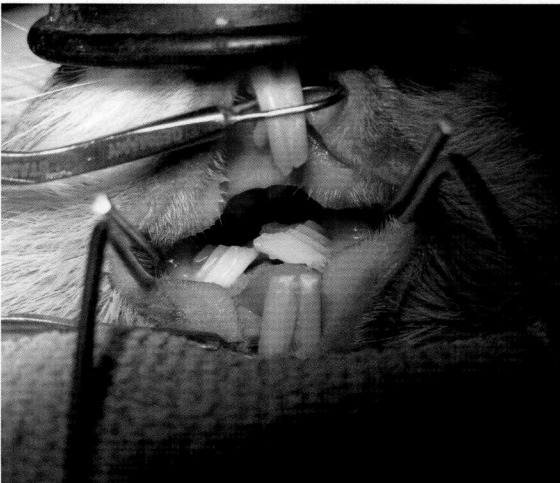

Fig. 14.11 Guinea pig – severe cheek tooth overgrowth (clinical presentation) The tongue is trapped by the mandibular cheek teeth.

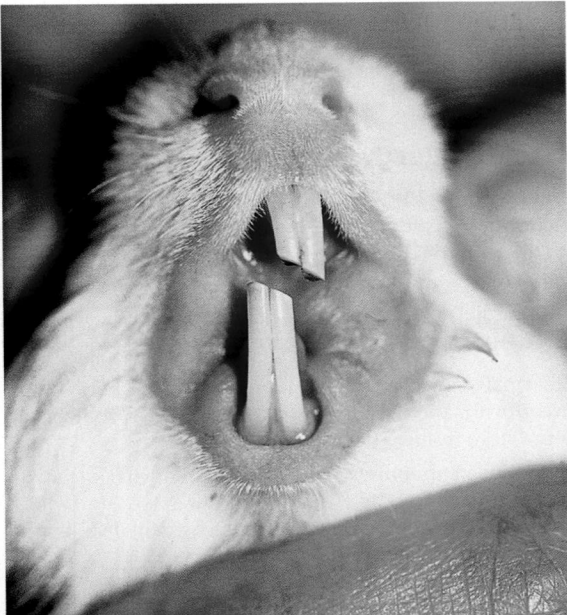

Fig. 14.12 Guinea pig – uneven wear of the incisor teeth (clinical presentation) The uneven wear of the incisor teeth was caused by overgrowth of the cheek teeth.

problems since collagen is necessary for anchoring the tooth in the socket (Schaeffer and Donnelly 1997; Brown and Rosenthal 1997a). A 'full body check' is mandatory in guinea pigs with dental disease. Dental problems are often secondary to disease in other organ systems, e.g. urolithiasis, ovarian cysts or gastrointestinal problems. The animals are usually presented when pathology is advanced and prognosis is usually poor. Restoring normal occlusion should be attempted. The maxillary cheek teeth should be trimmed almost level with the gingiva. They should be trimmed at a 30° angle, so that the crowns are shortest on the buccal side. The mandibular cheek teeth should also be trimmed at a 30° angle, this time shortest on the lingual side. The mandibular teeth should be trimmed so short that they do not entrap the tongue, i.e. almost level with the gingiva. The lingual tip of each tooth should barely touch the tongue. All dental spikes need to be identified and removed.

It is essential to check husbandry and ensure that the animal receives a sufficiently abrasive diet. Supplementation with vitamin C is generally beneficial.

CHINCHILLAS

Chinchillas are herbivorous rodents, with aradicular hypsodont teeth. Dental disease is extremely common in this species; one report mentions 35% of apparently healthy chinchillas showing cheek tooth elongation on examination (Crossley 2001a).

The healthy mouth

- Incisor enamel is orange-yellow in color
- Incisors are worn down in a chisel-shaped pattern
- The occlusal plane of the incisors is horizontal
- At rest, the mandible is held in a caudal position, and the incisor teeth are out of occlusion
- The mandible is wider than the maxilla
- The cheek teeth are upright in position, i.e. do not tilt as in guinea pigs
- The cheek teeth have a horizontal occlusal plane
- The palatine shelf and dorsal border of the mandible converge rostrally
- The crowns of the cheek teeth are almost level with the gingiva.

The radiographic features of a chinchilla with normal dentition and occlusion are depicted in Figure 14.14.

Incisor overgrowth

Primary incisor overgrowth is extremely rare. In a large survey (more than 700 animals were examined) investigating the incidence of dental disease in this species, only one animal with incisor overgrowth due to a maxillary brachygnathism was identified (Crossley 2001a). In contrast, secondary incisor overgrowth is common.

Cheek tooth overgrowth

Most pet chinchillas have some degree of cheek tooth elongation. They seem to cope well with simple elongation as long as no sharp spikes are formed on the occlusal surfaces, and as long as the process is not complicated by periodontal disease (Crossley 2001a).

Due to the upright position of the cheek teeth, even slight overgrowth of the visible crown will result in occlusal forces that exceed eruptive forces. The visible crown will stop erupting. Instead, continued tooth growth will proceed in an apical direction (retrograde eruption) and result in apparent 'root' elongation. In the mandible, swellings associated with the apical growth of the cheek teeth are readily palpated along the ventrolateral border even with minor overgrowth. This is a major difference between chinchillas and guinea pigs. Palpable swellings of the ventral mandibular border indicate early cheek tooth overgrowth in chinchillas. In guinea pigs, this clinical finding is evidence of advanced disease.

As cheek tooth overgrowth progresses, dramatic changes in the structure of the upper jaw and mandible occur (Figs 14.15, 14.16). In the upper jaw, the root elongation may present clinically as lachrymal overflow and/or eye

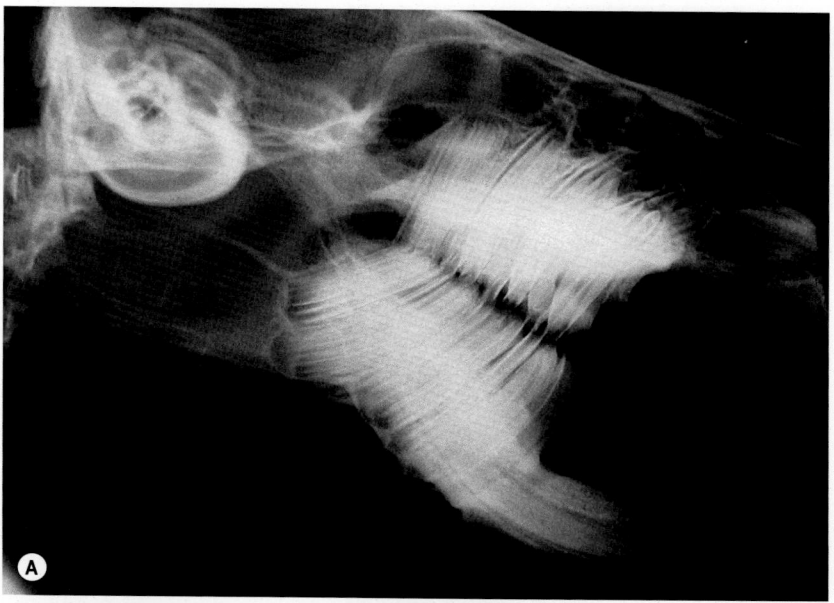

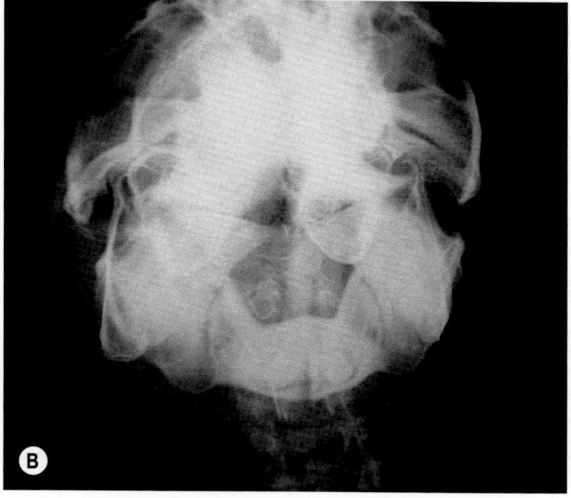

Fig. 14.13 Guinea pig – cheek tooth overgrowth (radiographic features) (A) Lateral view. The massive overgrowth of the cheek teeth is forcing the mouth open and the mandible is pushed rostrally. (B) Rostrocaudal view. This view is extremely helpful in guinea pigs. It allows visualization of dental spikes and shows the tipping of the teeth. Note also the good image of the TMJ obtained with this view.

protrusion. In the mandible, the cortical bone may be destroyed during the root elongation, resulting in perforation. Since apical growth of the teeth occurs as an early response to overgrowth, pathology is usually advanced before there is obvious elongation of the visible crowns on intraoral clinical inspection.

Radiographic features of cheek tooth overgrowth include:

- Occlusal irregularities
- Apparent root elongation
- Overgrowth of the clinical crowns
- Secondary incisor crown elongation.

Treatment consists of radical shortening of the cheek teeth, i.e. level with the gingival margin. Due to the insidious nature of cheek teeth overgrowth, many chinchillas are only presented for treatment when the pathology is

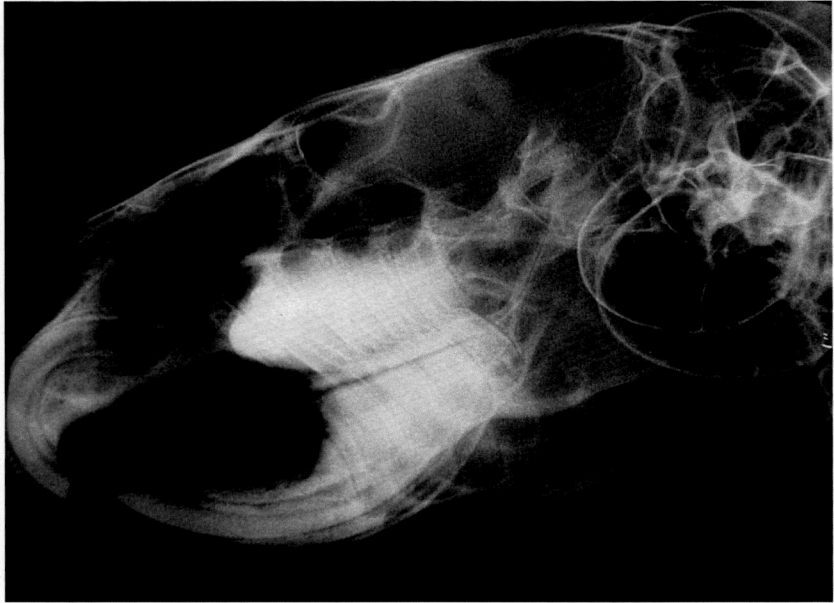

Fig. 14.14 Chinchilla – clinically healthy (radiographic features) Cheek teeth with short crowns and roots, smooth occlusal plane.

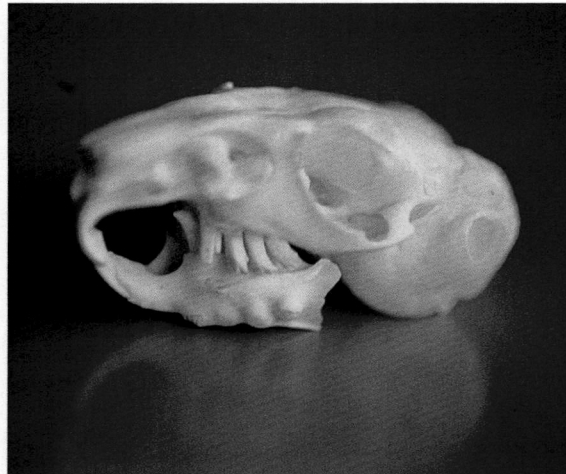

Fig. 14.15 Chinchilla skull – severe tooth overgrowth This is a very advanced case.

extensive and irreversible. In these animals, euthanasia is the only option (Crossley 2001a).

Other dental conditions

Loss of periodontal attachment is more often caused by food impaction triggering destruction of the periodontium rather than irritation from plaque accumulation.

Both caries and root resorption have been described in chinchillas (Crossley 2001a; Crossley et al. 1997). Starch and sugar are a significant proportion of the pet chinchilla's diet, and the diet is less abrasive than the diet in the wild. Therefore, incipient occlusal caries will not be worn down, as it would be in the wild animal.

PRAIRIE DOGS

Prairie Dogs belong to the squirrel-type rodent group. The two most common dental diseases in captive prairie dogs are periodontal disease of the brachyodont cheek teeth and so-called pseudo-odontoma of the incisor teeth (Fig. 14.17). The so-called pseudo-odontoma is a mass of dysplastic dental tissue, probably caused by abnormal pressure on the germinal tissues of the incisor teeth from repeated trauma, e.g. biting on cage bars, fractures, improper tooth trimming (Bennett 2007a; Capello 2011). Ultimately, this leads to severe apical dysplasia at the incisor teeth and tooth eruption ceases. In the maxilla, it presents as a calcified space-occupying mass obstructing the nasal cavity leading to respiratory problems. Intraorally the lesion can be seen as a protuberant mass on the hard palate. In the mandible, the incisors show intrusive growth of deformed, folded tooth structure further distal to the last molar than in the non-affected animal. The best treatment option consists of surgical extraction of the

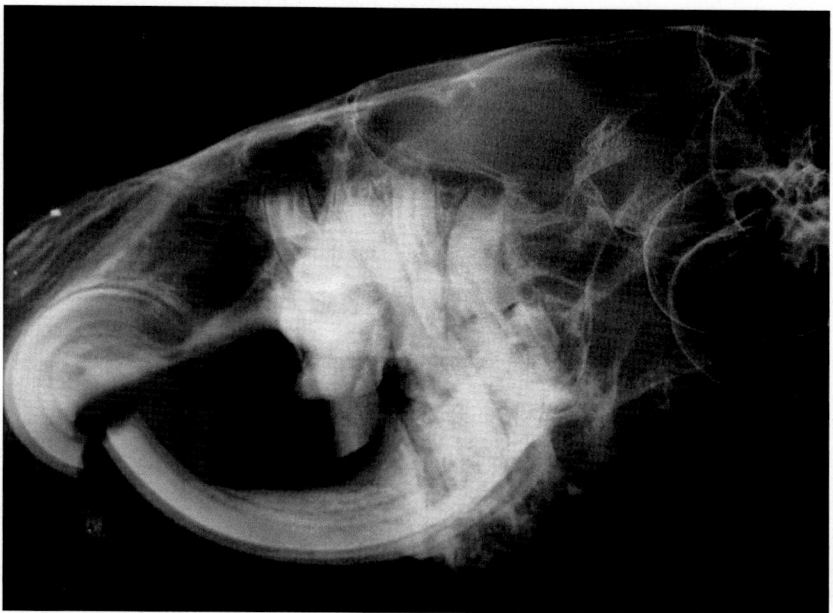

Fig. 14.16 Chinchilla – advanced cheek tooth pathology (lateral radiograph) Advanced cheek tooth problems. Root and crown elongation 'wavy' occlusal plane. Radical coronal reduction of the cheek teeth and change of feeding regimen resulted in clinical cure and weight gain. The same animal was represented 2 years later for recent weight loss because of dental disease that did not respond to treatment and he was euthanized.

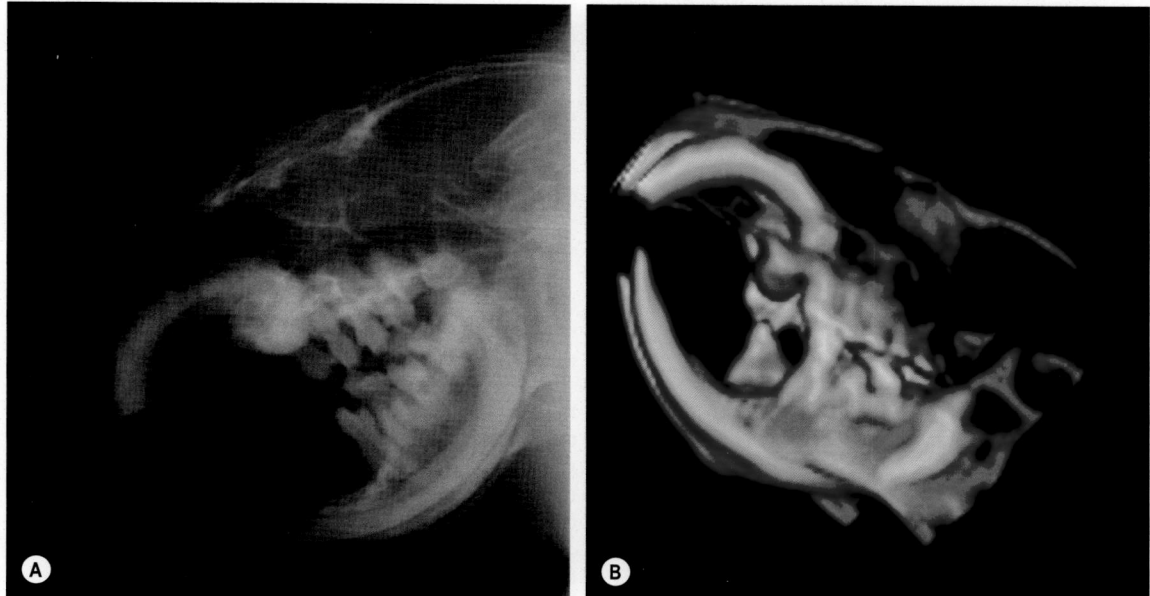

Fig. 14.17 Prairie Dog: Pseudo-odontoma (A) Lateral radiograph: The reserve crown of the upper incisors is severely irregular and folded. At the 'apical' part a large mass of dysplastic dental tissue can be seen that blocks the nasal cavity and deforms the palate. The mandibular incisors also show features of dysplasia particularly at the apical part, and show intrusive growth into the mandible. (B) 3D CT reconstruction. Disfigurement of the palate can be seen at the site of the pseudo-odontoma. Also note the bone expansion in the mandible due to intrusive growth of the lower incisors. (Courtesy of the CT-MR Unit, Department of Medical Imaging and Small Animal Orthopaedics, Ghent University, Belgium.)

incisors, though this is very complex and challenging surgery. Rhinostomy tubes placed distal to the mass to facilitate breathing in affected animals have also been used, but we consider this as a less humane treatment option, since nothing is done with the distorted teeth and the pressure they cause within the bone. In advanced cases, euthanasia may be the only humane treatment option.

RATS, MICE, HAMSTERS, AND GERBILS

Rats, mice, hamsters, and gerbils have brachyodont cheek teeth, sparing them from the severe malocclusion problems seen in guinea pigs and chinchillas.

Incisor overgrowth (Fig. 14.18) in these species is usually caused by lack of gnawing. They are usually fed a diet that requires minimal gnawing. Successful treatment

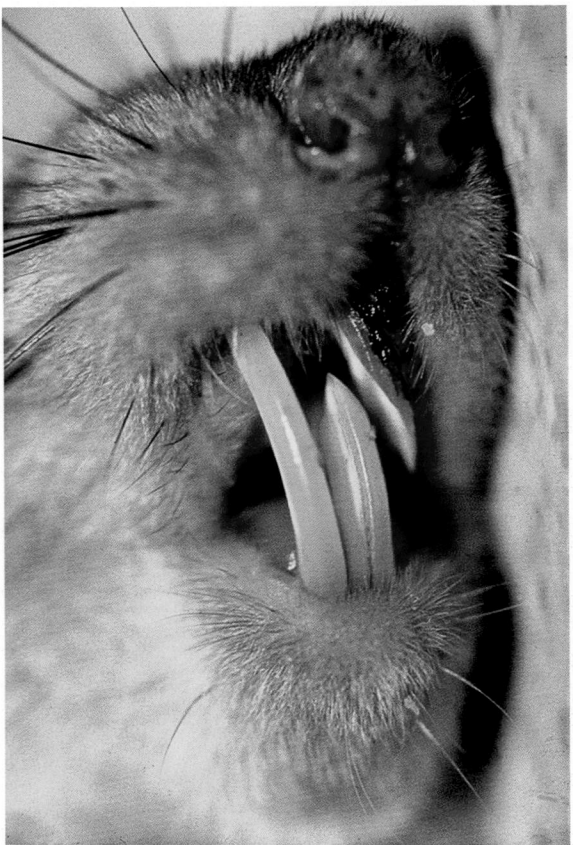

Fig. 14.18 Rat – incisor overgrowth (clinical presentation) Incisor overgrowth caused by lack of wear. One of the upper incisors is fractured due to excessive overgrowth.

is a combination of changing the diet and professional trimming of the teeth. These animals need to be presented with material to gnaw on, e.g. twigs of nontoxic trees such as fruit trees for the smaller species and whole nuts in the shell for the larger species.

Information in literature regarding susceptibility of these species to plaque-induced periodontal disease is conflicting. While some authors report it to be relatively uncommon (Wiggs and Lobprise 1995), others report it to be common in laboratory maintained animals (Miles and Crigson 1990). In our experience, periodontal disease is common in pet rodents. This will ultimately result in exfoliation of the affected tooth. Treatment is the same as in the dog and cat, namely professional periodontal therapy consisting of supra- and subgingival scaling, polishing, and extraction of severely affected teeth.

TRAUMATIC TOOTH INJURIES

The most common cause of 'traumatic tooth injuries' is probably the use of nail cutters (clippers) to shorten overgrown incisors. Apart from being an unpleasant procedure for the pet, the nail cutters shatter the tooth. The fracture may extend below the gingival margin and the pulp is often exposed. The resultant pulpal inflammation may be so severe that periapical abscessation develops and extensive treatment is required. *Nail cutters should not be used (either by the owner or the veterinarian) to shorten overgrown incisors.*

While the most common cause of tooth injuries may be iatrogenic, all the pocket pets are prone to traumatic injuries. They are often kept for small children who do not handle them as carefully as one might like. In fact, accidentally dropping to the floor is common. This type of trauma often results in tooth fracture (usually incisors), sometimes accompanied by jaw fracture.

Uncomplicated crown fracture (i.e. the pulp is not exposed to the external environment) requires no other treatment than smoothing of any sharp edges. Complicated crown fracture (i.e. the pulp is exposed) requires covering the exposed pulp with hard-setting calcium hydroxide cement (e.g. Dycal) and a layer of intermediate temporary restorative material. These patients are best referred to a specialist. The opposing tooth or teeth need to be trimmed regularly to compensate for the lack of wear until the fractured tooth is back in occlusion. In some cases, the trauma causes injury to the periapical germinal tissue. The injured tooth may cease to grow or may grow in the wrong direction. The tooth may also become malformed. In such cases, extraction of the damaged tooth and its opponent is indicated. Another option is trimming at regular intervals (usually every 3–5 weeks). The latter is more stressful for owner and pet. It is also more expensive for the owner in the long term.

TOOTH TRIMMING

Tooth trimming is the most commonly indicated procedure in lagomorph and rodent dentistry. The aim is to recreate normal, or near normal, occlusion. It is thus essential to know the normal occlusal pattern for each of the species. Improved husbandry, i.e. feeding an appropriately abrasive diet, will then help maintain normal occlusion as normal wear occurs.

Tooth trimming is a difficult and time-consuming procedure. It should be performed under general anesthesia. While trimming incisors without general anesthesia is possible, it is impossible to check and trim cheek teeth. The whole occlusion needs evaluation. It is rare that just the incisors need shaping. In fact, it is more common that the cause of the problem rests with the cheek tooth occlusion.

Practice is required to master the art of tooth trimming. It can be hazardous even in experienced hands. The space available to work in is limited and one 'slip' can have fatal consequences, e.g. accidentally severing major blood vessels. Good lighting is crucial and precision instruments must be used. The soft tissues must be protected at all times.

Equipment and instrumentation requirements (Figs 14.19, 14.20) include:

- Good lighting
- Mouth gag
- Cheek dilator(s)
- Spatulas for protection of soft tissues
- Slow-speed straight hand piece
- High-speed hand piece
- Selection of slow-speed burs (HP fissure and acrylic burs of different sizes)
- Selection of high-speed burs (fissure and possibly pear-shaped, of different sizes).

Incisor teeth

Incisors are best trimmed using a fissure bur in a high-speed hand piece. In our experience, diamond discs are potentially hazardous (soft tissue injuries) to both the operator and the patient, and should not be used. Using a fissure bur in a slow-speed hand piece will also do the job, but it does take a bit longer. The lips and tongue should be protected to avoid soft tissue damage.

A high-speed unit generates large amounts of heat on the tooth. This can lead to thermal injuries of the tooth and associated structures. The golden rule is thus that a high-speed unit should never be used without water cooling of the bur. Moreover, if a bur is run dry at high speed, it will become blunt within seconds. Therefore, if a high-speed unit is used to trim the incisors, the water cooling should not be turned off. It has been suggested that if a 'waltz-rhythm' (1 second of bur contact with the tooth, followed by 2 seconds off the tooth allowing it to cool down) is used, then the water can be turned off. The

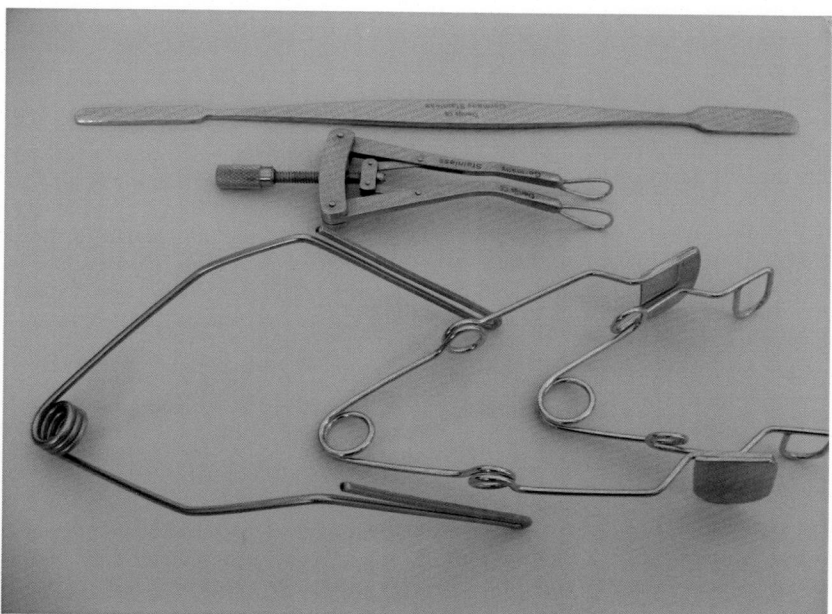

Fig. 14.19 Equipment 1 – gags and dilators From top to bottom: round-ended spatula; light model mouth gag; different types of cheek dilators.

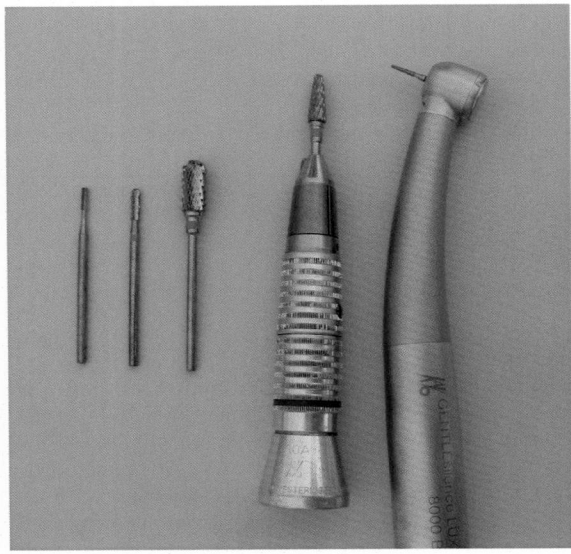

Fig. 14.20 Equipment 2 – burs and hand pieces From left to right: HP fissure bur; two types of HP acrylic bur; low-speed hand piece with acrylic bur; high-speed hand piece with FG fissure bur.

spatula is used to protect the tongue. Bur protectors are available. They lead to a false sense of security and have a sharp edge, which may injure the soft tissues if used without caution, especially when the mucosa is already ulcerated. We usually do not use them.

Overgrown cheek teeth need to be shortened radically – usually almost level with the gingiva. Moreover, the normal inclination of the occlusal surface should be recreated (almost horizontal in rabbits and chinchillas, 30° angle in guinea pigs). Recreating the normal occlusal inclination for the species is called 'occlusal equilibration'. A straight slow-speed hand piece is used. The choice of bur depends on the size of the animal and operator preference. Our preference is either an acrylic bur (stainless steel) or the HP cheek tooth bur (tungsten-carbide, 6 mm diameter). Moistening the teeth, e.g. wiping them with a wet cotton bud, facilitates smooth working of the bur. In addition, by wiping away enamel and dentine shavings, visualization is improved.

Laceration of soft tissues and consequent hemorrhage should be avoided. The tongue and the buccal mucosa distal to the last molar will bleed heavily if traumatized. It is easy to entrap the sublingual mucosa of a rabbit in the dental bur, and it is most difficult to stop the serious bleeding that results. Hemostasis can usually be achieved with continuous pressure. Suturing lacerated tissue is extremely difficult due to the lack of space in the long and narrow oral cavity.

After trimming, the mouth should be cleaned (to avoid inhalation of debris) and re-inspected.

EXTRACTION

Teeth affected by severe disease need extraction. In the pocket pets, there are rarely alternative treatments. Moreover, extraction may be preferable to trimming every few weeks.

The basic principles of extraction are similar to those used in other species. Extraction of teeth in dogs and cats is covered in Chapter 13.

Aradicular hypsodont incisor teeth

The most common indications for extraction of incisors are:

- Primary incisor overgrowth
- Periapical abscessation.

It is essential to evaluate the whole mouth and treat any cheek tooth disease. Preoperative lateral radiographs should be taken, to assess root structure and extent of pathology present.

Tooth extraction is a surgical procedure and should be performed in a clean mouth using sterile instruments.

evidence to show that this is safe is lacking. If this option were used, we would recommend keeping the teeth moist by dropping water over them intermittently.

For incisors that are in occlusion, the chisel-shaped wear pattern should be restored. In patients with primary incisor overgrowth (i.e. relative mandibular prognathism), the recreation of the normal wear pattern is not required since the teeth do not occlude anyway. Patients with primary incisor overgrowth will need regular trimming (usually every 3–5 weeks) for the duration of their life. Extracting the incisor teeth is probably the best treatment for these patients.

Pulp exposure is a common complication when trimming elongated incisor teeth. One study has shown that, while the tip of the pulp cavity in normal incisor teeth does not extend above the level of the interdental gingival papilla, it frequently extends supragingivally in elongated incisor teeth (Crossley 2001b). If the pulp is exposed, it needs to be covered with a hard-setting calcium hydroxide cement and an intermediate restorative material.

Cheek teeth

To access the cheek teeth, the mouth has to be opened wide and the cheeks held out of the way. The cheek dilators are often too short to keep the buccal mucosa safe from injury with the bur. We use a round-ended spatula between the cheek and the cheek dilator to keep the mucosa away even at the level of the last molar. A second

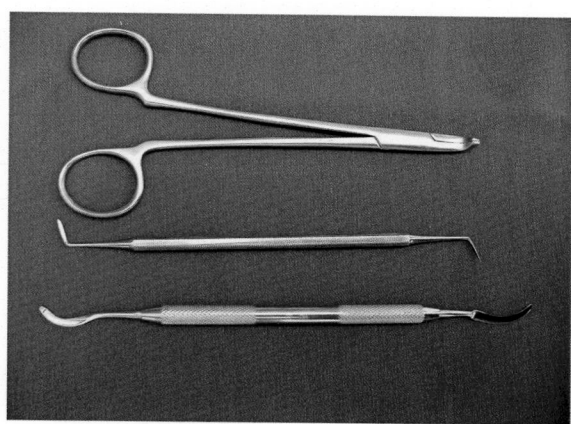

Fig. 14.21 Equipment 3 – extraction From top to bottom: molar extraction forceps; Crossley molar luxator; Crossley incisor luxator.

Specialized instrumentation is needed (Fig. 14.21), and with the increasing popularity of rabbits and rodents as pets, these instruments are now available (e.g. Crossley luxator). For very small animals, instruments may need to be custom-made by bending hypodermic needles of suitable size.

Extraction can be performed using a closed technique (i.e. without raising a gingival access flap) or using an open technique (i.e. raising a gingival flap for access to the alveolar bone). We use a closed technique in most instances. The procedure is as follows:

1. The gingival attachment is severed down to the level of the margin of the alveolar bone using a No. 11 scalpel blade in a handle, or with a sharp luxator.
2. The luxator is gently inserted into the periodontal space, alternatively on mesial and distal aspects of the tooth, holding tension by slight rotation for 10–20 s each time, stretching and tearing the periodontal ligament. The luxator is not used on the buccal and palatal/lingual tooth aspects as the strongest attachment is on the mesial and distal surfaces.
3. Alternate the luxator application between mesial and distal, working further apically each time, until the tooth feels loose in the alveolus. It is important to support the mandible while working; too much force can easily lead to mandibular fracture.
4. Once there is considerable mobility, longitudinal traction with extraction forceps can be applied until the tooth comes out.
5. The alveolus (especially the most apical portion) is thoroughly debrided with a spoon curette to destroy any germinal tissue at the apex, thus reducing the likelihood of the extracted tooth reforming. Even with complete removal of the tooth and curettage of the apical germinal tissue, an extracted tooth will occasionally regrow. The owner should be informed of this risk prior to the procedure.
6. The extraction socket may be left open to heal by granulation or the gingiva may be used to close the site and achieve primary healing. If the socket is sutured closed, ensure that there is no tension. We generally suture the gingiva across the alveolus. It helps control hemorrhage and keeps the coagulum in the socket.

We do not recommend inserting hemostatic packing materials into the extraction socket, as they may delay healing. While postoperative systemic antibiotics are generally not indicated, unless there was evidence of preoperative infection, good postoperative analgesia is mandatory.

If the tooth fractures during extraction, two basic options for management exist. The choice of method depends on the reason for the extraction. If the reason for extraction was infection, the root remnant must be removed to achieve healing. An open extraction technique is indicated as follows:

1. Raise a gingival flap to access the alveolar bone.
2. Remove alveolar bone (with a small round bur in either a high- or slow-speed hand piece).
3. Proceed with luxators as described in the previous section for closed extraction.
4. Debride the apical portion of the alveolus once the tooth has been removed.
5. Replace the gingival flap and suture the extraction socket closed.

If the reason for the extraction was not infection, e.g. elective extraction rather than frequent trimming, then the best option for management is to leave the root remnant in place and wait for a few weeks for the tooth to regrow. Once it has regrown, a second extraction procedure is performed.

Cheek teeth

Brachyodont

The pocket pets with brachyodont cheek teeth are spared the pathology associated with overgrowth of teeth. In our experience, the most common indication for tooth extraction is plaque-induced periodontal disease.

Extraction techniques for the brachyodont teeth of dogs and cats are covered in Chapter 13. The same techniques are used for rats, mice, gerbils and hamsters. The instruments need to be small. Hypodermic needles can be used as elevators. Due to the limited space, only mobile teeth are easy to remove.

Aradicular hypsodont

The most common indication for extraction of cheek teeth is that they are affected by endodontic or periodontic disease resulting in periapical abscessation. These teeth are difficult to extract. They have long submerged crowns and root elongation or deformity often further complicates extraction. Cheek teeth can be extracted using either an intraoral or extraoral approach, or a combination of both.

An intraoral approach is indicated when a tooth has lost a significant portion of its periodontal support and is mobile. The instruments used need to be thin, angled and sharp. A selection is available on the market. Bent hypodermic needles can also be used as elevators. The technique is a closed extraction. The elevator is inserted into the periodontal ligament space and worked around the whole circumference of the tooth until it loosens. Sometimes there is insufficient space to remove the long tooth in one piece. The crown can then be cut transversely into pieces as it is removed out of the alveolus.

If the tooth is not mobile, either an extraoral approach or a combination of extra- and intraoral access is usually required. Referral to a specialist is recommended. Although buccotomy incision facilitates extraction, it is associated with major disadvantages, e.g. significant risk of severe hemorrhage, complicated healing. We do not recommend the approach via buccotomy incision, unless there is a lesion (usually an abscess) that requires surgery at this site. Mandibular teeth can be extracted using a surgical extraoral approach from the ventrolateral aspect of the mandible, and repulsed into the mouth or extracted via the surgical incision.

Once a cheek tooth has been extracted, the patient will require long-term monitoring and regular trimming of the opposing teeth, as these will not wear down appropriately.

SUMMARY

◆ Dental problems in lagomorphs and rodents are very common.

◆ Most conditions are associated with incorrect husbandry and diet, and these issues must be addressed as part of the treatment.

◆ These species are often presented late in the disease process, with consequent poorer prognosis.

◆ Thorough intraoral examination requires general anesthesia and radiography. Even under optimal conditions, some pathology may be missed.

◆ Rabbits, guinea pigs, chinchillas, and degus with incisor overgrowth usually have a primary problem affecting the cheek teeth. Primary incisor overgrowth is considered rare except in young rabbits (less than 1 year of age).

◆ In guinea pigs, the problem is exacerbated by vitamin C deficiency. In chinchillas, it may be detected early by palpation of swellings on the ventral border of the mandible.

◆ Rats, mice and hamsters with incisor overgrowth are not being given suitable food or substrate materials for gnawing.

◆ Nail cutters are contraindicated for incisor shortening. As the problem is usually related to cheek teeth overgrowth, general anesthesia is indicated.

◆ Suitable equipment and instruments are needed for safe and effective tooth trimming in pocket pets.

◆ Closed extraction of incisors is the usual procedure, but extraction of the cheek teeth can be problematical and referral should be considered.

REFERENCES

Bennett, R.A., 2007a. Odontomas in Prairie Dogs. Small Animal and Exotics. Proceedings of the North American Veterinary Conference, Orlando, USA, pp. 1628–1629.

Bennett, R.A., 2007b. Rabbit abscesses and PMMA beads: the do's and don'ts. Small Animal and Exotics. Proceedings of the North American Veterinary Conference, Orlando, USA, pp. 1612–1615.

Brown, S.A., Rosenthal, K.L., 1997a. Self Assessment Colour Review of Small Mammals. Manson, London, pp. 77–78.

Brown, S.A., Rosenthal, K.L., 1997b. Self Assessment Colour Review of Small Mammals. Manson, London, pp. 63–74.

Capello, V., Gracis, M., Lennox A., 2005a. Endoscopy. In: Rabbit and Rodent Dentistry Handbook. Zoological Education Network Inc, Lake Worth, pp. 101–107.

Capello, V., Gracis, M., Lennox A., 2005b. Surgical treatment of periapical abscessation. In: Rabbit and Rodent Dentistry Handbook. Zoological Education Network Inc, Lake Worth, pp. 249–273.

Capello, V., 2011. We are not smaller rabbits, either. Dentistry of other rodent species and ferrets. Small Animal and Exotics. Proceedings of the North American Veterinary Conference, Orlando, USA, pp. 1681–1684

Crossley, D.A., 1995a. Clinical aspects of lagomorph dental anatomy: the rabbit (Oryctolagus cuniculus). Journal of Veterinary Dentistry 12(4), 137–142.

Crossley, D.A., 1995b. Clinical aspects of rodent dental anatomy. Journal of Veterinary Dentistry 12(4), 131–135.

Crossley, D.A., 2000. Rodent and rabbit radiology. In: DeForge, D.H., Colmery, B.H., III (Eds.), An Atlas of Veterinary Dental Radiology. Iowa State University Press, Ames, pp. 247–259.

Crossley, D.A., 2001a. Dental disease in chinchillas in the UK. Journal of Small Animal Practice 42(1), 12–19.

Crossley, D.A., 2001b. The risk of pulp exposure when trimming rabbit incisor teeth. Proceedings of the 10th European Veterinary Dental Society Annual Congress, Berlin, Germany.

Crossley, D.A., Dubielzig, R.R., Benson, K.G., 1997. Caries and odontoclastic resorptive lesions in a chinchilla (Chinchilla laniger). Veterinary Record 141(27), 337–339.

Crossley, D.A., Jackson, A., Yates, J., et al., 1998. Use of computed tomography to investigate cheek tooth abnormalities in chinchillas (Chinchilla laniger). Journal of Small Animal Practice 39(8), 385–389.

Flecknell, P.A., 1991. Guinea pigs. In: Beynon, P.H., Cooper, J.E. (Eds.), Manual of Exotic Pets. BSAVA, Cheltenham, pp. 52.

Harcourt-Brown, F.M., Baker, S.J., 2001. Parathyroid hormone, haematological and biochemical parameters in relation to dental disease and husbandry in rabbits. Journal of Small Animal Practice 42(3), 130–136.

Harcourt-Brown, F.M., 2002. Therapeutics. In: Textbook of Rabbit Medicine. Elsevier Science, Oxford, pp. 94–120

Klaus, P., Bennett, R.A., 1999. Management of abscesses of the head in rabbits. Proceedings of the North American Veterinary Conference, Orlando, USA.

Miles, A.E.W., Crigson, C., 1990. Colyer's Variations and Diseases of the Teeth of Animals, revised edn. Cambridge University Press, Cambridge, pp. 567–569.

Redrobe, S., 1997. Surgical procedures and dental disorders. In: Flecknell, P. (Ed.), Manual of Rabbit Medicine and Surgery. BSAVA, Cheltenham, pp. 129–133.

Remeeus, P.G.K., Verbeek, M., 1995. The use of calcium-hydroxide in the treatment of abscesses in the cheek of the rabbit resulting from a dental periapical disorder. Journal of Veterinary Dentistry 12(1), 19–22.

Schaeffer, D.O., Donnelly, T.M., 1997. Disease problems in guinea pigs and chinchillas. In: Hillyer, E.V., Quesenberry, K.E. (Eds.), Ferrets, Rabbits and Rodents: Clinical Medicine and Surgery. WB Saunders, Philadelphia, pp. 260–281.

Tyrrell, K.L., Citron, D.M., Jenkins, J.R., et al.; Veterinary Study Group, 2002. Periodontal bacteria in rabbit mandibular and maxillary abscesses. Journal of Clinical Microbiology 40(3), 1044–1047.

Van Caelenberg, A., De Rycke, L., Hermans, K., et al., 2010. Comparison of radiography and CT to identify changes in the skulls of four rabbits with dental disease. Journal of Veterinary Dentistry 28(3), 172–181.

Wiggs, B., Lobprise, H., 1995. Dental anatomy and physiology of pet rodents and lagomorphs. In: Crossley, D.A., Penman, S. (Eds.), Manual of Small Animal Dentistry. BSAVA, Cheltenham, Ch. 7, pp. 68–73.

Appendix

ENDODONTICS

This appendix is included for completeness. However, I do not recommend that these procedures are undertaken by the general practitioner for the following reasons:

- A substantial investment in specialist equipment is needed
- The procedures require expertise and experience to be successfully completed
- The procedures are time-consuming unless practiced regularly
- The likelihood of success in inexperienced hands is not good
- The consequences of an unsuccessful procedure are painful and potentially serious to the animal and will result in the need for further treatment.

Should there be an interest by a general practitioner in performing endodontics, then a practically based training course must be attended prior to undertaking any endodontic procedure on a patient.

Endodontics is the treatment of the pulp of the tooth (*endo*: inside; *-dontic*: tooth).

There are three pulpal treatments, each of which has specific indications. They are:

1. Pulp capping
2. Partial pulpectomy with direct pulp capping
3. Root canal therapy.

Conventional root canal therapy is the most commonly indicated type of endodontic treatment. It involves total removal of pulp tissue, i.e. total pulpectomy, cleaning and filling of the root canal, followed by tooth restoration.

Root canal therapy is indicated when there is, or may be, irreversible pulp pathology (e.g. generalized pulpitis or pulp necrosis, often in combination with periapical involvement) in the mature permanent tooth. Immature permanent teeth are a special consideration and are dealt with separately.

The objectives of conventional root canal therapy are:

- To clean and disinfect the pulp chamber and root canal(s)
- To fill the root canal(s) with a non-irritant, antibacterial material, thus sealing the apex
- To close the access and exposure sites with a suitable restorative material.

Many different methods are employed in the preparation and filling of root canals. In simple terms, root canal therapy involves removing the pulp, replacing it with an inert material and restoring the tooth. The inflamed or dead pulp is removed using special files. Once the pulp has been removed, the root canal is cleaned, both mechanically with files but also chemically with a disinfectant. The clean and disinfected root canal is then filled with inert material and the crown is restored with a suitable restorative material. The tooth is not restored to its original shape and size as the biting forces in dogs are much greater than those in humans and the restoration would be likely to fail if this was attempted.

The whole procedure is performed under general anesthesia and under strict radiographic control. It is time-consuming, as each step needs to be performed with meticulous detail to ensure successful outcome.

The outcome of conventional root canal therapy should be monitored radiographically for 6–12 months postoperatively. This will also require general anesthesia. Evidence of disease around the tip of the root at this time indicates the need for further endodontic therapy or extraction of the tooth. Further endodontic therapy usually consists of re-doing the root canal therapy, often in conjunction with surgical endodontics (usually removing the tip of the root and sealing the root canal from this direction as well).

Special considerations with immature teeth

A partial pulpectomy and direct pulp capping procedure is indicated for recent tooth crown fractures with pulp exposure in an immature tooth. An immature tooth has a thin dentine wall and an open apex, allowing a good blood supply to the pulp. Treatment is aimed at maintaining a viable pulp, as this is needed for continued root development.

A necrotic immature tooth requires endodontic treatment if it is to be retained. The procedure is an adaptation of conventional root canal therapy as already described for the mature permanent tooth. The necrotic pulp tissue is gently removed and the pulp chamber and root canal thoroughly cleaned. It is important to remove all the necrotic tissue, which usually extends slightly beyond the radiographically verifiable open apex. Sterile calcium hydroxide powder or paste is packed into the root canal, extending just beyond the apex. A degree of apexogenesis (normal root length and apex development) or apexification (treatment-stimulated root closure) can be achieved if this procedure is performed. The exposure site is sealed with a restorative material.

The tooth is monitored closely and the calcium hydroxide dressing is changed approximately every 6 months, as a fresh dressing is more effective in stimulating apexogenesis and apexification. When no further root development can be seen radiographically and if the apex is closed, a conventional root canal treatment should be performed. A conventional root canal treatment can only be carried out if the apex is closed. If the apex is still open and closure cannot be stimulated by repeated calcium hydroxide dressings, it may be possible to obtain an apical seal using a surgical approach and placing a root filling in a retrograde manner.

It must be noted that multiple general anesthesia episodes are required and thus, in most cases, extraction of an immature tooth with a necrotic pulp is the best course of action. Salvage procedure as described above is really only indicated for the strategic permanent teeth that have undergone some degree of maturation.

It should also be noted that immature teeth might well be present in the mature animal if trauma caused pulp necrosis during the developmental period. Treatment of such teeth is the same as for any immature permanent teeth, regardless of the actual age of the animal.

Glossary

Abrasion Wear of tooth surfaces that are not in contact with one another

Acrylic General name for methyl methacrylate and polymethyl methacrylate. Polymer material used in dental restoration, splinting and orthodontics.

Alveolar bone Bone forming the sockets for the teeth.

Alveolar mucosa Oral mucosa that covers the alveolar processes.

Alveolar septum The dense bone separating alveoli of adjacent teeth.

Alveolus Socket within bone and soft tissue in which a tooth is normally located.

Ameloblast Enamel-forming cell that arises from oral ectoderm.

Ameloblastoma Benign, but locally invasive, neoplasm originating from odontogenic epithelium.

Anelodont Teeth that develop a true anatomic root structure and do not continuously grow throughout life.

Anisognathism Having upper and lower jaws of differing widths. Normal in many species.

Ankylosis (Greek for 'immobile'). Fusion of bone and tooth substance along the root surface.

Anodontia The congenital absence of teeth.

Anterior Situated in front of. This term is commonly used to denote the incisor and canine teeth or the area toward the front of the mouth.

Anterior crossbite Reverse scissor occlusion of one, several or all of the incisors.

Apatite Calcium hydroxyapatite [Ca_{10} (PO_4)$_6$ (OH)$_2$], the main mineral component of dental hard tissues.

Apex Point or extremity of a conical object such as a tooth root.

Apexification Treatment-stimulated closure of the root apex.

Apexogenesis Normal root length and apex development.

Apical Direction toward the root tip or away from the incisal or occlusal surfaces.

Apical delta Fine branching channels at the root apex of many canine and feline teeth through which nerves, blood vessels and lymphatics pass.

Apical foramen A single opening at the root apex through which nerves, blood vessels and lymphatics pass.

Aradicular Without roots.

Aradicular hypsodont Dentition with long crowned teeth, without a true root structure, which are continually growing (e.g. lagomorphs, guinea pigs, chinchillas). Elodont.

Attached gingiva Tightly attached gingiva extending from the free gingiva to the alveolar mucosa.

Attachment epithelium Cells that attach the gingiva to the tooth.

Attrition Abnormal or excessive wear of occluding tooth surfaces.

Avulsion Separation by traction. The dislocation of a tooth from its alveolus.

Bifurcation Division into two parts or branches, as any two roots of a tooth.

Bisecting angle Technique of taking radiographs to minimize linear distortion by aiming the beam perpendicular to the line that bisects the angle formed by the long axis of the tooth and the film.

Biting force The pressure exerted by teeth when engaged by the muscles of mastication.

Body of the mandible Horizontal portion of the mandible, excluding the alveolar process.

Brachycephalic Having a short skull, e.g. Bulldogs, Pekinese.

Brachygnathism Having a short jaw.

Brachyodont Teeth that have a short crown : root ratio, with a true root.

Bruxism Abnormal grinding of the teeth.

Buccal Of, or towards, the cheek.

Buccal surface Surface of a posterior tooth positioned immediately adjacent to the cheek.

Bur A rotary instrument used for cutting and shaping teeth, bone, metal, etc.

Calcification Process by which organic tissue becomes hardened by a deposit of calcium salts within its substance. Literally, the term denotes the deposition of any mineral salts that contribute toward the hardening and maturation of tissue.

Calcium hydroxide Alkaline powder used as such or incorporated into pastes and cements for use as a direct or indirect pulp dressing.

Calcium hydroxide cement Alkaline dental cement popular for lining cavities.

Calculus Hard deposit which accumulates on the teeth. Mineralized plaque. Tartar.

Canines *See* Cuspids.

Caries Progressive dissolution of tooth structure by bacterial acid and enzyme action. Common in humans, less common in dogs and not described in cats.

Carnassial teeth The largest shearing teeth in the upper and lower jaws (upper 4th premolar and lower 1st molar in dogs and cats).

Caudal Towards the tail. Away from the nose/head.

Cavity An abnormal hole or depression in the surface of a tooth, e.g. caries cavities and feline resorptive lesion cavities.

Cementoblasts Cells that form cementum.

Cemento-dentinal junction (CDJ) Junction where the cementum and dentine contact.

Cemento-enamel junction (CEJ) The line between anatomic root and crown where enamel ends, meeting the cementum covering the root. Term usually only used when referring to brachyodont teeth.

Cementoid Term meaning cementum-like.

Cementum Bone-like connective tissue usually covering the surface of tooth roots and sometimes the crown. Consists of 65% mineral (calcium hydroxyapatite), 23% organic (mainly collagen), 12% water.

Cervical Of or towards the neck. Of that part of a tooth where root and crown meet.

Cervical line The cemento-enamel junction where root and crown of brachyodont teeth meet.

Cervix (neck) Narrow or constricted portion of a tooth in the region of the junction of crown and root.

Cheek teeth Term used to signify the premolar and/or molar teeth of herbivores as a functional unit.

Cheilitis Inflammation of the lips.

Chlorhexidine Chemical disinfectant often used for plaque control. Used as either the gluconate or acetate.

Cingulum The raised section or rudimentary cusp seen on the palatal or lingual surface of the crown of incisor teeth in humans and dogs.

Cleft lip Defect or gap in the upper lip, occurring during fetal development.

Cleft palate Lack of joining together of hard or soft palate.

Clinical crown That portion of the tooth protruding above the gingiva.

Clinical root That portion of the tooth below the gingiva.

Closed apex Natural constrictive closing of the tooth apex.

Closed curettage Root scaling and root planing of a periodontal pocket shallow enough to allow the apical extent to be reached with hand instruments.

Cold-cure acrylic Acrylic which cures when an amine activates the initiator without the application of heat. Self-curing.

Condyloid process That portion of the vertical ramus of the mandible that forms part of the temporomandibular joint.

Congenital Present at birth.

Contact point A point where two adjacent teeth touch.

Coronal Towards or pertaining to the crown of a tooth.

Coronally positioned flap Gingival flap that is placed at a point coronal to its original position.

Coronoid process Bony projection at the upper anterior portion of the vertical ramus. It is the attachment location for the temporal muscle.

Cortical plate Dense bone on the outer buccal and lingual surfaces of the alveolar bone.

Crown 1 That part of a tooth that is normally situated within the oral cavity or above alveolar bone and usually covered by enamel.

Crown 2 A prosthetic reconstruction of the coronal part of a damaged tooth.

Curette Dental instrument used for removing plaque and calculus from the subgingival surface of tooth roots. Also used for root planing.

Cusp A raised or pointed portion of a tooth crown.

Cuspids (canine teeth, fang teeth) Four pointed teeth situated one on each side of both jaws, immediately distal to the corner or lateral incisors.

Cyst Sac of fluid lined by epithelial cells. Cysts may grow to varying sizes.

Deciduous teeth Those teeth which are normally shed and replaced in diphyodont dentitions. Temporary, puppy, kitten, milk, baby or primary teeth.

Deglutition Action of swallowing.

Dental abrasion Wear from the friction of an externally applied force, such as brushing.

Dental attrition Wear or loss of tooth substance due to normal masticatory forces, i.e. teeth that are in contact.

Dental luxator Instrument with a wider, but more delicate blade than an elevator that is used in the periodontal space to sever the periodontal ligament attachment.

Dentigerous Containing or associated with teeth, e.g. dentigerous cyst – a cyst that forms around an unerupted tooth.

Dentine (dentin) Hard connective tissue forming main bulk of most teeth. Consists of 70% mineral (calcium hydroxyapatite), 18% organic (mainly collagen), 12% water.

Dentino-enamel junction (DEJ) Juncture within the crown of the tooth where the dentinal and enamel walls meet.

Dentition Name used to signify the characteristics, arrangement and function of teeth, e.g. carnivorous, herbivorous and omnivorous dentition.

Developer Solution to make the latent image on an exposed X-ray film visible.

Developmental Of, or relating to, formation, e.g. developmental groove – a linear depression in the surface of a tooth usually originating from the fusion of separate parts during the formation of the tooth.

Diastema A natural gap or space between teeth in the same jaw. Examples include the space between the incisors and cheek teeth in lagomorphs and rodents, and the space between maxillary incisors and canine teeth in carnivores.

Dilaceration Deformity of a tooth root or crown. Usually used to refer to sharp angulation of a tooth root.

Diphyodont Dentition where one set of teeth (the deciduous dentition) is shed, being replaced by a second set (the permanent dentition).

Disclosing agents Organic dyes capable of indicating the presence of plaque.

Disinfectants Agents that remove or kill microorganisms.

Distal Furthest away from. Away from the median point of the dental arch. The actual direction varies along the dental arch.

Distal surface Surface of a tooth facing away from the median line following the curve of the dental arch.

Dolichocephalic Having a long skull, as seen in Rough Collies and Dobermans.

Dysplasia Abnormal development, e.g. enamel dysplasia.

Elodont Teeth that grow throughout life. Aradicular hypsodont teeth.

Enamel Very hard outer layer of tooth crown in humans and carnivores. Consists of 96% mineral (calcium hydroxyapatite), 2% protein (enamelin), 2% water.

Enamel hypoplasia Condition in which the enamel layer is thin or reduced.

Endodontic Of, or pertaining to, the tissue within a tooth, i.e. the pulp/dentine unit.

Endodontic filling materials Means of obturating pulp chamber after extirpation and disinfection.

Endodontic sealers Materials used to create a seal between endodontic filling materials and the wall of the pulp chamber.

Endodontics Study and treatment of the dental pulp.

Epiglottis Mucosal-covered cartilage that helps cover the laryngeal opening.

Epulis Clinical descriptive term to denote mass on the gingiva.

Eruption Movement of a tooth as it emerges through surrounding tissue so that the clinical crown gradually appears longer.

Exfoliation Shedding or loss of a primary tooth.

External resorption Destruction of dental hard tissue that commences at the external root surface.

Extirpation Complete surgical removal of a part, such as a pulp.

Extract To pull out or remove.

Extrusion Over-eruption or extension of a tooth from its socket.

Facet A flattened surface worn on a tooth, usually caused by contact with an opposing tooth.

Facial The outward facing, i.e. labial and buccal, surfaces of the teeth.

Fauces Space between the left and right palatine tonsils, i.e. medial to the palatoglossal folds.

Filling *See* Restoration 1.

Filling materials Restorative materials used to obturate cavities, e.g. those left after the removal of caries.

Fissure A developmental fault seen as a deep fold or cleft in the occlusal or buccal surface of a tooth.

Fixer solutions Used to preserve and enhance the latent image on the radiographic film.

Fluorapatite The acid-resistant form of hydroxyapatite.

Fluoride agents Sources of fluoride ions that are suitable for use in the mouth.

Follicle A small sac or cyst.

Follicular cyst Dentigerous cyst or dilation of the follicular space around the crown of a tooth that is unerupted or impacted.

Fossa A shallow depression, e.g. the depression between the cingulum and incisal edge of certain incisor teeth.

Frenectomy Excision of the frenulum.

Frenoplasty Excision of part of the frenulum to alter its contours.

Frenulum Fold of alveolar mucosa forming a noticeable ridge of attachment between the lips and gums.

Frenum Fold of skin or lining tissue that limits the movement of an organ (e.g. tissue under the tongue).

Fulcrum Centre of rotation of the tooth, usually occurring approximately at the junction of the middle and apical thirds of the root.

Functional occlusion Active tooth contacts during mastication and swallowing; also called dynamic occlusion.

Furcation Forking or branching point. Bifurcation or trifurcation: the area where the roots of multirooted teeth meet.

Fusion The joining of two or more teeth each retaining its own structure.

Gemination The partial splitting of a tooth giving the appearance of a double crown whilst having a single root structure.

Gingiva Oral mucosa that surrounds the teeth.

Gingival Of, or pertaining to, the gingiva.

Gingival crest Most occlusal or incisal extent of gingiva.

Gingival fibers Periodontal fibers in the gingival connective tissue.

Gingival fluid Tissue fluid that exudes through the sulcular epithelium.

Gingival hyperplasia Proliferation of the gingiva.

Gingival margin Crest of gingiva around the tooth.

Gingival papilla Gingival tissue in the interproximal space between two adjacent teeth.

Gingival pocket Abnormal, pathologic space extending down a tooth root from the gingival sulcus.

Gingival sulcus Gap or potential space situated between the free gingiva and the tooth surface.

Gingivectomy Excision of excessive gingival tissues to create a new gingival margin.

Gingivitis Inflammation of the gingiva.

Gingivoplasty Periodontal surgery used to correct gingival deformities of contour not associated with pocketing.

Gnathic Of the jaw. In general use refers to the mandible.

Groove Shallow linear depression on the surface of a tooth. There are two common types:

1. *Developmental groove:* Marks the boundaries between adjacent cusps and other major divisional parts of a tooth.
2. *Supplemental groove:* An indistinct linear depression, irregular in extent and direction, that does not demarcate major divisional portions of a tooth.

Gum In common usage. Gingiva.

Halitosis Unpleasant breath odor.

Hard palate Bony vault of the oral cavity proper covered with soft tissue.

Hemisection A tooth being cut in half generally through the furcational area.

Hereditary Term describing traits received from ancestors that produce specific characteristics.

Heterodont Dentition comprising teeth of different shapes and functions.

High-speed Used to describe air driven turbine mechanisms capable of rotation at over 100 000 rpm. Typical high-speed hand pieces rotate burs at around 300 000 rpm.

Homodont The feature of having all teeth of the same general shape or type, although size may vary, as in fish, reptiles and sharks.

Horizontal fibers Alveolodental periodontal ligament fibers running from the cementum to the alveolar crest to resist horizontal tooth movements.

Horizontal ramus That portion of the jaw composed of the body and symphyseal area of the mandible.

Hydroxyapatite Form of calcium phosphate, the basic mineral of enamel, dentine and cementum. *See* Apatite *for formula.*

Hypersialism Excessive salivation or drooling.

Hypocalcified enamel Condition in which there is either an insufficient number of enamel crystals or insufficient growth of the crystals.

Hypodontia Condition in which some teeth are missing.

Hypoplastic enamel Thin enamel, commonly seen in conjunction with enamel hypocalcification.

Hypsodont Dentition comprising long crowned teeth, radicular or aradicular.

Impacted tooth A tooth that cannot erupt, or complete its eruption, due to contact with an obstruction such as another tooth.

Incipient caries First indication of enamel demineralization seen as a chalky white spot.

Incisal Coronal portion or direction in incisors.

Incisal bone The premaxilla, rostral-most area of upper jaw, that accommodates the maxillary incisors and is formed solely by the medial nasal process; also known as the primary plate.

Incisor Center teeth in either arch that are essential for cutting.

Infrabony pocket Periodontal pocket that has its base apical to the alveolar crest; also known as intrabony pocket.

Interceptive orthodontics Generally considered to be the extraction or recontouring (crown reduction) of primary or permanent teeth that are contributing to alignment problems of the permanent dentition.

Interdental Situated between adjacent teeth, e.g. interdental wiring.

Interdental papillae Projection of gingiva between the teeth.

Interdental septum Bone between the roots of adjacent teeth.

Internal resorption Loss of the dentinal structure internally.

Interproximal Between adjoining surfaces of adjacent teeth.

Interproximal space Space between adjoining teeth.

Interradicular fibers Alveolodental periodontal ligament fibers in multirooted teeth that go from the interradicular crestal bone to cementum.

Intraradicular septum Bone between the roots of multirooted teeth.

Intrusion Movement of the tooth further into the alveolus.

Irreversible pulpitis Inflammation of the pulp that cannot be resolved, leading to the death of the vital pulp.

Isognathism Condition of having equal jaw widths, in which the premolars and molars of opposing jaws align with the occlusal surfaces facing each other, forming an occlusal plane.

Junctional epithelium Epithelium that acts to hold mucosa in the base of the gingival sulcus to the tooth.

Labial Of, towards, or pertaining to, the lips.

Labial surface Surface of an anterior tooth positioned immediately adjacent to the lip.

Lamina dura Radiographic term denoting the cribriform plate, bundle bone and the dense alveolar bone surrounding a root.

Level bites When the incisor teeth meet edge on edge or the premolars or molars occlude cusp to cusp.

Lingual Of, towards, or pertaining to, the tongue.

Lingual surface Surface of a tooth immediately adjacent to the tongue.

Low-speed Dental engines or hand piece capable of providing rotation up to 30 000 rpm.

Luxation Dislocation of a joint. Partial or complete separation of a tooth from its alveolus.

Macrodontia Having larger teeth than normal.

Malar abscess Facial abscess of dental origin.

Malocclusion Abnormal tooth positioning.

Mandible Lower jaw.

Mandibular Pertaining to the lower jaw.

Mandibular condyle Rounded top of the mandible that articulates with the mandibular fossa.

Mandibular symphysis Point at which the mandibular processes merge, forming the mandible.

Mastication Act of chewing or grinding.

Maxillae Paired main bones of the upper jaw.

Maxillary Pertaining to the upper arch.

Medial/median Toward/at the midline of the body.

Mental foramen Foramen on the lateral side of the mandible, below the premolars.

Mesial Towards the point of the dental arch situated in the median plane.

Mesial surface Surface of a tooth facing toward the median line, following the curve of the dental arch.

Mesocephaly Condition marked by a balanced facial profile, somewhere between dolichocephalic and brachycephalic, as in German Shepherds.

Microdontia Having smaller teeth than normal.

Milk teeth Those teeth that are normally shed and replaced in diphyodont dentitions. Primary, temporary, deciduous, puppy, kitten or baby teeth.

Mixed dentition The feature of having primary and permanent teeth in the dental arches at the same time.

Molars Teeth with occlusal surface that can be used to grind food or break it down into smaller pieces.

Monophydont Having one set of teeth, i.e. permanent only.

Mucogingival junction The line between attached gingiva and oral mucosa.

Occluding Contacting opposing teeth.

Occlusal Of, or pertaining to, the surface of a tooth which meets a tooth in the opposite jaw, e.g. the occlusal surfaces of molar teeth.

Occlusal equilibration The recontouring of abnormal occlusal surfaces of teeth to improve function, most often necessary in herbivores with continually erupting teeth.

Occlusal surface Surface of a premolar or molar within the marginal ridges that contacts the corresponding surfaces of antagonists during closure of the posterior teeth.

Occlusal trauma Injury caused by malocclusion.

Occlusion Coming together. The relationship of upper and lower teeth.

Odontoblast Dentine-forming cell that originates from the dental papilla.

Odontoclasts Multinucleated cells responsible for destroying cementum, dentine and enamel.

Odontogenic cysts or tumors Lesions arising from cellular components of the developing tooth structure.

Odontoma Mixed odontogenic tissue tumor containing both epithelial and mesenchymal cells. It may be either compound (disorganized mass) or complex (with denticles).

Oligodontia Having fewer teeth than normal due to their failure to develop.

Open bite Failure of teeth to come into occlusion, an abnormal gap remaining between opposing teeth when the jaw is closed.

Open curettage Therapy and root planing of an area that has been exposed by a flap for additional visualization.

Operculectomy Excision of an operculum to allow further eruption and crown exposure.

Operculum Persistence of a thick, fibrous gingiva over a partially or even fully erupted tooth.

Oral epithelium Lining membrane of the oral cavity consisting of stratified squamous epithelium.

Oral mucosa Stratified squamous epithelium running from the margins of the lips to the area of the tonsils and lining the oral cavity; also known as oral mucous membrane.

Oropharynx Section between the tonsils and the base of the tongue.

Orthodontics Study and treatment relating to restoration of normal tooth position and jaw relationships.

Osteoblasts Cells that form bone.

Osteoclasts Multinucleated cells responsible for destroying bone.

Palatal Pertaining to the palate or roof of the mouth.

Palatal surface Lingual (medial) surface of maxillary teeth.

Palate Roof of the mouth.

Peg teeth The small 2nd maxillary incisors, located behind the large 1st maxillary incisors, in lagomorphs.

Pellicle Amorphous coating of salivary proteins and glycoproteins attached to exposed tooth surfaces in the mouth.

Periapical Around the tip of a tooth root.

Periodontal Around or surrounding teeth and their roots. Of, or pertaining to, the periodontium.

Periodontal disease Plaque-induced inflammation of the periodontium.

Periodontal membrane or ligament Collagen fibers attached to the tooth roots and alveolar bone, serving as an attachment of the tooth to the bone.

Periodontitis Plaque-induced inflammation of the periodontal tissues, resulting in irreversible loss of periodontal ligament and alveolar bone.

Periodontium Periodontal tissues. Tissues adjacent to, surrounding and supporting the tooth and its roots. Alveolar bone, periodontal ligament, cementum and gingiva.

Permanent teeth Final or lasting set of teeth that are typically of a very durable and lasting nature (opposite of deciduous).

Physiologic mobility Degree of tooth movement that can be considered normal.

Pit A small developmental depression usually in the occlusal surface of a tooth.

Plaque Biofilm that accumulates on teeth, composed of mucin, food residues, desquamated epithelial cells, leukocytes, bacteria and their products including mucopolysaccharides.

Posterior Situated toward the back, such as premolars and molars.

Posterior crossbite Condition in which the cusps of a posterior tooth (premolar, molar) in one arch exceed the normal cusp relation of those in the opposing arch, bucally or lingually.

Pre-eruptive stage Period of time when the crown of the tooth is developing.

Premaxilla Bony area of the upper jaw that includes the alveolar ridge for the incisors and the area immediately behind it in primates.

Premolars Permanent teeth that replace the primary molars, designed to help hold and carry, like cuspids, and break food down into smaller pieces, like molars; also known as bicuspids.

Primary teeth *See* Deciduous teeth.

Prognathism Having a longer or protruding jaw, e.g. relative mandibular prognathism.

Proxima Close to or toward the center or midline.

Proximal surface Surface of a tooth facing toward an adjoining tooth in the same arch (e.g. both mesial and distal surfaces are proximal surfaces).

Pseudopockets False gingival pockets in which gingival height is increased due to hyperplasia, resulting in increased periodontal probing values although there is no real attachment loss.

Ptyalism Excessive salivation, usually with excess drooling from mouth (slobbers).

Pulp Soft tissue within a tooth; contains odontoblasts, nerves, blood vessels, lymphatics and connective tissue.

Pulp canal Root canal. The space within a tooth root running from the apex to the pulp chamber.

Pulp cavity The pulp canal and chamber.

Pulp chamber The space within a tooth crown occupied by pulp tissue.

Pulp-dentine unit The sensitive tissue of the tooth.

Pulp dressing Calcium hydroxide-containing pastes and cements are used as pulp dressings and protectants. They are used as indirect pulp capping agents when there is only a very thin layer of dentine remaining after cavity preparation. The hard-setting cements may be used as liners beneath surface restorations.

Pulpal exposure Unnatural opening of the pulp chamber by pathologic or mechanical means.

Pulpal necrosis Partial or total pulpal death.

Pulpectomy Extirpation of the entire pulp.

Pulpitis Inflammation of pulp tissue – may be caused by thermal, chemical, infective or traumatic insults.

Radicular Of, or pertaining to, the (tooth) root.

Radicular ankylosis Loss of part or all of the periodontal ligament, resulting in fusion of root cementum and socket bone.

Radicular hypsodont Dentition with long crowned teeth having short, distinct, closed root structure: continuously erupting but not continually growing (e.g. equines). Anelodont.

Ramus of the mandible Vertical portion of the mandible.

Ranula Salivary retention cyst (sialocele) located under the tongue, caused by blockage of the sublingual duct or gland.

Recession Migration of the gingival crest in an apical direction, away from the crown of the tooth.

Reparative dentine Dentine deposited because of injury or irritation to the pulp. Tertiary dentine.

Resorption Physiologic removal of tissues or body products, as of the roots of deciduous teeth or of some alveolar process after the loss of the permanent teeth.

Restoration 1 The placed restorative materials, i.e. a filling.

Restoration 2 Act of placing restorative materials, e.g. filling a tooth cavity.

Restorative agent A material used to fill a cavity or rebuild tooth structure (amalgam, composite, glass-ionomer, etc.).

Restorative dentistry The study of, or treatment involving, the replacement of lost or missing tooth structure.

Root That part of tooth normally contained in the alveolus.

Root bifurcation That point at which a root trunk divides into two separate branches.

Root exposure Uncovering or exposing of root surfaces due to periodontal tissue loss.

Root planing Procedure for smoothing the cementum of the root of a tooth.

Root trifurcation That point at which a root trunk divides into three separate branches.

Rostral Toward the nose. Away from the tail.

Rugae Small ridges of tissue extending laterally across the anterior of the hard palate.

Scaler Dental instrument used for the removal of plaque and calculus from the crowns of teeth. Hand scaler, ultrasonic scaler, sonic scaler.

Scissor bite Normal relationship of the maxillary incisors overlapping the mandibular incisors whose incisal edges rest on or near the cingulum on the lingual surfaces on the maxillary incisors.

Secondary dentine Dentine deposited after the eruption of a tooth.

Self-cure acrylic Acrylic caused to set by the action of chemicals without external heat.

Self-curing filling materials Filling materials caused to set by the action of chemicals rather than light.

Slobbers Ptyalism causing fur to be wet and matted around the mouth, jaw and ventral neck, particularly in chinchillas.

Soft palate Unsupported soft tissue that extends back from the hard palate free of the support of the palatine bone.

Stomatitis Inflammation of the soft tissues of the oral cavity or mouth.

Subgingival curettage Removal of diseased soft tissue within a periodontal pocket.

Subluxation Incomplete dislocation of a joint, such as the temporomandibular joint or a tooth.

Submandibular Referring to the region below the mandible; a group of lymph nodes around the mandibular gland.

Supernumerary teeth Extra teeth, above the normal number. Often seen in the incisor region in brachycephalic dogs and the premolar region of dolichocephalic dogs.

Tartar *See* Calculus.

Temporary teeth Deciduous teeth.

Temporomandibular joint Joint composed of the condylar process of the vertical ramus of the mandible and the mandibular fossa of the temporal bone of the skull.

Tertiary dentine Dentine deposited as a result of injury or irritation to the pulp. Reparative dentine.

Toothbrushing Mechanical means of removing dental plaque.

Version Angulation: bucco-, linguo-, labio-, palato-version; Angulation of a tooth or teeth with the crown deviated toward the cheek, tongue, lip, palate.

Vestibule That part of the mouth between the teeth and the lips/cheek.

Wet dewlap Moist dermatitis on the ventral neck of rabbits from ptyalism due to malocclusion, stomatitis or other oral inflammation. Slobbers.

Xerostomia Dry mouth, due to lack of salivary secretion.

Index

Page numbers followed by 'f' indicate figures, 't' indicate tables, and 'b' indicate boxes.

A

Abbreviations, 65, 65t
Abrasion, 87, 89–90
  preventive dentistry, 124
Abscesses
  facial, 198–200, 200f
  periapical, 90–91
  periodontal, 105f
Actinomyces viscosus, 98
Adrenaline, 20
Advancement flap, 143f
Air polishing, 6
Airway obstruction, 18
Airway security, 15
Allodynia, 19
Alveolar bone, 40
  destruction, 100
American Veterinary Dental College, 52
Amino-alcohols, substituted, 34
Amoxicillin, 32
Amoxicillin-clavulanic acid, 32
Ampicillin, 32
Analgesia, 18–27
  pain pathway, 19, 19b
  see also Local anesthesia (LA)
Anesthesia, 15–18
  brachycephalic patients, 17–18
  general *see* General anesthesia
  geriatric patients, 17
  local *see* Local anesthesia (LA)
  long periods, 16
  maxillofacial trauma, 18
  patient monitoring, 17, 17b
  principles, 15–17
Ankylosis, 133–134, 133f
Anodontia, 81
Anterior crossbite, 46–47, 50f

B

Antibiotics, 31–34
  delivery, 33–34
  impregnated beads, 199–200
  periodontal disease, 32–34
  preventive use, 31–32
  therapeutic use, 32
    principles, 32
Antimicrobial agents, 33
Antiplaque agents, 34
Antiseptics, 34
Aradicular hypsodont teeth, extraction, 191, 208–210, 209f
Attachment loss, 103–104, 103f
Attrition, 87, 87f, 89–90
  preventive dentistry, 124
Autoimmune disorders, 98t
Autologous transfusion, 16
Avulsion, 155f–156f, 156–157

B

Bacteremia, treatment-induced, 31
Bactericidal antibiotic, 32
Benzathine penicillin, 200
Biofilms, 33
Bisecting angle technique, 74–75, 76f–77f
Bite
  level, 45
  mandibular brachygnathic, 46, 48f
  mandibular prognathic, 44–45, 47f
  reverse scissor, 45
  see also Crossbite
Blood loss, 16–17
Brachycephalic breeds, 44, 46f, 54
  anesthesia, 17–18
Brachyodont teeth, 191
  extraction, 209
'Bumper bar' technique, 164–165
Bupivacaine, 20
Burs, 8, 11f
Butorphanol, 18

C

Calcification, pulp, 90, 90f
Calculus, 99–100
  forceps, 6
Canine teeth, 44, 44f
  bonding upper/lower, 166, 167f
  extraction, 186
  fixation, 158f–159f
  mandibular *see* Mandibular canines
  maturation, 38f
  maxillary *see* Maxillary canines
  occlusion, 51, 52f
  malocclusion, 47
Carbide blades, 4
Caries, 87–88, 88f–89f
  preventive dentistry, 124
Cats
  chronic gingivostomatitis (CGS), 114–116
  occlusion, normal, 44, 45f
  radiographic views, 78
  record sheets, 63f–65f
  resorptive lesions (RL), 130f, 133–134, 135f
  tooth extraction, 186–187
  upper airway obstruction, 18
  see also Dentition
Cemento-enamel junction (CEJ), 103–104, 103f
Cementum, 39–40
Central hypersensitivity, 19
Cerclage/hemicerclage techniques, 163–165
Cheek teeth
  extraction, 209–210
  rabbits, 195
  trimming, 208
Cheek teeth overgrowth
  chinchillas, 202–204, 204f
  guinea pigs, 201, 201f–203f

lagomorphs/rodents, 208
  rabbits, 196–198, 198f–200f, 199b
Cheeks, examination, 58b
Chemical plaque control, 124
Chews, dental hygiene, 123–124
Chinchillas, 202–204
  cheek teeth overgrowth, 202–204, 204f
  dental conditions, 204
  healthy mouth, 202
  incisor overgrowth, 202
Chlorhexidine gluconate, 34
  mechanical plaque control, 34
Chronic gingivostomatitis (CGS), 114–117
  clinical signs, 114–115
  diagnosis, 115–116
  dogs, 116–117
  treatment, 116, 116f, 117b
Cleaning, hand instruments, 12–13
Cleanliness, degrees of, 1
  see also Hygiene, oral
Client education, 121–122, 122b
Clinical attachment level (CAL), 61
Columbia curettes, 5
Common conditions, 81–95
  caries, 87–88, 88f–89f
  developmental see Developmental disorders
  eruption/shedding disorders, 86–87, 86f
  hard tissue wear, 87, 87f
  oral tumours, 92f–93f, 93–94
  osteomyelitis, 93
  pulp/periapical disease, 89–93
  root resorption, 94, 94f
Compressed air driven units, 8, 9f–10f
  care, 12
Compressors, care of, 12
Congenitally missing teeth, 81, 82f
Coronal amputation, 136, 137f–138f
Crossbite
  anterior, 46–47, 50f
  posterior, 49, 50f
Cross-matching blood, 16
Crown fractures, 147–149, 150f, 152f
  root and, 147, 149, 151f
Curettes, 4–5, 5f–6f
  sharpening, 9–10, 12f
Cysts, periapical, 90–91

D

Debridement, subgingival, 110f
  closed, 111–112, 111f
  open, 111–112, 112f
Degrees of cleanliness, 1
Dental prophylaxis, 106
Dentine, 38–39

Dentistry and Oral Surgery Service, Veterinary Medical Teaching Hospital, University of California, 32
Dentition, dogs/cats, 37, 38b, 38t
  anatomy, 37–39, 38f
  permanent, 54
  see also Primary dentition
Developmental disorders, 81–86
  number/size/shape anomalies, 81–83
  structural anomalies, 83–86
Diets, dental, 123–124
Digital radiography, 67–68, 70–71
  direct, 67, 69f–70f, 70–71, 73f
  handling/mounting images, 72, 73f
  indirect, 67, 69f, 70, 73f
Dilators, 207f
Diphyodont, defined, 37
Dogs
  caries, 88, 124
  chronic gingivostomatitis (CGS), 116–117
  occlusion, normal, 43–44
  prairie, 204–206, 205f
  record sheets, 62f–63f
  tooth extraction, 184–186, 186f
  see also Dentition
Dolichocephalic breeds, 44, 47f, 52
Double overlapping flap technique, 144–145, 145f
'Dough' technique, 168

E

Ectodermal dysplasia, 81
Education, client, 121–122, 122b
Elective tracheotomy, 28
Elevators, 7, 174–176, 174f–175f, 180f, 181
  periosteal, 7, 9f
  sharpening, 10
Emergencies, 141–170
  conditions, 141, 142f
  soft tissue trauma, 141–147
Emphysema, 188
Enamel, 37–38
Enamel hypoplasia (dysplasia), 83–86, 84f–85f
Endodontic lesions, combined periodontic, 91–93
Endodontic treatment, 152–154
Endotracheal intubation, 1
  brachycephalic patients, 18
  maxillofacial trauma, 18
Endotracheal tubes, 15–16, 18
Enzymes, mechanical plaque control, 34
Epulis, 93
Equipment, 1–13
  ergonomic considerations, 1, 2f
  extraction, 7–8, 209f

maintenance, 8–13
  operator considerations, 1
  oral/dental examination, 2–4
  overview, 1
  patient considerations, 1
  periodontal therapy, 4–7, 108f
  radiography, 67–72, 68b, 69f
  tooth trimming, 207f–208f
Eruption disorders, 86–87, 86f
Esophagostomy tubes, 28
Essential oils, mechanical plaque control, 34
Ethical considerations, 54
European Standard (EN), Document 556 (cleanliness), 2
European Standard (EN)/International Organization for Standardization (ISO)
  Document 14937 (cleanliness), 2
  Document 15883 (cleanliness), 2
European Veterinary Dental College (EVDC), 52, 65–66
Examination see Oral examination
Explorers, 3, 3f
External fixation, 164–165
External root resorption, 94f, 129
  inflammatory (EIRR), 130–131
Extraction, 171–189
  aradicular hypsodont teeth, 191, 208–210, 209f
  closed, 172, 174–180
  complications, 187–188
  contraindications, 172
  equipment, 7–8
  forceps, 7
  indications, 171
  lagomorphs/rodents, 208–210
  open, 172–173, 180–186, 182f–186f
  persistent primary teeth, 125
  radical, 116, 116f
  resorptive lesions (RL), 136
  techniques, 172–187, 173f
  types, 172
Extraktor, 7, 7f–8f, 173, 173f–176f, 176, 180f, 181
  sharpening, 10, 12f
Eye protection, 16

F

Facial abscess, rabbits, 198–200, 200f
Faucitis, 115, 115f
Feeding tubes, 28
Feline calicivirus (FCV), 114–116
  isolation, 116
Feline immunodeficiency virus (FIV), 114–116
Feline leukemia virus (FeLV), 114–116
Fixation, wire, 157, 157f

Fluoride
  mechanical plaque control, 34
  topical application, 86
Foramina, radiography, 79
Forceps
  calculus, 6
  extraction, 7
Fractures *see* Jaw fractures; Teeth, fractures
Full mouth radiographs, 78, 78f
Furcation involvement, 60–61, 61f, 61t
Fusion, 82–83
Fusobacterium spp, 98

G

Gags, 207f
Gemination, 82–83
General anesthesia, 1
  oral examination, 58, 58b
Gerbils, 206
Geriatric patients, anesthesia, 17
Gingiva
  anatomy, 39–40, 39f–40f
  hyperplasia, 99f, 101–102, 102f,
    113–114, 113f
  index, 59–60, 60t
  inflammation, 131f
  overgrowth, 131f
  recession, 60, 62f–63f, 103f, 104,
    148f–149f
Gingivitis, 97, 99f
  antibiotics, 33
  assessment, 59–60, 60t
  calculus, 99–100
  clinical signs, 101, 102f
  consequences, 101–102
  diagnosis, 101–102
  etiology, 97
  pathogenesis, 100–101
  plaque, 98
  with stomatitis, 114–115, 115f
  stomatitis with, 115, 115f
  treatment, 106, 106b, 107f
  see also Periodontal disease
Gingivoplasty, 113–114, 113f
Gracey curettes, 4–5, 5f
Grafting techniques, 143f
Granuloma, periapical, 90–91
Guinea pigs, 201–202
  cheek tooth overgrowth, 201,
    201f–203f
  healthy mouth, 201, 201f
  incisor overgrowth, 201
  vitamin C, 193

H

Halothane, 18
Hamsters, 206

Hand instruments
  cleaning/sterilization, 12–13
  extraction, 7
  scaling, 4–5, 5f–6f
Hard palate, examination, 58b
Hard palate defects, 142–145, 142t
  repair options, 142–143
  surgery, principles, 142–145
Hard tissue
  resorption, 129–131
  treatment, 171
  wear, 87, 87f
Hemicerclage techniques, 163–165
Hemorrhage, 16–17
  extractions, 188
Hemostasis, 17
Horizontal bone loss, 100, 104, 104f
Hygiene, oral, 121–124
  dental chews, 123–124
Hyperalgesia, 19
Hypersensitivity, 98t
  central, 19
  peripheral, 19
Hyperthermia, 16
Hypodontia, 81
Hypothermia, 16
Hypsodont teeth, 191
  aradicular, extraction, 208–210, 209f

I

Iatrogenic injuries, 162f–163f
Idiopathic feline external root
    resorption, 133–134, 135f
Immune system disorder, 98t
Incisor teeth
  aradicular hypsodont, 208–209, 209f
  occlusion, 45, 51, 52f
  malocclusion, 51
  overgrowth, 195–196, 197f, 201–202,
    206f
  rabbits, 195
  scissor bite, 44, 44f
  trimming, 207–208
Indwelling nasogastric intubation, 28
Infiltration anesthesia, 19–20, 21f–24f
Inflammatory diseases, oral, 98t
  pain, 19
  root resorption, 130
Infraorbital nerve block, 21–26, 25f
Instrumentation *see* Equipment
Interceptive orthodontics, 125
Interdental fixation, 166–169
  ligature/splints, 166–168, 168f–169f
Interferon, 116
Interlock, dental, 52f
Interlock-induced abnormalities, dental,
    51
Intermaxillary fixation, 165–166

Internal root resorption, 129
International Organization for
    Standardization *see* European
    Standard (EN)/International
    Organization for Standardization
    (ISO)
Intraoral acrylic splints, 166–168,
    168f–169f
Intravenous fluid therapy, 16
Intubation techniques, 27–28
  feeding tubes, 28
Isoflurane, 18

J

Jaw fracture, 157–169, 159f–161f
  biomechanics, 159, 161f–162f
  complications, 169
  extractions, 188
  indications, 159–160
  interdental fixation, 166–169
  intermaxillary fixation, 165–166
  orthopedic techniques, 163–165
  postoperative care, 168–169
  repair
    methods, 160–163, 162f–163f
    principles, 160
  tooth-borne appliances, 165
Jaw length, 47f

L

Lagomorphs/rodents, 191–211
  dental anatomy, 191–192, 192b,
    192f–193f
  examination, 193–195
    face/oral cavity, 194, 194b
    further scans, 195
    radiographic, 194–195
  extraction, 208–210
  husbandry, 192–193
  prairie dogs, 204–206, 205f
  rats/mice/hamsters/gerbils, 206, 206f
  tooth trimming, 207–208, 207f–208f
  tooth types, 191
  traumatic tooth injuries, 206
  see also Chinchillas; Guinea pigs;
    Rabbits
Langenbeck technique, 143–144, 144f
Lidocaine, 20
Lips
  examination, 58b
  injuries, 141–142, 143f
L-noradrenaline, 20
Local anesthesia (LA), 19–27, 21f
  complications, 26–27
  indications, 27
Löe and Silness gingival index, 60, 60t
Lower canines, medial displacement, 47

Index

Luxation, 154–156, 155f–156f
Luxators, 7, 7f, 174–176, 174f–175f, 181
  sharpening, 10

M

Malignant neoplasms, 93
Malocclusion, 43, 46–49
  classification, 52–54
  dental, 43, 46–49
  extraction, 172
  lagomorphs/rodents, 193
  management, 54–55
  mandibular canines, 49–50
  maxillary canines, 50–51, 50f
  persistent primary teeth, 49
  preventive dentistry, 54–55, 125–126
  skeletal, 43–46
  treatment, 54–55
Mandible, narrow, 46, 50f
Mandibular brachygnathic bite, 46, 48f
Mandibular canal, 69f, 79
Mandibular canines
  extraction procedure, 183–184, 185f–186f
  malocclusion, 49–50
Mandibular fracture, 157, 159, 160f–161f, 165
  horizontal ramus, 164, 164f–165f
  symphyseal, 163, 163f–164f
Mandibular molars, extraction technique, 184–186
Mandibular nerve block, 21, 23–26, 26f
Mandibular prognathic bite, 44–45, 47f
Maxillary alveolus, 145–147
Maxillary canines
  extraction procedure, 181–183, 182f–184f
  malocclusion, 50–51, 50f
  rostral displacement, 47
Maxillary molars, extraction technique, 184–186
Maxillary premolars, extraction technique, 184–186
Maxillofacial trauma, 18
Mechanical scaling instruments, 5–6
Membrane-stabilizing agents, 20
Mental nerve block, 26, 27f
Mepivacaine, 20
Metronidazole, 32
Mice, 206
Micromotor unit, 8
Mirrors, 3
Missing teeth, congenitally, 81, 82f
Molar teeth
  extraction, 184–186, 187f
  mandibular, 184–186, 187f
  maxillary, 184–186

occlusion, 44
  malocclusion, 49, 50f
  premolar relationship, 44, 45f
Monocryl® sutures, 11
Morphine, 18
Mouth
  floor, examination, 58b
  full mouth radiographs, 78, 78f
  gags, 16
Mucous membranes
  examination, 58b
  ulceration, 103f
Multi-rooted teeth, 176–180, 177f–178f
  extraction procedure, 179–180, 179f–180f, 186–187, 187f

N

Nail cutters, 206
Nasogastric intubation, indwelling, 28
Neoplasms, oral, 93–94, 93f
  malignant, 93
Neuropathic pain, 19
Nonspecific plaque hypothesis, 98
Non-steroidal anti-inflammatory drugs (NSAIDs), 19
Nutrient canals, radiography, 69f, 79

O

Occlusal equilibration, 208
Occlusion, 43
  classification, 52–54
  evaluation, 51, 51f–52f, 52b, 57, 58b
  normal, 43–44, 53f
  see also Malocclusion
Odontoma, 92f, 93
Oligodontia, 81
Opioids, 19
Oral examination, 57–61
  conscious, 57, 58b
  equipment, 2–4
  general anesthesia, 58, 58b
  periodontium, 58–61, 59f
Oral hygiene see Hygiene, oral
Oral inflammatory diseases see Inflammatory diseases, oral
Oral neoplasms, 93–94, 93f
  malignant, 93
Oronasal communication, 188
Oronasal fistulae, 142–147, 147f
  single layer repair, 146–147, 147f
  double layer repair, 147, 147f–149f
Oropharynx, examination, 58b
Orotracheal intubation, 28
Orthodontic devices, 125–126, 126f
Orthodontic movement, 55
Orthopedic techniques, traditional, 163–165, 163f

Osteomyelitis, 93
Overcrowding/supernumerary teeth, 82, 82f, 172
Overgrowth, tooth, 193
  cheek teeth, 196–198, 198f–204f, 199b, 201–204
  incisor teeth, 195–196, 197f, 201–202, 206f
'Overshot', 46
Oxygen, 16
Oxygenating agents, mechanical plaque control, 34
Oxymorphone, 18

P

Pain pathway, 19, 19b
Pain relief
  non-pharmacologic methods, 27
  see also Analgesia
Palatine artery, 142, 175f
Parallax effect, 75–78
Parallel technique, 74, 75f
  radiographs, 104
Particle blasting, 6
Pedicle flaps, 143–145, 143f
Pellicle, 98
Penetration, oral mucosa, 2
Peptostreptococcus spp, 98
Periapical lesions, 85f, 89–91, 89f, 91f, 148–149, 152f–153f
Periodontal attachment level (PAL), 61, 103–104
Periodontal disease, 97–119
  antibiotics, 32–34
  combined endodontic lesions, 91–93
  diagnosis, 101–106
  etiology, 97–100
  oral examination, 101
  overview, 97, 98t, 99f
  pathogenesis, 100–101
  preventive dentistry, 121–124
  professional therapy, 108–114, 108f
  surgery, 107, 113–114
  treatment, 106–107
  see also Chronic gingivostomatitis (CGS)
Periodontal ligament (PDL), 40, 133–134, 133f–134f
Periodontal probe, 3, 3f
  probing depth (PPD), 60, 60f, 103–104, 103f
Periodontal therapy, equipment, 4–7
Periodontitis, 102–106
  advanced, 171
  antibiotics, 33
  clinical signs, 102, 103f
  consequences, 106
  diagnosis, 101–106, 103f

etiology, 97
  with horizontal bone loss, 99f
  jaw fracture, 159f
  treatment, 106–107, 107b
  with vertical bone loss, 99f
  see also Periodontal disease
Periodontitis-associated genotype
    (PAG), 101
Periodontium
  anatomy, 38f, 39–40
  damage, 154–157, 155f–156f
    procedure, 157
  oral examination, 58–61, 59f
Periosteal elevators, 7, 9f
Peripheral hypersensitivity, 19
Peripheral inflammatory root resorption
    (PIRR), 130–133
Peripheral sensitization, 19
Permanent dentition, malocclusion, 54
Persistent primary teeth
  extraction, 125, 171–172
  malocclusion, 49
  maxillary canines, 50f
Pharyngeal packing, 1, 2f, 16
Pharyngotomy, 27–28
Photostimulatable phosphor plate, 69f,
    70
Plaque, 97–98, 100f
  control, 122–124
    mechanical, 33–34
  treatment, 98b
Polishing, 6–7, 112, 113f
Porphyomonas spp, 98
Posterior crossbite, 49, 50f
Power equipment, 2, 8
  care, 11–12
  scalers, 108, 109f
Prairie dogs, 204–206, 205f
Premolar teeth
  interdigitation, 44, 44f, 51, 53f
  maxillary, 184–186, 186f
  molar relationship, 44, 45f
  occlusion, 44, 51, 52f
  malocclusion, 49, 50f
Preventive dentistry, 121–127
  caries, 124
  excessive wear, 124
  malocclusion, 125–126
  periodontal disease, 121–124
  tooth fracture, 124–125
Prevotella spp, 98
Primary dentition
  extraction, 186
  malocclusion, 54
Procaine hydrochloride, 20
Procaine penicillin, 200
Prodenta program, 66
Prophy paste, 6–7
  cup/brush, 6

Prosthesis (silicone/acrylic), 145
Pseudo-odontoma, 204–206, 205f
'Pseudopocketing', 60
Pulp disease, 148–149, 152f–153f
  necrosis, 149
  reactions, 89–90, 90f

Q

Quaternary ammonium compounds,
    mechanical plaque control, 34

R

Rabbits, 195–201
  cheek tooth overgrowth, 196–198,
    198f–200f, 199b
  dental conditions, 200–201
  examination, 194f
  facial abscess, 198–200, 200f
  healthy mouth, 195
  incisor overgrowth, 195–196, 197f
  radiographic features, 195, 196f
  skull, 192f
Radiography, 67–80
  anatomical landmarks, 79
  diagnostic view, 69f
  non-diagnostic view, 68f
  equipment/materials, 67–72, 68b
  full mouth, 78f
  interpretation, 78–79
  intraoral techniques, 73–78, 74f
  lagomorphs/rodents, 194–195
  overview, 67
  patient preparation, 72
Rats, 206
  incisor overgrowth, 206f
  skull, 193f
Records
  oral examination, 57, 61–66, 65t
  record sheets, 4, 62f–65f
Regional blocks, 19–26, 24f–25f
Reimplantation, 157
Replacement resorption, 130
Resorptive lesions (RL), 129–140
  diagnosis, 130f, 135, 135f
  epidemiology, 131–132
  etiology/pathogenesis, 132–134, 132f
  overview, 129, 130f–131f
  surface, 133–134, 133f
  treatment, 135–136, 172
Rinn box, 71f
Rodents *see* Lagomorphs/rodents
Roots
  abnormalities, 83, 83f–84f
  planing, 109–112
  type 1, 132, 132f
Root fractures, 147, 152, 152f
  crown and, 147, 149, 151f

Root resorption, 94, 94f
  external, 94f
Ropivacaine, 20
Rotation flap, 143f
'Rubber toy' technique, 125–126, 126f

S

'Salt and pepper' technique, 167–168
Sanguinarine, mechanical plaque
    control, 34
Scalers, sharpening, 9–10, 11f–12f
Scaling
  equipment, 4–6, 108f
  subgingival, 109–112, 110f
  supragingival, 108–109, 109f
Scalpel blades, 10–11
Scissor bite, reverse, 45
Seal of acceptance system (VOHC®),
    124
Sensors, 69f, 70–71
Sevoflurane, 18
Sharpening equipment, 8–9
Shedding disorders, 86–87
Sickle scaler, 5f
Single-rooted teeth, 174–176
  extraction procedure, 174–176, 186
Skeletal malocclusion, 43–46, 46f–47f
Skull
  chinchilla, 204f
  guinea pig, 201f
  rabbit, 192f
  rat, 193f
SLOB rule (Same direction Lingual,
    Opposite direction Buccal), 75–78
Soft muzzles, 165–166
Soft palate defects, 145
  double layer repair, 145, 146f
Soft tissue trauma, 141–147
Sonic scalers, 6, 108–111
Specific plaque hypothesis, 98
Spirochetes, 98
Splints, intraoral acrylic, 166–168, 168f
Split palatal U-flap technique, 145, 146f
Sterilization, hand instruments, 12–13
Stomatitis, 97, 98t
  with gingivitis, 115, 115f
  gingivitis with, 114–115, 115f
  see also Chronic gingivostomatitis
    (CGS)
Streptococcus sanguis, 98
Subgingival scaling, 109–112, 110f
  scalers, 6f
Sublingual oedema, 188
Subluxation, 154, 155f–156f
Substituted amino-alcohols, mechanical
    plaque control, 34
Suction, 11, 16
Sulcular lavage, 112–113

Supernumerary teeth, 82, 82f, 172
Supragingival scaling, 108–109, 109f
  scalers, 6f
Surface resorption, 129–130
Suture kits/material, 11
Symmetry, head, face, neck, 51, 51f
Syringes, 21f

T

Tape muzzle, 165–166, 166f
Teeth
  examination, 58b
  extraction *see* Extraction
  fractures, 147–152, 150f–152f, 172,
    188
    preventive dentistry, 124–125
  mobility, 61, 62t
  multi-rooted *see* Multi-rooted teeth
  overgrowth *see* Overgrowth, tooth
  radiography *see* Radiography
  sectioning, 176–180, 177f–179f
  single-rooted *see* Single-rooted teeth
  supernumerary, 82, 82f, 172
  traumatic injuries, 147–157, 172, 206
  trimming, 207–208
  see also Dentition
Thermal bone injury, 187–188
Tongue, examination, 58b
Tooth-borne appliances, 162–163, 165
Toothbrushing, 122–123
  frequency, 123
  technique, 123, 123f

toothbrushes, 122–123
  toothpaste, 122–123
Topical chlorhexidine, 34
Topical fluoride application, 86
Tracheotomy, elective, 28
Transposition flap, 143f
Trauma
  maxillofacial, 18
  soft tissue, 141–147
  tooth injuries, 147–157, 172, 206
Treatment-induced bacteremia, 31
Triadan system, modified, 62, 65t
Triclosan, mechanical plaque control,
  34
'Tub-tank', 1
Tumours, oral, 92f–93f, 93–94

U

Ulceration, mucous membrane, 103f
Ultrasonic scalers, 6, 108–111, 109f
'Undershot', 44–45
Universal curettes, 5f
Upper airway obstruction
  brachycephalic patients, 17–18
  cats, 18

V

Vasoconstrictors, 20
Veau–Wardill technique, 144, 144f
Vertical bone loss, 99f, 105f
Vestibular flap, 145

Veterinary Medical Teaching Hospital,
  University of California, 32
Veterinary Oral Health Council
  (VOHC®), 124
Viral infections, 98t
Vitamin C, 193
Vitamin D, 134

W

Wear, excessive
  hard tissue, 87, 87f
  preventive dentistry, 124
Wiring, orthopedic, 163–165
Wry bite, 46, 48f–49f, 54

X

X-ray film, 69–70, 70f
  exposure settings, 71t, 72f
  handling/mounting, 71–72, 72f
  interpretation, 78–79
  orientation, 70
  placement, 74–75, 77f
  processing, 71f–72f
X-ray unit, 68, 70f
  see also Digital radiography

Printed in the United States
By Bookmasters